THE CESAREAN BIRTH

Editor-in-Chief

Ranjit Akolekar

Associate Editors

Suchitra N. Pandit

Sanjay B. Rao

THE NATIONAL BOOK DEPOT

First Edition Reprint 2023

Published by

Vaidehi Shah

THE NATIONAL BOOK DEPOT

Opp. Wadia Children's Hospital,
Parel, Mumbai - 400 012.
Tel : +91-22-2413 1362 | 2413 1354
Mobile: 9757001960 | 9757001961
E-mail: nationalbook55@gmail.com
Website: www.nationalbookdepot.com

ISBN : 978-81-87540-39-7

Printed by : Neel Graphics

Dedicated To
All Those People
Who Made
Cesarean Birth Possible.....

FOREWORD

It gives me a great pleasure to write the foreword for this book. Cesarean delivery is one of the commonest operations done in Obstetrics and Gynecology. This surgery has become safer in the recent years due to the safety of blood transfusion, advent of powerful antibiotics and improvement in anesthesia & surgical techniques. As the surgery became safer, its use has increased. The indications for cesarean section have increased over the years due to various reasons viz. improved neonatal care, revision of certain obstetric policies during conduct of labor, pregnancies following assisted reproductive techniques and lastly due to medico legal considerations. This rise in the incidence of cesarean section has raised concern worldwide, and there has been a systematic effort directed to curb the rising cesarean trends.

Recently, there has been a strong focus on evidence based medical practice. Several randomized trials have been conducted on various aspects of cesarean delivery. It is worthwhile to be aware about the recent developments in the discipline so that a good practice of medicine is followed.

This book exhaustively deals with various issues relating to cesarean birth. There has been a focused effort to look at the operation of cesarean delivery from a modern, evidence-based perspective. The selection of the contributors is particularly good and they contributed the chapters well.

The editors have done an excellent job and I congratulate them for preparing such an exhaustive manuscript. Dr. Ranjit Akolekar is one of the promising and young Obstetricians in Mumbai and has a keen interest in academics. Dr. Suchitra Pandit is the Chairperson of the young talent promotion committee of FOGSI and has been involved with various academic activities over the years.

The book deals with a wide variety of issues and should prove to be good reading for all the postgraduates and clinical practitioners.

Sadhana K Desai

DR. SADHANA DESAI
President, FOGSI.

MESSAGE

Cesarean birth is an important part of obstetric care. It therefore becomes imperative to adopt an evidence-based approach, which will offer the patient the best possible care.

The art of obstetrics can be learnt and skills can be honed with constant efforts being made over the years. A correct attitude towards acquiring skills and knowledge is something one finds with difficulty.

I am extremely happy that Ranjit Akolekar, a committed and dynamic member of my committee took up the initiative to write, compile and edit such an exhaustive manuscript on cesarean birth. Sanjay Rao, a dedicated and enthusiastic member of my committee also contributed in editing the manuscript.

I am confident that every chapter in this monogram would voice contemporary opinions related to the subject. This would be particularly useful to all postgraduate students and practicing obstetricians who wish to update their knowledge and understanding.

This book covers a wide variety of subjects related to childbirth – with special emphasis to anesthesia, neonatal care and medicolegal aspects of cesarean section, which are an important part of contemporary obstetric practice.

S Pandit

DR. SUCHITRA N. PANDIT
Chairperson
Young Talent Promotion committee
FOGSI

ACKNOWLEDGEMENT

A manuscript of this nature is seldom an individual enterprise. This exhaustive manuscript, likewise, has also been possible due to the collective involvement of few people, whom I acknowledge with a deep sense of gratitude.

I sincerely thank the FOGSI President, Dr. Sadhana Desai and the managing committee for allowing me to publish this book under the aegis of FOGSI. In the same context, I also thank Dr. Suchitra Pandit for giving me the opportunity to publish the book through her committee. I sincerely appreciate the constant encouragement given to me by Dr. Suchitra Pandit. She motivated me to complete the manuscript at a time when doing so seemed difficult as I was busy pursuing my Fellowship in Fetal Medicine. I also thank her for helping me to edit the text.

I have a similar sense of appreciation for the constructive criticism given by Dr. Sanjay Rao during preparation of this book and acknowledge his help during making of this manuscript. I acknowledge the efforts made by my colleague, Dr. Nagendra Sardeshpande, in formatting the diagrams into the text, apart from contributing well-written chapters.

This text would not have been possible without the participation of all the authors who have contributed excellent chapters. I appreciate all the effort made in authoring of such detailed and comprehensive chapters. I thank Ms. Tanvi Jakhi for contributing the line diagrams in the text.

My interest in Obstetrics would not have been so intense without the excellent training I received as a resident at LTMG hospital in Mumbai. I am particularly grateful to my teachers Dr. V.R. Ambiye and Dr. V.D. Patkar for allowing my interest to grow and blossom.

I thank my father, for his invaluable advice and criticism, which I always look forward to. I am particularly indebted to him for teaching me what pleasure lies in studying science and medicine.

This manuscript would not have been possible without the constant support, inspiration, motivation and understanding of my best friend and wife, Deepika.

I specially thank my publisher Mr. Raju Shah, who encouraged me to write this book. I also thank Mr. Viren Shah for doing an excellent job of printing the text.

PREFACE

Childbirth is a natural phenomenon. It is nature's way of ensuring that a species procreates and survives. As childbirth is a nature's creation, laws of nature therefore, govern it. If we look at the other creations of nature around us, we realize that not all of them are beautiful; few are unsightly and some even dangerous. And so is childbirth; it can be the most wonderful experience in the lifetime of a woman or at times the most dangerous one.

But being the most intelligent species on the planet, we have advanced in ways unimaginable and incomprehensible by most other species. We have the ability to intervene in nature and we have extended it to manage and assist childbirth. We have invented the cesarean birth. Cesarean birth has made it possible for babies to be born and be alive who otherwise would never have seen the light of the day. Likewise, it has made some women, healthy mothers, who had never hoped they could be mothers and healthy too. Cesarean delivery has revolutionized childbirth for human beings.

But as is true for all good things in life, it is at times overindulged in. Therefore, we have at the crux, the issue of concern over rising cesarean delivery trends. Cesarean delivery is a mode of childbirth for women who are unable to deliver vaginally or who are at a certain risk if they do so. Cesarean birth was not invented so that it could be offered to women as an alternative option to the natural childbirth. To do so, would constitute an abuse of this wonderful procedure.

As we continue to progress each day, new information is assimilated and older views are revised. It is happening everywhere, in science, in medicine and in obstetrics. As obstetricians, to be able to manage a patient in the best possible way, it is obligatory to be aware of the recent trends and advances.

This manuscript gives an overview into various aspects of cesarean birth. It is not only designed to meet the needs of a postgraduate resident who wants to be introduced to cesarean birth in a proper way but is also for the clinical practitioner who can use this as a ready reckoner.

Ranjit Akolekar

LIST OF CONTRIBUTORS

Ranjit Akolekar
MD, DNBE, FCPS, DGO
Obstetrician and Gynaecologist
Clinical Fellow, Department of Fetal Medicine,
Mediscan Prenatal Diagnosis And Fetal Therapy Center

Sarita Bhalerao
MD,DNB,FCPS,DGO,DFP,MRCOG
Asst. Hon. Professor, Bandra Bhabha Municipal Hospital
Consultant, Guru Nanak Hospital, Mumbai

Nikhil Datar
MD,DNB,FCPS,LLB,DHA
Obstetrician And Gynaecologist
Medicolegal Consultant, Mumbai

Sejal Desai
MD,DGO,DNB,FCPS
Senior Registrar,
LTM Medical College and Hospital, Mumbai

Sanjay Gupte
MD,DGO
Senior Vice President (elect), FOGSI 2004
Obstetrician And Gynaecologist,
Sanjeevani Maternity Hospital, Pune

Sarbjit Kaur
MBBS, DGO
Registrar,
K J Somaiya Medical College and Hospital, Mumbai

Grace Korula
MD, DA
Professor & Head, Department Of Anaesthesia
Christian Medical College, Vellore

Sankaranarayana K
MD,DM,DCH
Registrar,
Department Of Neonatology
LTM Medical College and Hospital, Mumbai

Trishala Meghal
MD,DNB,DGO
Obstetrician and Gynaecologist, Mumbai

J A Mondkar
MD,DCH
Professor & Head, Department Of Neonatology
LTM Medical College and Hospital, Mumbai

Pallavi Naik
MBBS, DGO
Registrar,
BYL Nair Charitable hospital & TN Medical college, Mumbai

Suchitra N Pandit
B Pharm,MD,DNB,DFP,MRCOG,FICOG
Assoc. Professor and Unit Chief,
LTM Medical College and Hospital, Mumbai
Chairperson, Young Talent Promotion Committee, FOGSI

Trupti Pai
MD,DNB,FCPS, DGO
Lecturer,
Wadia Maternity Hospital, Mumbai

Mandakini Parihar
MD,DGO
Assoc. Hon. Professor
K J Somaiya Medical College & Hospital, Mumbai.
Hon. Joint Secretary, FOGSI

Rohan Potdar
MBBS,DGO
Registrar,
K J Somaiya Medical College and Hospital, Mumbai

Sanjay B Rao
MD,DNB,DGO,FCPS,MICOG
Lecturer,
LTM Medical College and Hospital, Mumbai

Nagendra Sardeshpande
DNB,DGO,FCPS,DFP
Obstetrician And Gynaecologist,
Brahman Sabha Hospital, Mumbai

Nozer Sheriar
MD,DNB,FCPS,DGO,FICOG
Obstetrician And Gynaecologist,
Holy Family Hospital & Masina General Hospital, Mumbai
Chairperson MTP committee, FOGSI

Reena J Wani
MD,DNB,FCPS,DGO, DFP, MRCOG
Assoc. Professor, BYL Nair Charitable hospital &
TN Medical college, Mumbai

CONTENTS

1 | CHAPTER

Introduction

Ranjit Akolekar

Cesarean delivery is one of the most commonly performed operations today. As medical science and especially obstetrics has evolved over the recent years, there has been a parallel and steady increase in the rate of cesarean births. From times when childbirth was an event not necessitating medical attention to the present times when concerns are voiced about high cesarean delivery rates, obstetrics has for sure, traveled a long way.

This evolution in obstetrics has paralleled the cultural and social advance that society has witnessed over the last few decades. What has changed the whole vista of childbirth is the social emphasis on gender equality and economic freedom for women. With economic freedom came a participation in decision-making, especially in nuclear families. Women always had opinions, but now they were voiced and valued. Because obstetrics is essentially about giving care to the laboring woman, it evolved rapidly in the backdrop of a changing social milieu.

The operation of 'cesarean delivery' has also witnessed this evolution; from it being done in desperate situations as a postmortem surgery to save the unborn child to the present times when one of the most common indications for cesarean delivery is a previous cesarean birth.

The indications for cesarean delivery have been undergoing a gradual change over the last few decades. This change has been in the form of an increase in the number of indications rather than anything else, as cesarean births have become safer. This is not to imply that they have become safer than normal uncomplicated vaginal deliveries but that they have become more safe than they used to be. The major contributors to making cesarean delivery 'safer' were improvement in techniques of anesthesia, advent of powerful and effective antibiotics, availability of blood transfusion and last but not the least, improvement in surgical techniques and operative skills. What has also contributed to broadening the spectrum of indications is the tremendous advance made in neonatal intensive care. The initial list of indications for cesarean delivery included conditions where it was done mainly for maternal interest when a further trial of labor was considered hazardous. More recently, however, the health of the fetus has played a significant role in making the decision for a cesarean birth. This has become increasingly pronounced after the advent of high-resolution ultrasound, Doppler ultrasound and electronic fetal monitoring. What contributed to the increasing list of indications for cesarean section was the safety of cesarean birth in certain high-risk pregnancies. There also has been a definite trend in some centers towards a planned cesarean birth for women who have conceived following assisted reproductive techniques. Of late, the safety of an elective cesarean birth has prompted some obstetricians in the developed world to consider and allow for the feasibility of an elective cesarean section based on maternal request.

Most of this and especially the advance made in operative techniques was possible because of the constant urge and will on part of the medical and obstetric fraternity to improve and evolve. Scientific progress requires critical analysis, introspection and continuous audit. It is imperative that a sense of appreciative inquiry is maintained all through the professional career even by individual clinicians, regarding management protocols and operative techniques. This concept is an important part of learning medicine and should be imbibed by all trainees and resident doctors who aspire to be good clinicians and surgeons.

In the present parlance, a sound practice of obstetrics would also require a continuous updating of knowledge, as every day brings forth new information. It is imperative that both trainers and trainees should update knowledge on a regular basis so that the best practice of medicine is followed. Especially in the last few decades, various facts about obstetric decision-making have changed and lots of them have been revisited. Continuing medical education should not just be the norm, but the rule.

Modern clinical practice needs to be evidence based; what forms the gold standard for this evidence-based practice is knowledge from randomized clinical trials. There have been several randomized controlled trials regarding many aspects of cesarean delivery, the results of many of which are quite interesting, as they are informative. It is not only important but also necessary to embrace this information for a contemporary and evidence-based medical practice.

This information explosion has brought about newer perspectives and approaches involving obstetrics in general and cesarean birth in particular. It has created controversies too.

In India, the obstetric practice in the urban vis-a-vis rural setting presents a glaring dichotomy, possibly due to lack of necessary infrastructure in the rural sector. It may take some more time for the health planners to equip our primary and district health centers with better infrastructural facilities. To bridge the dichotomy, what would go a long way in improving obstetric care is having update knowledge and correct attitude.

Women have been bearing children for thousands of years but it is only in the last couple of hundred years that a cesarean birth has been possible. Cesarean birth has been definitely instrumental in decreasing the maternal and perinatal morbidity and mortality. Even though cesarean birth has become safer than it used to be, still it is not without morbidity. Therefore, the decision for the mode of delivery must be made with judicious caution.

A sincere effort has been made to collate the necessary information regarding 'cesarean delivery in contemporary practice'. Few issues may have remained unadrressed in order to remain concise. Critical opinions would be highly appreciated.

2 | CHAPTER

The Need For Abdominal Childbirth In Human Beings

Ranjit Akolekar

FRAMEWORK

- Introduction
- The evolutionary perspective
    - Primate childbirth
    - Childbirth in Homo Sapiens
    - Becoming Biped
    - Becoming intelligent
    - Summary

INTRODUCTION

Obstetrics is a wonderful discipline. It permits an insight into the fundamental biological processes leading to human creation. The phenomenon of birthing is simply the climaxing of those processes. It is all the more fascinating and fulfilling when an obstetrician is able to assess, modulate and intervene when required, to counter the adversities of nature, thus ensuring the safe delivery of the baby.

Obstetric patients too, are a very special class of patients. They do not come to see the doctor because of some illness but they come and see the doctor so that they can be assisted with the wonderful process of childbirth. Childbirth is such a profound event that it instills a unique sense of awe in all those who witness the event.

Obstetricians witness and assist in childbirth on a very regular basis. But the beauty of the event does not cease to amaze us. Medicine and science have advanced tremendously, but there are many facets of childbirth, which still persist as riddles. This awesome event in the lifetime of an individual is so profound that it makes us acknowledge the beauty and power of nature. It is just so amazing and stupefying how nature designed the most efficient allograft. It is just so wonderful how this symbiosis between the mother and the fetus develops and proceeds upto a predestined time when the biological clock says, its time, to deliver.

There are many aspects of childbirth which science has been able to explain but there remains an equally long list of events, which still remain to be explained. We can have painless childbirth, but we still fail to completely understand why human labor is so inherently painful. We know that human gestation has an average time frame of 40 weeks but we do not know why it is 40 and not shorter or longer, especially when there are other mammals with much shorter or longer gestations. We still do not know what causes the onset of labor. Many scientists have analyzed it and we still do not know the answer in black and white.

We do not understand why childbirth in human beings is so inherently painful and potentially dangerous. We can only wonder as to why this is so.

But as the most dominant species on the planet, we are intelligent. We designed a way to circumvent difficult labors. We designed a way to avoid the resultant fetal & maternal morbidity, and sometimes mortality. We devised an alternative mode of delivery. We devised the abdominal childbirth. And we call it 'the cesarean birth'.

In the subsequent text it is discussed whether the need to have an abdominal childbirth was a necessary evolutionary sequelae that was unavoidable or whether it was an ingenious invention that our species made. The process of childbirth has been compared in Homo sapiens, who we are, to the process in other primate species. Also addressed is the issue whether the need to be biped was responsible for the change in our birthing process.

These are some issues, which have always interested me. I do understand that the subsequent text might not appeal to all the readers but for the few readers whose attention I have managed to catch, I can say that this is an interesting, albeit different perspective to understanding childbirth.

THE EVOLUTIONARY PERSPECTIVE

Most women, who are mothers, would agree that pushing a baby through the birth canal is not an easy task. To understand why it is so, we ask ourselves a question: was it always so difficult? Our static view of the universe might tempt us to think that yes, it has always been so. But the evidence is quite to the contrary.

Some believe that childbirth was easy and painless once upon a time but that changed after Eve ate the forbidden fruit in the Garden of Eden. She enjoyed eating the fruit but was cursed to deal with a painful and difficult childbirth from then on. Whether the latter part of the statement is a fact or fiction is debatable but what is correct for sure is that human childbirth was not always so difficult. At least that is what study of human evolution tells us.

We have evolved as a species from subhuman primates. The evolutionary path was a long one and passed through various stages of mental and physical development. Without going into the details of our evolutionary history, I would briefly mention that once upon a time we were quadruped subhuman primates, and then evoled into biped subhuman primates. It is the latter species which evolved in the following sequence: Australopithecine, Homo erectus, Neanderthal, Homo sapiens and now Homo sapiens sapiens, who we today are. If evolution is a continuous process, whom will we be in the years to come, what will we look like and what will be our form? One can only wonder.

It is believed that the birth process in our earlier species was not so difficult. This has been studied and analyzed as a part of paleo-anthropology. There are two major reasons for the relative ease of childbirth: one, the wider and more robust pelves' and second the small cranial size of our ancestors.

These two important evolutionary events are discussed in the later part of the text but first let us study the process of childbirth in our ancestors and how it changed as our species evolved. The closest approximation to studying the process of childbirth as it happened in our ancestors is to study the process in our closest evolutionary relative, the primates. We have evolved from a common ancestor and primate body architecture closely approximates that of our ancestors.

PRIMATE CHILDBIRTH

To be able to be born the fetus has to pass through the birth canal, which is formed by the pelvic bones. The two innominate bones are joined together to form the pelvis. The pelvis has an inlet, a cavity and an outlet. The dimensions of the pelvis are more spacious in lower primates than they are in Homo sapiens.

Non-human primates, who walk quadruped i.e. on four limbs, have relatively short labors, and many primates give birth in isolation and do not require assistance from others. The pelvic opening is large and there is plenty of room for the fetus to deliver.

To understand primate childbirth, the birthing process in monkeys provides a good example. In the monkey pelvis, the pelvic inlet, the mid-cavity and the outlet maintain the same cross section throughout i.e. they are antero-posteriorly oval, the posterior part being wider than the anterior part. This is different from that in Homo sapiens in whom these subdivisions of the pelvis are oriented in a different fashion.

The monkey fetus enters the pelvis in a cephalic presentation and engages in an occipito-posterior position, with the broad back of the skull against the spacious back of the mother's pelvis. The fetus just glides downwards with the uterine contractions and effortlessly delivers as the head does not have to negotiate any narrow pelvic segments and it does not have to undergo rotation. The need for rotation is not there as all the three pelvic segments are aligned antero-posteriorly.

Monkeys usually give birth either squatting or crouching on all fours. First hand observations of monkey's birthing process have revealed that the fetus delivers in occipito-posterior position and as the fetus is delivering, the mother reaches down to guide it out of the birth canal and towards her nipples. In many cases, she also wipes mucus from the baby's mouth and nose to aid its breathing process. The monkey infants are strong enough at birth to take part in their own deliveries. Once their hands are free, they grab the mother and pull themselves out.

CHILDBIRTH IN HOMO SAPIENS

The process of childbirth in human beings is somewhat similar with some modifications. The modifications enable human fetuses to deliver vaginally, in spite of their evolutionary differences.

The human pelvis is structurally similar but architecturally different i.e. it has different dimensions. The human pelvis can also be divided into the inlet, cavity and outlet. The inlet is more or less round. However, it is more broad than long meaning that its transverse diameter is more than its antero-posterior diameter. Whereas the pelvic outlet is more long than broad i.e. its antero-posterior diameter is more than its transverse diameter. This has important implications for human birth. The head usually enters the pelvis in the transverse diameter i.e. occipito-transverse but to be able to deliver through the pelvis it will have to undergo a twist of 90° so that the outlet can be negotiated. This requires the human fetus to undergo an obligatory rotation, which is referred to as the 'internal rotation'. Moreover, the fetal head delivers commonly in the occipito-anterior position, which makes it difficult for the mother to assist birth. Assisting her own childbirth is otherwise also not possible, as she is busy with the formidable task of pushing her baby through the birth canal.

The childbirth is made more difficult because of the large size of the fetal head, which just barely negotiates the pelvis.

This difficulty is complicated more by the fact that all pelves' in human beings are not the same. There is a certain amount of diversity, although some types are more common than the other (Gynecoid pelvis is commonest type). But the fact remains that diversity exists.

But why was there a need to develop a different pelvic architecture when the process of childbirth was efficient when we were primates? The need was there because we invited it. We invited this need in two ways: one by becoming bipedal from quadrupeds and second by becoming more intelligent and thereby increasing our cranial size.

How and why these two important evolutionary events occurred and how they changed childbirth forever is discussed below.

BECOMING BIPED

It is an evolutionary fact that once we were quadruped. What evolutionary forces were at play, which drove our ancestors to become bipedal, is an important question. It had to occur for some evolutionary advantage if we are to believe Darwinism ('Survival of the fittest').

There are numerous theories trying to explain the evolutionary benefit of the erect posture that ultimately led to hominid species becoming the most dominant species on the planet. The most logical theory is that the freeing of hands for purposeful manipulation of tools provided an increased ability to defend itself and to acquire food. These factors could have contributed to the evolutionary benefit in terms of competition with other species.

Becoming bipedal certainly benefited us in evolutionary terms but it definitely had an influence on the pelvic architecture.

Pelvic architecture changed because with bipedalism the pattern of weight transmission changed. The innominate bones became important structures in weight transmission.

In bipedal hominids, the pelvis assumes a broad, shallow, bowl-like shape with a widened but shortened ilium, thus bringing the sacrum closer to the acetabulum. These changes, together with forward curvature of the lower spine and further flattening of the thoracic cage, help transmit weight of the trunk directly to the legs, producing a balanced center of gravity along a vertical axis.

Bipedalism is quite an unusual development, as any superficial observation of the animal kingdom will confirm. Bipedalism also caused problems with the size of the pelvis. A balance had to be found between a more efficient, thus narrower pelvis (the faster you could run, the more likely you were to survive) and a pelvis of adequate size to allow birth. This balance between efficiency and adequacy was a critical development in human evolution and this was what Magnus Murphy called "the mechanical imperative".

The upright posture of humans brought with it a number of other problems as well. When we look around the animal kingdom, we find in most mammals that the pelvic "floor" is not a floor at all. Since the usual primate posture is for the body to be horizontal, the brunt of the intra-abdominal weight does not fall on this structure at all, but rather onto the anterior abdominal wall. In the upright human, the pelvic floor became an important support structure for the pelvic and abdominal contents. The full force of gravity had to be counteracted by the pelvic floor. This became another structure, which the fetus had to negotiate during the process of childbirth.

The initial change in pelvic architecture did not have a significant effect on the process of childbirth. This is because even though pelvic dimensions changed, the fetal head was still not large enough to cause difficulties in childbirth. It is only with further evolution of the species that the cranial size increased with increasing intelligence.

BECOMING INTELLIGENT

About 2-3 million years ago, primate brain size and complexity increased, more than doubling from australopithecines to Homo sapiens. This increase is called encephalization. Various evolutionary processes and especially the development of speech led to a massive increase in the brain capacity. Development of speech is one of the theories to explain the evolutionary fitness of Homo sapiens. It is speech that made communication and thus development of culture possible. The development of speech led to a massive increase in certain parts of the brain, particularly the frontal and temporal lobes. Various evolutionary processes, for instance the complex, manual manipulations requiring fine neural control, as well as the development of speech, led to a massive increase in brain capacity. (Average cranial capacity for modern humans is in the order of 1400 ml).

The large brain size obviously creates problems for the birthing process since the fetus survives best if it is large, but with obvious consequences for the mother. The birthing process can be likened to a competitive interaction between the mother and her fetus, with some common ideals (for instance the survival of both), but also some divergent goals, i.e. to personally come from the experience in as good a shape as possible. Infants with large heads (and their mothers) were at increased risk during birth simply because there was greater chance of prolonged and obstructed labor, leading to birth asphyxia and possibly death. Natural selection favored infants with small heads and immature brains at birth. The human brain at birth is only one-quarter the size of an adult's. (In monkeys, the newborn's brain is one-half the size of an adult's). Because human infants are relatively helpless at birth, the first three months of life are considered by many anthropologists to be essentially a fourth trimester. The infant's brain develops rapidly, so that by age 3 the brain is three-quarters adult size. This trait not only makes birth safer and relatively easier, but also ensures that much behavior is based on learning rather than instinct.

SUMMARY

With evolution of a more advanced hominid species, two important events occurred. They were: bipedalism and encephalization. These two events made human childbirth inherently risky. Bipedalism changed the pelvic architecture and introduced a constraint on the dimensions of the pelvis. At the same time, encephalization resulted in an enlarged cranial size. The end result was that the fetal head just snuggly fitted and passed through parts of pelvis just barely.

Moreover, the change in pelvic architecture requires the fetus to undergo rotation during delivery to be able to pass through it.

At the same time, enough force has to be generated and enough uterine work has to be done to help the fetus to negotiate the narrow pelvis. A lot of uterine work is required to cause internal rotation and for stretching of the pelvic diaphragm.

Therefore, human childbirth is a prolonged, difficult and laborious process compared to other primate species where childbirth is simple and short.

Because of all the above reasons, childbirth in human beings is potentially dangerous. Prolonged labor, especially with a disparity in size of the fetal head and maternal pelvis can spell doom for the fetus. A prolonged labor is associated with an effort on part of the mother to force the fetus through the birth canal. This results in the uterus contracting more strongly which leads to a decreased blood supply to the fetus.

Until such a time that the option of abdominal delivery was not available, the neonatal, perinatal and maternal morbidity/mortality statistics were high. Advances in obstetrics and other allied branches has made it possible to perform an abdominal childbirth for those women who are at risk for fetal and maternal morbidity/mortality.

Magnus Murphy in his article on 'Choosing Cesarean birth: An alternative to today's crisis in Natural childbirth' says "Our ability to deliver babies safely by cesarean section in cases of obstructed labor has revolutionized our ability to intervene in nature. This ability has not only removed the necessity for an adequate pelvis, but also the impediment to possible further evolutionary brain-size development. The question has been asked whether evolution as a species shaping force, is still active in humans. As a result of our intellectual ability to subject nature to our collective will, many of the selection pressures of the Darwinian model are not valid in our species anymore. By safely delivering and helping babies who would otherwise have died to survive, we have escaped the tyranny of raw natural selection. This is not only the result of modern medicine but our whole society has a role to play here. Whether selection still plays a subtle role in the human race however, is an interesting question with no definite answer".

Science cannot be viewed in isolation. Advances made in software technology, molecular biology and genetics have revolutionized our view of science and medicine. As our understanding of biological processes and medicine becomes more and more profound each day, our narrow way of looking at a discipline has broadened. None of the individual scientific disciplines should be viewed mutually excusive of the other; progress in one discipline has implications for other disciplines. It is when science is viewed in this particular context, that it appears more meaningful and interesting.

Difficult labors and potentially dangerous childbirth was what nature gave us in turn for a place in the fast lane of evolution. By devising an alternative mode of childbirth, we have definitely intervened in the natural process of evolution. But if we also believe that evolution is a continuous process and that it is happening this very minute, then one can only wonder where our species will go from here and more interestingly how will 'natural childbirth' be like?

REFERENCES

1. Wenda Trevathan, Human Birth: An Evolutionary Perspective. New York: Aldine de Gruyter, 1987.
2. Dana Walrath Rethinking Pelvic Typologies and the Human Birth Mechanism Current anthropology Volume 44, Number 1, February 2003.
3. Abitbol, M. M. The shape of the female pelvis. Journal of Reproductive Medicine 1996; 41:24250.
4. Berge Christine. Obstetrical interpretation of the australopithecine pelvic cavity. Journal of Human Evolution 1984; 13:57387.
5. Choosing Cesarean Birth: An alternative to today's Crisis in Natural Childbirth?: Magnus Murphy, MD: on www.obgyn.net.
6. Bruzek, Jaroslav. Degree of pelvic sexual dimorphism in human populations: A Greene t-test application. Human Evolution 1996; 11:18389.
7. Hunt, K. The evolution of human bipedality. Journal of Human Evolution.1993; 26:185-202.
8. Leakey, R. In:The Making of Mankind. Eds. 1981. New York: The Rainbird Publishing Group Limited
9. Strickberger, M. In: Evolution. Eds. 1990. Boston: Jones and Bartlett Publishers, Inc.
10. Anthropologist researches skeletons for secrets of childbirth evolution. Update. University of Delaware. Vol. 21, (7), May 2002.

3 | CHAPTER

The History of Cesarean Delivery

Ranjit Akolekar

FRAMEWORK

- Introduction
- The early times
- The middle ages
- After the dark ages
- Conclusion

INTRODUCTION

"History is the study of past events. It is a systematic attempt to learn about and verify past events and to relate those events to one another and to the present".

If we make an attempt to study the history of cesarean birth, we reach as far back as the earliest known civilized human habitations and we realize that there have been anecdotal references to abdominal childbirth even in those times. These references to abdominal childbirth date back to as far as 2000 BC. These references to abdominal childbirth have been dealt with in the text below but it is important to note that the word 'cesarean' has not been a part of scientific literature before middle ages.

There is considerable confusion regarding the origin of this particular phrasing of abdominal childbirth. Pliny, a historian, first stated that Julius Ceasar was delivered by an abdominal incision. This is however, not true. This myth was preserved through middle ages in many manuscripts, e.g. in the first printed version of 'The twelve ceasers' written in the second century AD by Suetonius and printed in 1506. The text written by Suetonius includes a woodblock print that is claimed to be a picturization of the first cesarean section (Fig. 2).

Another probability is that the term originated from the Lex Regia or Lex Caesara, ascribed to Numa Pompilius in 716 BC. This law dictated the performance of abdominal delivery of the fetus from a mother who was dying or dead, as an attempt to save the child for a state wishing to increase its population.

As if the confusion about the origin of the word 'Caesarean' was not enough, there is an equal confusion about the origin of the second part of the phrase i.e. section. Etymologists are fascinated by this term because it represents a unique word formation. The use of the term 'Cesarean section' is called a pleonasm. A pleonasm is a phrase, which uses two words with similar meanings. Most probable origins for this elusive pleonasm are from some form of Latin words meaning 'to cut' or 'to kill'. The Latin verb caedo, caedere, cecidi, or ceasum means to cut or to kill. The second part of the phrase probably arose from the verb seco, secare, secui, or sectum meaning to cut. The noun for this verb is section.

It is stated that Rousset first used the phrase in his book but this has been debated. Bauhin, who published Rousset's book a year later, used the phrase Caesarea Sectio, in the index of the book for the first time. Later, Guillemeau in 1598 used the phrase 'cesarienne section' in his French manuscript. Modern version is an anglicized version of the French spelling cesarienne and thus our modern literature is provided with the words "cesarean section".

THE EARLY TIMES

Cesarean delivery has been a part of human culture since ancient times and there are tales in both western and non-western cultures of this procedure resulting in live mothers and offspring. Numerous references to cesarean delivery appear in ancient Hindu, Egyptian, Grecian, Roman, and other European folklore. Yet, the early history of cesarean delivery remains shrouded in myth and is of dubious accuracy.

According to Greek mythology Apollo removed Asclepius, founder of the famous cult of religious medicine, from his mother's abdomen.

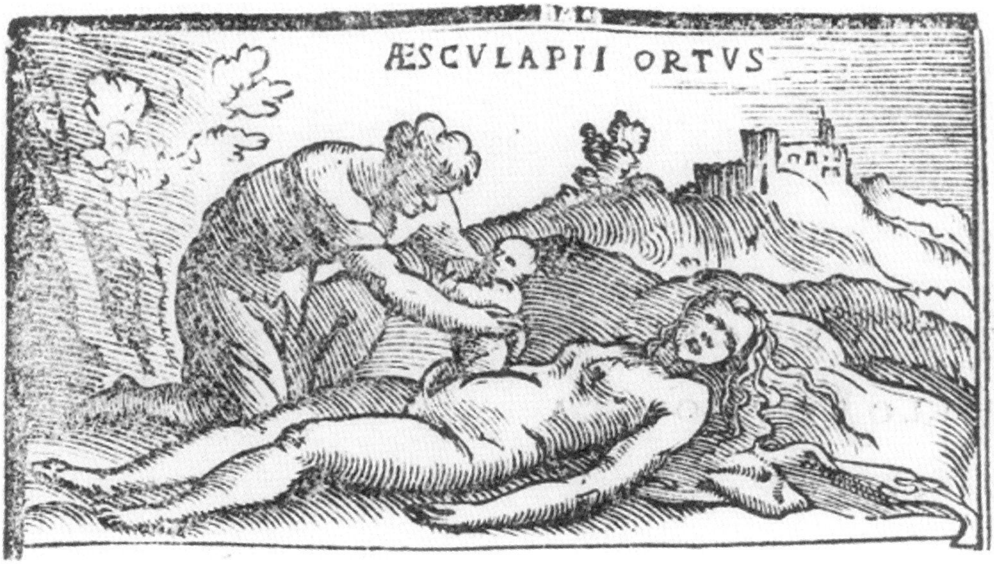

Fig. 3.1 The extraction of Asclepius from the abdomen of his mother Coronis by his father Apollo. Woodcut from the 1549 edition of Alessandro Beneditti's De Re Medica. Courtesy: National Library of Medicine, USA.

The earliest record, however, of performance of cesarean delivery is from Sumer, where it was reported that the operation was performed on slaves in the second millennium BC. Most of the abdominal deliveries during these times were performed on dead women as a part of religious belief. The document and seals from Sumer also have reference to surgical instruments and delivery by abdominal means. These artifacts establish the fact that the operation was done earlier than 2000 BC.

There is considerable ambiguity regarding the origin of the word 'cesarean' and the birth of Julius Caesar. It was said that the word 'cesarean' owed its origin to Julius caesar, who was born by an abdominal delivery. This myth was preserved through middle ages in many manuscripts e.g. in The Faits dex Romains in the 1300s and in the first printed version of The Twelve Caesars written in second century AD and printed in 1506. This picture below is a woodblock print that purports to be the first picturization of a cesarean birth, but this is an error.

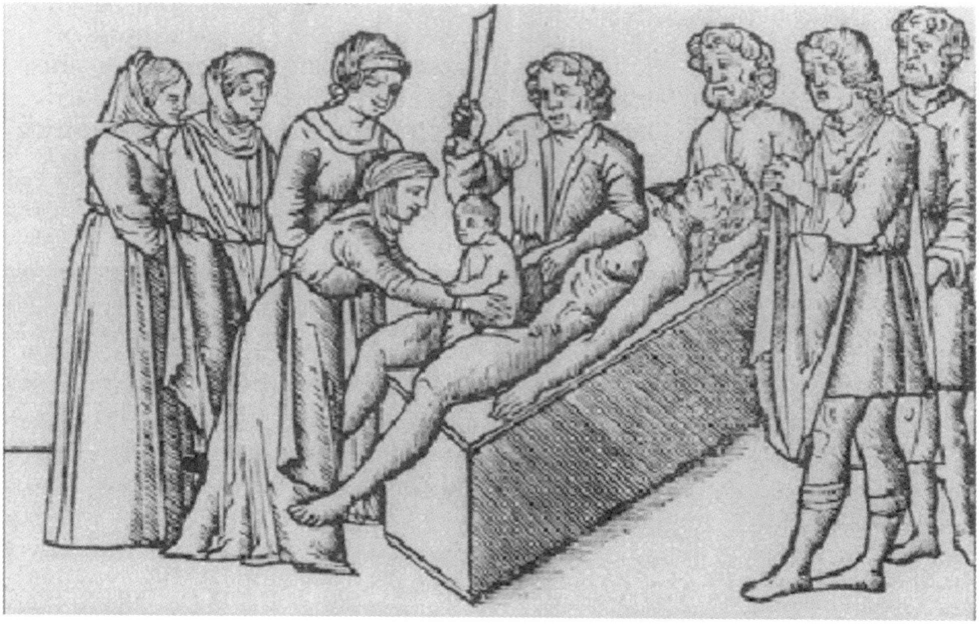

Fig. 3.2 One of the earliest printed illustrations of Cesarean section. Purportedly the birth of Julius Caesar. A live infant being surgically removed from a dead woman. From Suetonius' Lives of the Twelve Caesars, 1506 woodcut. Courtesy: National Library of Medicine, USA.

The surgical birth of Julius Ceasar seems unlikely since his mother Aurelia is reputed to have lived to hear of her son's invasion of Britain. At that time the procedure was performed only when the mother was dying or dead, as an attempt to save the child for a state wishing to increase its population. So, it is highly unlikely that she would have survived an abdominal childbirth.

There are also references in Chinese literature about a cesarean delivery being preformed at around 120 AD by a surgeon in the Han Dynasty. This surgery was again mentioned in the Chinese scriptures in the Tang Dynasty as a post mortem procedure. The first reference to a cesarean delivery on a live woman is made in the Hindu scripture, Sushruta samhita.

THE MIDDLE AGES

There are few records of the cesarean operation being done from 120 AD to 1115 AD e.g. Gebhart, the Bishop of Constance, was delivered in 919 AD; Count Linsgow, was delivered by the abdominal route in 949 AD. Both these were postmortem deliveries of premature infants, and the children were placed in the abdomen of a newly killed pig because the pig fat stayed warm and moist for a longer time than any other animal. These served as excellent rural incubators.

During the 12th century, a brave Spanish nobleman delivered the Mayer of Navarre when the latter's mother was killed during war. The nobleman saw the child's arm protruding through the mothers abdomen, pulled it free, and it lived and breathed at once, it is said. In the 16th century, one of the more controversial royal deliveries concerned the birth of Edward VII. Because of a failed labor, the king was questioned as to whether such an operation should be done, as it was usually fatal. The king presumably replied, "Proceed, for it is easier to find another wife than a son and heir".

During its evolution, cesarean delivery has meant different things to different people at different times. The indications for it have changed dramatically from ancient times to present times. During ancient times, the purpose essentially was to retrieve the infant from a dead or dying mother; this was conducted either in the rather vain hope of saving the baby's life, or as commonly required by religious edicts, so the infant may be buried separately from its mother. It was a measure of last resort, and the operation was not intended to preserve the mothers life. It was not until late middle ages that such a possibility really came within the grasp of the medical profession.

While the middle ages have been viewed largely as a period of stagnation in science and medicine, some of the stories of cesarean delivery actually helped to develop and sustain hopes that the operation could ultimately be accomplished. The first written record of a mother and a baby surviving a cesarean delivery comes from Switzerland in 1500 when a pig gelder, Jacob Nufer, performed the operation on his wife. After several days in labor and help from thirteen midwives, the woman was unable to deliver a baby. Her desperate husband eventually gained permission from the local authorities to attempt a cesarean delivery. By dint of his work in animal husbandry, Nufer also possessed a modicum of anatomical knowledge, which came handy during the surgical childbirth he attempted on his wife. The mother lived and subsequently gave birth normally to five children, including twins. Since this story was not recorded until 82 years later, the historians question its accuracy.

AFTER THE DARK AGES

The first unquestioned successful cesarean delivery performed by a physician was by Trautmann and Seest in 1610 AD in Wittenberg. From this time the operation was rarely used, but, as time passed, its use increased in spite of high maternal mortality. Cesarean delivery of a live woman is truly an operation of the late 1800s and the 1900s.

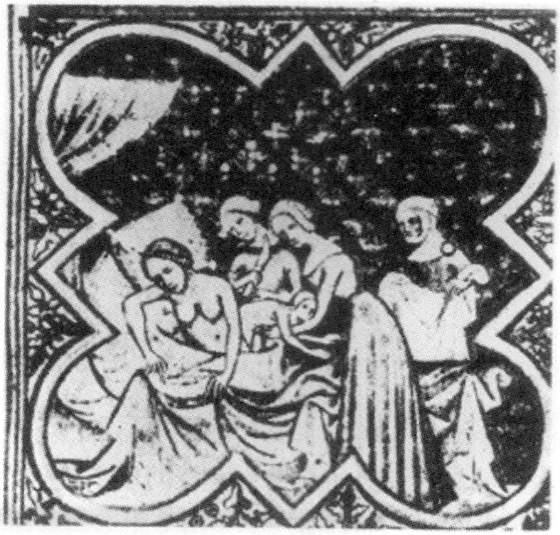

Fig. 3.3. Cesarean section performed on a living woman by a female practitioner. Miniature from a fourteenth-century "Historie Ancienne". Courtesy: National Library of Medicine, USA.

In the 18th century, the cesarean delivery operation had undergone many influences affecting its use. Until this time, female midwives gave majority of assistance during childbirth and medical care during childbirth was not in vogue. After the advent of obstetrical forceps, men's claims to authority over such instruments assisted them in establishing professional control over childbirth. In the western society, women for the most part were barred from carrying out cesarean deliveries until the late 19th century, because they were denied admission to medical schools. A woman, however, conducted the first recorded successful cesarean in the British Empire. Sometime between 1815 and 1821, James Miranda Stuart Barry performed the operation while masquerading as a man and serving a physician to the British army in South Africa. While Barry applied Western surgical techniques, nineteenth century travelers in Africa reported instances of indigenous people successfully carrying out the procedure with their own medical practices.

In 1879, for example, one British traveler, R W Felkin, witnessed cesarean delivery performed by Ugandans. The healer used banana wine to semi-toxicate the woman and to cleanse his hands and her abdomen prior to surgery. After the delivery, he massaged the uterus to make it contract but did not suture it; the abdominal wound was pinned with iron needles and dressed with a paste prepared from the roots.

The patient recovered well, and Felkin concluded that this technique was well developed and had clearly been employed for a long time. Similar reports come from Rwanda, where botanical preparations were also used to anesthetize the patient and promote wound healing. While many of the earliest reports of cesarean delivery issue from remote parts of Europe, the United States and from places far removed from the latest developments in medicine, it was only with increased urbanization and the growth of hospital that the operation began to be performed routinely.

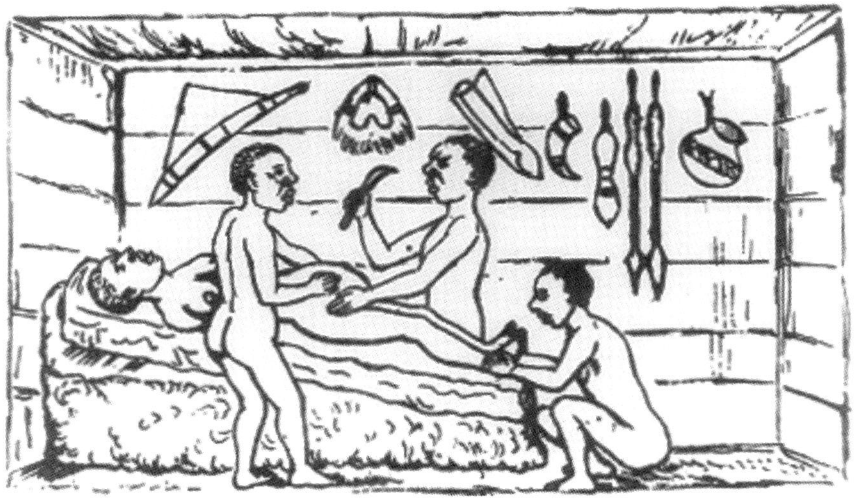

Fig. 3.4. Successful Cesarean section performed by indigenous healers in Kahura, Uganda. As observed by R. W. Felkin in 1879. Courtesy: National Library of Medicine, USA.

The majority of physicians employed in obstetric care were strongly opposed to the employment of cesarean except in the obviously moribund or recently expired woman. The few who advocated the use of cesarean when the mother was alive and in good condition were severely castigated by their peers but nevertheless persisted in their attitude. Of these pioneers, Levret and Baudelocque in France were the leading protagonists for cesarean delivery.

As a serious abdominal operation, the development of cesarean delivery reflected changes within general surgery. In the early 1800s, when surgery still relied on age-old techniques, its practitioners were dreaded and viewed by the public as little better than barbers, butchers, and tooth pullers. Well into the 1800s surgery continued to be barbarous and the best operators were known for the speed with which they could operate.

During the 19th century, however surgery was transformed – both technically and professionally. A new era in surgical practice began in 1846 at Massachusetts General Hospital when William T G Morton used diethyl ether while removing a facial tooth. The medical application of anesthesia spread rapidly but in obstetrics, though, there was opposition to its use based on the biblical injunction that women should sorrow to bring forth children in atonement for Eve's sin. This argument was substantially demolished when the head of Church of England, Queen Victoria, had chloroform administered for the birth of two of her children. Subsequently, anesthesia in childbirth became popular among the wealthy and practical in cases of cesarean delivery.

While doctors and patients alike were encouraged by anesthesia, mortality rates for cesarean delivery continued to remain high due to septicemia and peritonitis accounting for a large percentage of post-operative deaths. This changed with introduction of antiseptic methods using carbolic acid by Joseph Lister, a British surgeon in mid 1860s. By the end of the century antisepsis and asepsis gradually were making inroads into the problems of surgical infections.

Unfortunately, surgical techniques of those times also contributed to the appallingly high maternal mortality rates. Surgeons were afraid to suture the uterine incision because they thought internal stitches, which could not be removed, might set up infections and cause uterine rupture in subsequent pregnancies. They believed the muscles of uterus would contract and close spontaneously. The search for a safer operation continued, and it was at this time that the Italian professor Eduardo Porro did one of the first and most dramatic surgeries in 1876. He advocated hysterectomy in concurrence with cesarean delivery to control uterine hemorrhage and prevent systemic infections. There were several additions to the Porro operation, but the fact that it was considered mutilating made its use as a routine procedure unacceptable to many surgeons. Davis in 1920s advocated hysterectomy with exteriorization of cervical stump after the cesarean delivery. In spite of these technical changes, the morbidity and mortality of the cesarean delivery did not appreciably change.

This, however, was soon to change. A major technical advance in the cesarean delivery was made with the introduction of uterine sutures for control of hemorrhage. Uterine suture was a controversial matter in 1882 when two German surgeons, Kehrer and Sanger, introduced adequate and entirely useful methods for closure of uterine wound. This contributed greatly in reducing the morbidity of cesarean birth.

In the 19th century, obstetrics, gynecology and general surgery all began to proliferate and prosper because of the solution to the three absolute requirements for successful surgery: these were control of bleeding – hemostasis; control of pain – anesthesia and control of infection - asepsis.

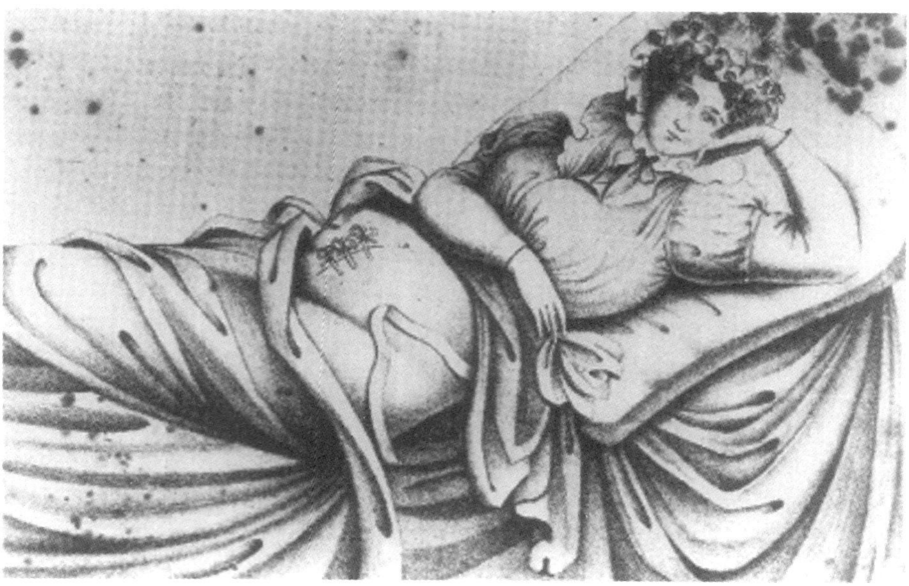

Fig. 3.5. A Cesarean patient prior to dressing the wound, 1822
Courtesy: National Library of Medicine, USA.

As surgeons' confidence in the outcome of their procedures increased, they turned their attention to other issues, including where to incise the uterus. Between 1880 and 1925, obstetricians experimented with transverse incisions in the lower segment. Along with the use of sutures to close the uterine wound in 1882, Kehrer also had performed the lower segment operation at around the same time but failed to report it.

In the early 1900s, extraperitoneal cesarean delivery was first described by Frank (1907) and subsequently modified by Latzko (1909) and Waters (1940). Pfannensteil in 1908 failed to perform an extraperitoneal cesarean delivery; he then did the cesarean delivery transperitoneally and entered the lower uterine segment and successfully delivered a baby.

Delee gives Osiander credit for being the originator of the low segment cesarean delivery. Osiander decided that there were many advantages to making an incision in the dependant portion of the uterus and performed such an operation in 1915. Various modifications were introduced for the lower segment cesarean delivery but finally, Kerr (1926) developed and popularized this approach, which is most commonly employed throughout the world today.

Over the years, other technical advances were made as cesarean delivery became a safer and therefore a more frequently performed surgical procedure.

CONCLUSION

This exhaustive account of the history of cesarean delivery is not only interesting but is equally important. What is most striking is the astounding and tremendous advance made in the management of childbirth especially in the last 200 years, when systematic human civilizations have been known to exist for at least last 2500 years. Introduction of cesarean delivery as a part of managed childbirth has not only been instrumental in making labor safe and decreasing the staggering mortality associated with it, but more recently, it has been responsible for contributing to lowering of perinatal morbidity and mortality especially in high risk pregnancies.

REFERENCES

1. Ackerknecht, Erwin H., A Short History of Medicine, Baltimore: The Johns Hopkins University Press, 1982.
2. Boley, J.P., "The History of Cesarean Section", Canadian Medical Association Journal, Vol. 145, No. 4, 1991, pp. 319-322.
3. Donnison, Jean, Midwives and Medical Men: A History of the Struggle for the Control of Childbirth, London: Historical Publications Ltd., 1988.
4. Eastman, N.J., "The Role of Frontier America in the Development of Cesarean Section", American Journal of Obstetrics and Gynecology, Vol. 24, 1932, p. 919.
5. Gabert, Harvey A., "History and Development of Cesarean Operation", in Obstetrics and Gynecology Clinics of North America, Vol. 15, No. 4. 1988, pp. 591-605.
6. Miller, Joseph M., "First Successful Cesarean Section in the British Empire", Letters, Vol. 166, No. 1, Part 1, p. 269.
7. Oakley, Ann, The Captured Womb: A History of the Medical Care of Pregnant Women, Oxford: Basil Blackwell Ltd., 1984, 1986.
8. Wertz, Richard W. and Dorothy C. Wertz, Lying-In: A History of Childbirth in America, New Haven: Yale University Press, 1989.

   Willson, J. Robert, "The Conquest of Cesarean Section-Related Infections: A Progress Report", Obstetrics and Gynecology, Vol. 72, No. 3, Part 2, September 1988, pp. 519-532.

4 | CHAPTER

Surgical Anatomy For Cesarean Delivery

Trishala Meghal

FRAMEWORK

- Introduction
- The abdominal wall
  - Skin
  - Subcutaneous tissue
  - Musculo-aponeurotic layer
  - Fascia transversalis
  - Parietal peritoneum
  - Visceral peritoneum
  - Blood supply
  - Nerve supply
  - Lymph drainage
- The uterus
  - Size and shape
  - Attachments
  - Relations
  - Parts of the uterus
  - Layers of the wall
  - Blood supply
- The vagina
- The ovary
- The fallopian tube
- The internal iliac artery
- The urinary bladder
- The ureter
- Suture materials
  - Absorbable sutures
  - Non-absorbable sutures
- Wound healing
  - Inflammation
  - Repair
  - Remodeling
- Conclusion

INTRODUCTION

Over the years, the knowledge of anatomy has increased, and so has its application to surgical techniques. Greater awareness of anatomical structures and tissue planes has helped in improving the techniques of surgical practice. Better surgical techniques along with safety of blood transfusion, and advent of effective antibiotics have reduced the mortality due to cesarean delivery from almost a hundred percent to less than 1 per 10,000 in the modern era.

It is extremely worthwhile to be aware of the normal anatomy of the abdominal wall, the female reproductive organs and the pelvic organs to be able to perform a cesarean section and deal with the complications of the same. This chapter discusses the relevant details of anatomy pertinent to performance of the cesarean delivery.

THE ABDOMINAL WALL

Cesarean delivery is defined as the birth of the fetus through an incision in the abdominal wall and uterine wall. Knowledge of the layered structure of the abdominal wall permits the surgeon to enter the abdominal cavity during cesarean delivery with maximum efficiency and safety.

The summary of the abdominal wall layers is provided in following box.

Skin

Subcutaneous Layer

- Camper's Fascia
- Scarpa's Fascia

Musculo-aponeurotic Layer

- Rectus sheath
- Rectus Abdominis muscle
- External oblique muscle
- Internal oblique muscle
- Transverse abdominal muscle

Transversalis Fascia

Peritoneum

As the incision for the caesarean section is made, the above layers are incised, each of which will be discussed in detail with the relevant applied anatomy[1, 2, 3, 4, 5].

Skin

The skin consists of two distinct elements: epidermis and dermis. The epidermis is composed of stratified squamous epithelium and the deeper layer i.e. the dermis is composed of dense connective tissue containing blood vessels, lymphatics and nerve fibres. The dermis tends to be thinner on the abdomen than on the back.

Since most of the bundles of collagen fibers in the dermis are arranged in parallel rows, surgical incisions made along the skin creases heal with minimum scarring. Conversely, an incision made across the rows of collagen results in formation of an unsightly scar. These skin creases are known as the cleavage lines, originally described by Langer in 1861. They tend to run longitudinally in the limbs and circumferentially on the abdomen.

Cutaneous nerve supply (Fig. 4.1)

The cutaneous nerve supply to the anterior abdominal wall is derived from the anterior rami of the lower six thoracic and first lumbar nerves i.e. the intercostals nerves seven to eleven, the subcostal nerves (T12), the iliohypogastric nerves (T12 and L1) and the ilioinguinal (L1) nerves. After giving off a lateral cutaneous branch, each intercostal nerve pierces the lateral border of the rectus sheath. There it provides a lateral branch that ends in the rectus muscle. The anterior branch passes through the muscle and perforates the rectus sheath to supply the skin as the anterior cutaneous branch.

The first lumbar nerve has a similar course, but it does not enter the rectus sheath. It is represented by the iliohypogastric nerve, which pierces the external oblique aponeurosis above the superficial inguinal ring, and by the ilioinguinal nerve, which emerges through the ring. They end by supplying the skin just above the inguinal ligament and the symphysis pubis. The lateral branch of the last thoracic nerve crosses the iliac crest to supply the skin of the buttocks. The dermatome of T7 is located in the epigastrium over the xiphoid process, T10 includes the umbilicus and that of L1 lies above the inguinal ligament and the symphysis pubis.

Minimal loss of skin sensations can result from any abdominal incision. Numbness below a transverse incision frequently occurs due to interruption of the nerve supply to the skin. Elevation of the rectus sheath off the muscle during the pfannensteil incision stretches the perforating nerve, which if ligated during hemostasis can result in cutaneous anesthesia.

Blood Supply (Fig. 4.1 and 2)

The skin near the midline is supplied by the branches of the superior epigastric artery (branch of the internal thoracic artery), the inferior epigastric artery (branch of the external iliac artery) and the superficial epigastric artery, which is a branch of the femoral artery. The superficial arteries accompany the cutaneous nerves. Those that accompany the lateral cutaneous nerves are branches of the posterior intercostal arteries, while those that travel with the anterior cutaneous nerves are derived from the superior and inferior epigastric vessels. The superficial inferior epigastric vessels run a diagonal course in the subcutaneous tissue from the femoral vessels toward the umbilicus, beginning as a single artery which branches extensively as it nears the umbilicus. The skin of the flanks is supplied by branches from the intercostals, lumbar and deep circumflex iliac arteries.

The venous blood is collected by a network of veins that radiate from the umbilicus. The network above the umbilicus drains via the lateral thoracic vein & the axillary vein into the superior vena cava and below the umbilicus via the superficial epigastric & great saphenous veins into the femoral vein, and finally into the inferior vena cava. A few small veins, the paraumbilical veins, connect the network through the umbilicus and along the ligamentum teres to the portal vein.

Lymphatic Drainage

The lymphatic drainage of the lower abdomen drains in to the superficial inguinal nodes and then into the iliac nodes.

When an incision is placed in the lower abdomen, the lymphatic drainage of the abdominal wall above the incision site is interrupted. Some tissue swelling may develop temporarily until collateral lymphatic drainage is established.

Subcutaneous tissue

In the subcutaneous tissue, the fat is contained in loculi, whose fibrous walls connect the overlying dermis to the underlying deep fascia. In the more superficial part of the subcutaneous layer, the fat predominates. This is the Camper's fascia which contains blood vessels and nerves.

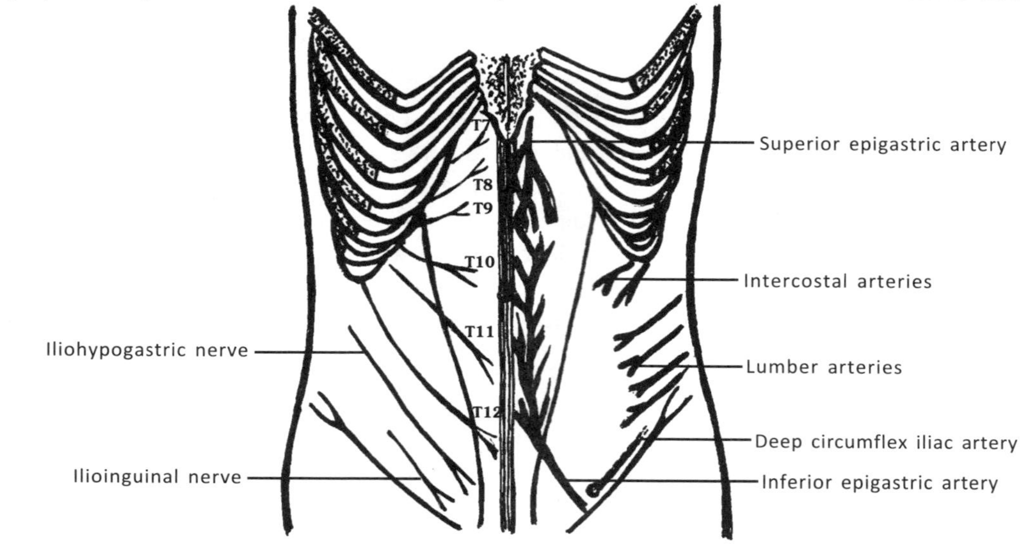

Fig. 4.1 Innervation and blood supply of anterior abdominal wall

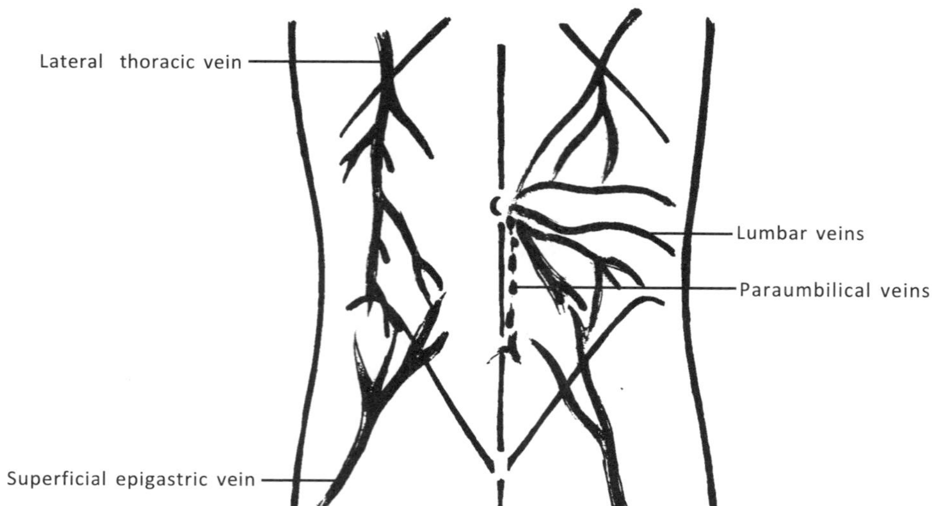

Fig. 4.2 Venous drainage of anterior abdominal wall

Closer to the rectus sheath, fibrous tissue predominates and this is the Scarpa's fascia (deep membranous layer). The Camper's and Scarpa's fasciae are not discrete or well-defined layers but represent a region of the subcutaneum. The Scarpa's fascia is best developed laterally and is not seen as a well-defined layer during vertical incisions. Superiorly, it becomes continuous with the superficial fascia of the back and thorax. Inferiorly it forms a sheath for the clitoris. Below in the perineum, it enters the wall of the labia majora. From there it passes to be attached on each side to the margins of the pubic arch, where it is referred as Colle's fascia. Posteriorly, it fuses with the perineal body and the posterior margin of the perineal membrane. Approximation of the Scarpa's fascia provides the tensile strength for appropriate healing of the caesarean section wounds.

The deep fascia in the anterior abdominal wall is merely a thin layer of connective tissue covering the muscles. It lies immediately deep to the membranous layer of superficial fascia.

Musculo-aponeurotic layer

The abdominal wall muscles work synergistically with the muscles of the back to flex, extend and rotate the trunk and pelvis. They act as efficient protectors of the abdominal viscera and by their tonicity they maintain the intra-abdominal pressure and help keep viscera in place. They are also the muscles of respiration since their contraction causes them to press upon the abdominal viscera, forcing them upward and thus elevating the diaphragm. There are two groups of muscles: the vertical muscles and the oblique flank muscles.

The vertically running muscles are the rectus abdominis on either side of the midline and the paired pyramidalis muscle, which is located just above the pubis. The recti are the muscles of locomotion and posture.

The flat flank muscles include the external oblique, the internal oblique and the transversus abdominis. Their fibers run diagonally or transversely. The tendons of these muscles unite to form a broad sheet like aponeuroses that unites with the corresponding member of the opposite side, forming a covering for the rectus abdominis muscle called the rectus sheath.

The vertical muscles (Fig. 4.3)

The Rectus Abdominis muscle is a long strap muscle that extends along the whole length of the anterior abdominal wall. It lies in the midline and the Linea Alba separates the pair from each other.

It arises by two heads, the medial head from in front of the symphysis pubis and the lateral head from the pubic crest. It courses superiorly and inserts into the 5th, 6th and 7th costal cartilages and the xiphoid process. Its upper insertion is 3 times as broad as it's pubic attachment. When it contracts, its lateral margin forms a curved ridge that can be palpated and often seen and is termed the linea semilunaris. It extends from the pubic tubercle to the costal margin of the 9th costal cartilage. The muscle has three or four transverse tendinous intersections. One is at the level of the umbilicus and two intersections are usually halfway between the umbilicus and the insertion at the xiphoid process. The tendinous intersections are tightly adherent to the anterior rectus sheath.

The paired Pyramidalis muscles arise from the crest of the pubic symphysis and inserts into the lower linea alba. It is often absent. Preservation of the Pyramidalis muscles is not essential when making incisions. The midportion of this muscle usually has an avascular raphe that can easily be incised for adequate exposure of the space of Retzius.

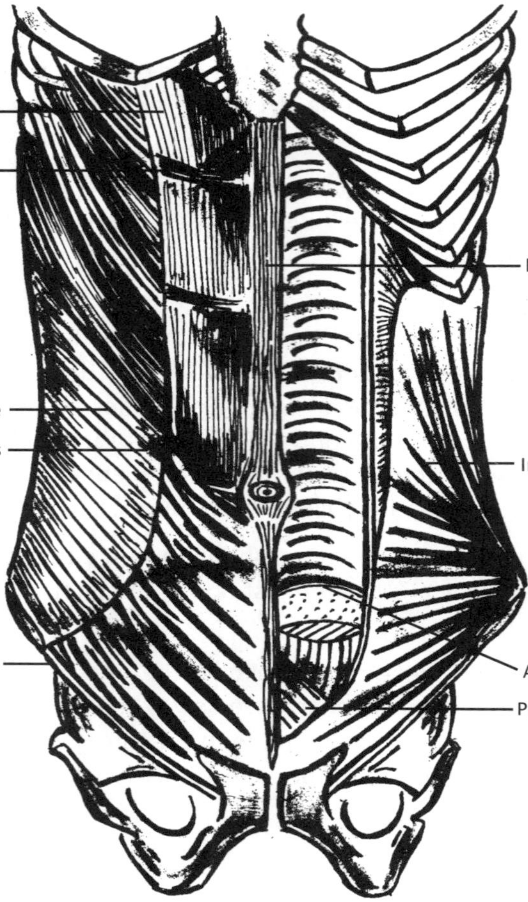

Fig. 4.3 Anterior view of the rectus abdominis muscle and its relations

The oblique muscles (Fig. 4.4)

The external oblique muscle and its aponeurosis form the anterior most layer of the flat muscles. The external oblique muscle originates from the lower eight ribs and fans out to be inserted into the xiphoid process, the linea alba, the pubic crest, the pubic tubercle and the anterior half of the iliac crest. Superiorly the fibers of this muscle run transversely and inferiorly they assume an oblique downward course. The muscle also forms a broad fibrous aponeurosis that passes anteriorly to the rectus muscle.

The internal oblique originates primarily from the anterior two thirds of the iliac crest, the thoraco-lumbar fascia and the lateral two thirds of the inguinal ligament. The muscle runs an upward oblique course and gives rise to the aponeurosis of the internal oblique. The aponeurosis splits at the lateral border of the rectus, forms a sheath around the rectus muscle and then inserts in the midline to form the linea alba. The muscle is inserted into the lower borders of the lower three ribs and their costal cartilages, the xiphoid process, the linea alba and the symphysis pubis.

The transverse abdominis is a thin sheet of muscle that lies deep to the internal oblique, and it's fibers run horizontally forward. It arises from the lower 6 costal cartilages, thoraco-lumbar fascia, the anterior two thirds of the internal lip of the iliac crest and the lateral third of the inguinal ligament. It has a transverse course. The lowest tendinous fibers join similar fibers from the internal oblique to form the conjoint tendon, which is fixed to the pubic crest and the pectineal line.

The line of demarcation between the muscular and the aponeurotic portions of the external oblique muscle in the lower abdomen occurs along a vertical line through the anterior superior iliac spine. The internal oblique and transversus abdominis muscles extend farther toward the midline, coming closest at their inferior margin, at the pubic tubercle. The fibers of the internal oblique are found underneath the aponeurotic portion of the external oblique muscle during a transverse incision. Hence, a layer by layer sharp dissection is carried out in order to avoid injury to the internal oblique. In addition, it is between the internal oblique and transverse abdominal muscles that the nerves and blood vessels of the flank are found and their injury may be avoided by careful dissection.

The Rectus sheath (Fig. 4.5)

The rectus sheath is a long fibrous sheath that encloses the rectus abdominis and the pyramidalis muscle and contains the anterior rami of the lower six thoracic nerves, the superior and inferior epigastric vessels and lymph vessels.

The aponeurosis of the internal oblique splits into anterior and posterior layers to enclose the rectus muscle. The external oblique aponeurosis fuses with the anterior layer to form the anterior layer of the sheath, and the transverses aponeurosis fuses with the posterior layer to form the posterior layer of the sheath. An inch below the umbilicus, this arrangement ceases and from this level downwards all the aponeuroses pass in front of the muscle and then inserts into the linea alba. There is thus, a free lower margin to the posterior sheath; it is concave and called as the arcuate line (semicircular line of Douglas).

There is an excellent fascial support anterior and posterior to the rectus muscles above the arcuate (semicircular) line. The lower half of the lower abdominal wall is weakened below the arcuate line, where the posterior division of the rectus sheath disappears. It is in this weakened section of the lower abdomen that most of the incisional hernias occur after cesarean section through lower midline incisions. In the lower abdomen the force required to approximate edges of a vertical incision is 30 times greater than the force required to approximate edges of a transverse incision.

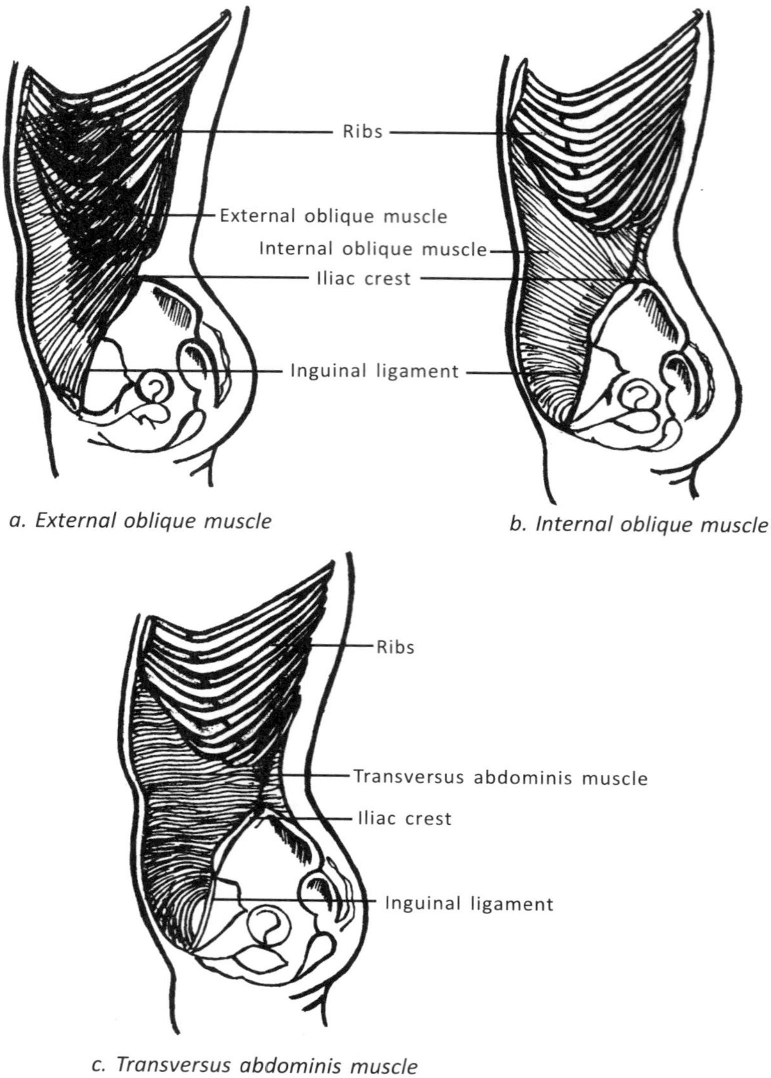

Fig. 4.4 Oblique and transversus muscles of the anterior abdominal wall.

The major function of the flat muscles is to assist in increasing intra-abdominal pressure. Each time these muscles contract, they pull at the linea alba. Because the linea alba represents the six major abdominal muscles (three on each side), cutting it, as with lower midline incisions, interrupts the major portion of the insertion of these muscles. Thus, contractions of these muscles in the postoperative period can result in considerable tension on the suture line. It is for the same reason that considerable care should be taken in suturing the fascial tissues after an abdominal surgery, especially with an incision in the lower abdomen.

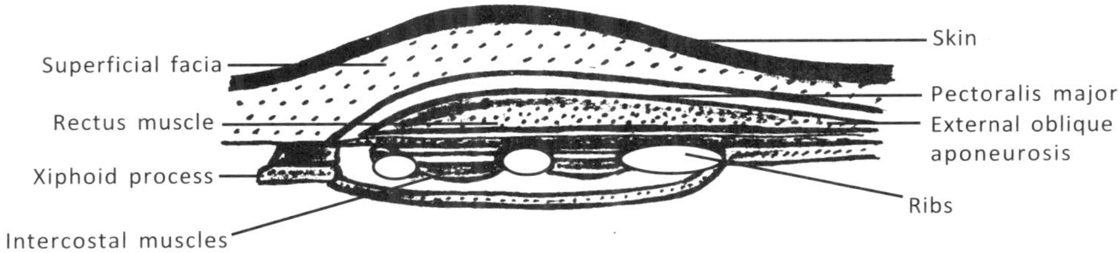

a. Above the costal margin

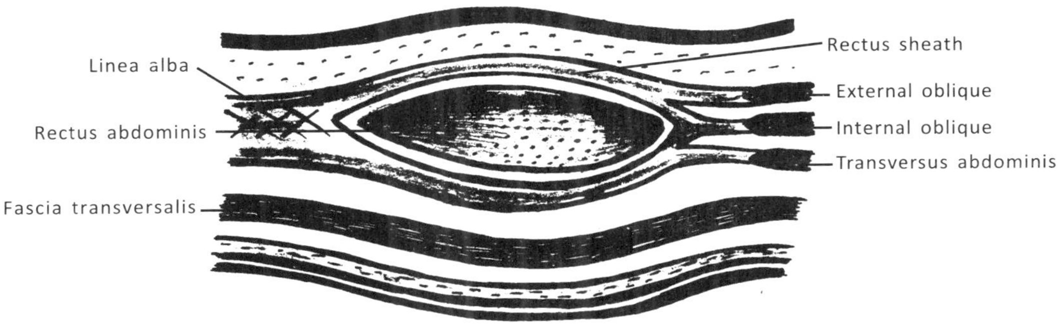

b. Between the costal margin and the arcuate line

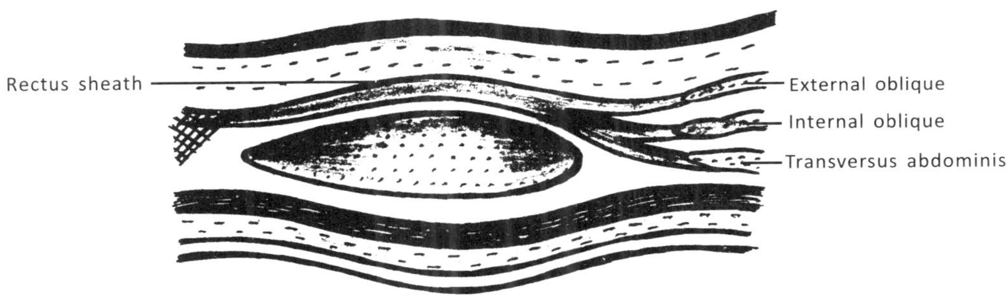

c. Below the arcuate line

Fig. 4.5 The rectus sheath

Fascia transversalis

The fascia transversalis is a thin layer of fascia lining the transversus abdominis muscle.

Extraperitoneal fat

The extraperitoneal fat is a thin layer of connective tissue that contains a variable amount of fat and lies between the fascia transversalis and the parietal peritoneum.

Parietal peritoneum

Parietal peritoneum is a serous membrane made up of a single layer of flattened mesothelial cells. It lines the walls of the abdominal cavity, the undersurface of the diaphragm and the pelvic cavity.

Below the umbilicus, there is a central fold of peritoneum with a pair of folds on either side. The central fold is the median umbilical fold containing the obliterated remains of the urachus. Lateral to this are the paired medial umbilical folds containing the obliterated umbilical arteries that connected the internal iliac vessels to the umbilical cord in fetal life. Farther laterally are the lateral umbilical ligaments containing inferior epigastric vessels. The reflection of the bladder on to the anterior abdominal wall is triangular in shape, with its apex blending with the median umbilical ligament. Since the apex is highest in the midline, incision in the peritoneum is made at the highest point and continued laterally to the midline to avoid bladder injury.

The peritoneum is supplied by the nerves of the overlying muscles i.e. the intercostal and the lumbar nerves.

Visceral peritoneum

It is the continuation of the parietal peritoneum, which leaves the posterior wall of the abdominal cavity and invests therein. The uterus is draped by this adherent fold of peritoneum that is continued laterally on each side to be attached to the sidewall of the pelvis; this reflection is the broad ligament. Anteriorly the peritoneum passes from the anterior abdominal wall on to the dome of the bladder, and then passes over to the base of the bladder. It then runs directly on to the anterior surface of the uterus till the level of the internal os. This is the uterovesical fold. The peritoneum then passes over the anterior surface of the body and fundus of the uterus and then downward over the posterior surface. It continues downward and covers the posterior surface of the vagina where it forms the pouch of Douglas. The visceral peritoneum is insensitive to pain. The visceral peritoneum forms a loose fold where it reflects over the posterior surface of the bladder. This is at level of the internal os and thus it helps to identify the lower segment, which is just above the level of the loose fold[6].

Closure of parietal peritoneum was advocated previously to establish normal anatomical relations, to prevent adhesion formation between the intestines and fascia or between the uterus and fascia, to reduce the risk of infection and to reduce the risk of herniation or dehiscence. However, the advantages of this technique have been disproved by prospective randomized trials. [7,8,9] In fact, suture tends to cause tissue ischemia, necrosis, inflammation and foreign body reactions to suture materials. These factors slow down the healing process and are considered important precursors for adhesion formation.

Blood supply of the abdominal wall

The main arterial supply of the abdominal wall consists of the superior epigastric, musculophrenic, deep circumflex iliac and inferior epigastric vessels.

The medial part of the abdominal wall receives blood from the epigastric arteries, while the musculophrenic and deep circumflex iliac arteries supply the lateral wall. The lateral wall is also supplied by the lower intercostal and lumbar arteries (T8 to T12 and L1). This freely anastomosing vascular system provides one continuous arterial and venous channel on both sides of the anterior abdominal wall, extending from the subclavian vessels cephalad to the external iliac vessels caudal. The linea alba is relatively bloodless. The limited vascular supply in this area of fascial fusion can impair wound healing when lower midline incisions are used. Thus, a secure closure is mandatory in such incisions.

The Superior epigastric artery, one of the terminal branches of the internal thoracic artery, enters the upper part of the rectus sheath. The artery descends behind the rectus muscle, supplying the upper central part of the anterior abdominal wall and anastomoses with the inferior epigastric artery.

The inferior epigastric artery is a branch of the external iliac artery just above the inguinal ligament. It runs upward and medially along the medial side of the deep inguinal ring. It pierces the fascia transversalis to enter the rectus sheath anterior to the arcuate line. It ascends behind the rectus muscle, supplying the lower central part of the anterior abdominal wall and anastomoses with the superior epigastric artery.

The deep circumflex iliac artery is a branch of the external iliac artery just above the inguinal ligament. It runs upward and laterally towards the antero-superior iliac spine and then continues along the iliac crest. It supplies the lower lateral part of the abdominal wall. The lower two posterior intercostal arteries, branches of the descending thoracic aorta and 4 lumbar arteries, branches of the abdominal aorta, pass forward between the muscle layers and supply the lateral part of the abdominal wall.

The epigastric vessels are subject to injury, particularly when a muscle splitting incision is used. Also, the deep circumflex or musculophrenic vessels can be injured when an extraperitoneal approach is chosen.

The venous blood from the skin is connected in to a network of veins that radiate from the umbilicus. The network drains above into the axillary vein via the lateral thoracic vein and below into the femoral vein via the superficial epigastric & great saphenous veins. A few small veins, the paraumbilical veins, connect the network through the umbilicus and along the ligamentum teres to the portal vein. They form a clinically important porto-systemic venous anastomosis.

The superior epigastric, inferior epigastric, and deep circumflex iliac veins follow the arteries of the same name and drain into the internal thoracic and external iliac veins. The posterior intercostal veins drains into the azygous veins and the lumbar veins drain into the inferior vena cava.

Nerve supply of the abdominal wall

The muscles of the anterior abdominal wall are supplied by the lower 6 thoracic nerves and the iliohypogastric and ilioinguinal nerves (L1).

The intercostal nerves pass behind the costal margin between the transversus abdominis and the internal oblique muscle and pass around to pierce the posterior rectus sheath. Each nerve is accompanied by its collateral branch in the neuro-vascular plane, but only the main nerve gives off a lateral cutaneous branch that supplies the skin.

The external oblique is muscular in only its upper part and is supplied segmentally by the 7th to the 11th intercostal nerves. The other two muscles are supplied by the lower 6 thoracic nerves (7th to 12th) inclusive and also by L1 via both iliohypogastric and ilioinguinal nerves, the later supplying the lower border of each muscle where it fuses into the conjoint tendon. Hence if the ilioinguinal and iliohypogastric nerves get damaged at the level of the antero-superior iliac spine, a weakening of the normal canal controlling mechanism can occur predisposing the patient to inguinal hernia.

Each nerve contains fibers from the last 2 or 3 intercostal nerves. A transverse incision is least likely to cause injury to the nerves. A vertical incision passing lateral to the rectus muscle or through the rectus muscle itself can denervate the medially lying muscle causing weakening of the muscle predisposing to incisional hernia formation. A midline incision in the linea alba or a transverse incision does not interfere with the motor innervation of the abdominal musculature. A minimal loss of the skin sensation can result from any abdominal incision, usually the paramedian incision. The iliohypogastric and ilioinguinal nerves are sensory in function. The injury to the iliohypogastric nerves can result in sensation changes in the skin over the mons, whereas injury to the ilioinguinal nerves can result in sensation changes to the labia majora. A wide transverse incision can result in numbness of the skin over the anterior part of the thigh.

Lymph drainage of the anterior abdominal wall

The cutaneous lymph vessels above the level of the umbilicus drain upwards into the anterior axillary lymph nodes. The vessels below this level drain downwards into the superficial inguinal nodes. The deep lymph vessels follow the arteries and drain into the internal thoracic, external iliac, posterior mediastinal and para aortic nodes[1,2,3,4,5].

THE UTERUS[13,14,15,16]

The uterus is a pear shaped muscular organ that is intermediate in position between the bladder, the rectum and the broad ligament.

Size and shape

In the adult nulliparous state, it is flat antero-posteriorly and piriform, with its narrow end postero-inferior in position. It is about 7.5 cm in length, 5 cm in breadth and 2.5 cms thick in its widest part. It weighs 30-40 grams.

During pregnancy, the uterus undergoes remarkable growth and weighs about 1100 grams at times. It elongates up to 35 cms and occupies a total volume of 5 liters.

Attachments

The broad ligaments are two wing-like double folds of peritoneum extending on either side of the uterus up to the lateral pelvic wall. Each broad ligament has a superior, inferior, lateral and medial margin. The inner two–third of the upper margin of the broad ligament is free forming the mesosalpinx that encloses the fallopian tube. The mesovarium consists of a fold of peritoneum containing the ovary and the ovarian ligament. The upper part of the lateral edge extends superolaterally to the ovary as the suspensory ligament of the ovary or the infundibulopelvic ligament, forming a raised fold of peritoneum due to underlying ovarian vessels and lymphatics. The ovarian and the uterine vessels run between the leaves of the broad ligament.

The round ligaments of the uterus are 10–12 cm long true ligamentous fibromuscular cords extending from the superolateral angle of the uterus through the deep inguinal ring, inguinal canal and the external inguinal ring to finally insert into the labium majus of the vulva. They lie in the anterior layer of the broad ligament below the uterine tube. Due to differential growth of the body of the uterus the insertion of the round ligament appears to be at the junction of the upper and middle thirds of the organ. Each round ligament is supplied by a branch of the ovarian artery in the broad ligament and by a branch from the inferior epigastric artery in the inguinal canal.

The uterosacral ligaments are two short fibromuscular cords that pass backward from the posterior aspect of the upper end of the cervix on each side of the rectum and then get attached to the sacrum. The uterosacral ligaments and the bases of the broad ligaments rise up to the pelvic brim with a resultant deepening of the pouch of Douglas The area underneath the broad ligament and the lateral pelvic wall is filled with loose vascular connective tissue. They are best palpated on rectal examination. They keep the cervix braced backwards against the forward pull of the round ligaments on the fundus and so maintain the body of uterus in anteversion.

The Mackenrodt's ligaments (cardinal or transverse cervical ligaments) extend from the cervix and vaginal fornix laterally to the sidewall of the pelvis. They are continuous on each side with the corresponding uterosacral ligaments. They extend laterally and merge with the fascia covering the obturator internus.

The ovarian ligament is a rounded fibromuscular ligament passing between the two layers of the broad ligament from the lower pole of the ovary to the lateral aspect of the uterus.

Relations

The bladder lies anteroinferior to the uterus and is separated from it by the uterovesical fold of the peritoneum and the underlying pubovesicocervical fascia.

Posteriorly, the uterus is in relation with the rectum and the sigmoid colon from which it is separated by the fold of peritoneum, the pouch of Douglas, which contains coils of small intestine.

Parts of the uterus

The uterine corpus or body is the part of the uterus extending between the isthmus and to a plane connecting the two fallopian tube insertions. The part of the uterus above the level of the insertion of the fallopian tubes and ovarian and uterine ligaments is the fundus.

After the first three months, the uterus becomes globular in shape. In late pregnancy, due to rapid elongation it assumes an ovoid shape. The uterus becomes an abdominal organ beyond 12 weeks. This enlargement is asymmetrical and is more marked at the fundus. The part of the uterus surrounding the placental site enlarges more rapidly.

The isthmus, in the non-pregnant state, is a 0.5 cm wide band of tissue between the body and the cervix. It is the area of transition from the cervical mucosa to the endometrium. During pregnancy and labor it enlarges to a 7.5–10 cm, long, thin walled portion called as the "the lower uterine segment". The upper uterine segment is quite firm and hard while the consistency of the lower uterine segment is much less firm. During labor, the upper segment contracts, retracts, and expels the fetus. In response to these contractions, the lower uterine segment and cervix dilate and form a greatly expanded thinned out fibromuscular tube for extrusion of the fetus.

The level at which the visceral peritoneum fuses with the uterus is approximately at the upper limit of the isthmus. Below this, the peritoneum is loose areolar tissue separating the bladder and the cervix. At term, this tissue becomes dense and covers the entire lower uterine segment fusing with the junction of the upper and lower segments along with the peritoneum.

After the disappearance of the anatomical internal os and incorporation of the isthmus into the body in the third month of pregnancy, there is gradual incorporation of the intra–abdominal portion of the cervix into the enlarging uterine body contributing to the lower uterine segment.

The uterine cervix is about 2.5 cm in length. It is narrower than the body, is cylindrical and is widest at its midlevel. The cervix bulges into the anterior vaginal wall and is divided into vaginal and supravaginal portions.

The supravaginal cervix is separated anteriorly from the bladder by pelvic cellular tissue (parametrium). The uterine arteries flank the cervix and the ureters pass about 2 cm lateral to it. Posteriorly, the supravaginal cervix is covered by the peritoneum that passes onto the posterior vaginal wall and is then reflected on to the rectum forming the rectouterine pouch or recess (the pouch of Douglas).

The vaginal part of the cervix projects into the anterior vaginal wall forming grooves called the vaginal fornices.

The canal of the cervix is continuous with the cavity of the body at what is commonly called the internal os. The lower opening into the vagina is called the external os. This is circular in nulliparous women but usually forms a transverse slit after childbirth. The external os is normally on a level with the ischial spines.

In the upper two-thirds, the cervical mucosa consists of numerous, deep glandular follicles secreting clear, viscid, alkaline mucus. The mucosa of the lower half of the canal has numerous papillae. Near the external os, the mucosa becomes non-keratinised stratified squamous type and is contiguous with the mucosal lining of the vagina.

During pregnancy, there is pronounced softening and congestion of the uterus along with increased vascularity, edema, hypertrophy and hyperplasia of the cervical glands. Also, at term, here is a marked reduction in strength of the collagen rich connective tissue. The cervical canal is filled with tenacious mucus (mucus plug), which is expelled during the prelabour phase (bloody show).

Layers of uterine wall

The uterus has an external serosal, middle muscular and an internal mucosal layer.

The serosa : It is the peritoneum, which posteriorly covers the body and supravaginal cervix.

The myometrium: At term, the walls of the body of the uterus are 1.5 cm or less in thickness. The dense, firm, grayish myometrium consists of spindle–shaped smooth muscle fibers arranged in three layers.

i) Outer Longitudinal: These fibers are arranged over the fundus like a hood and extend to the round ligaments.

ii) Inner circular: They form a sphincter like arrangement around the tubal orifices and the internal os.

iii) Intermediate: This is the most prominent layer consisting of crisscross fibers which also surround the blood vessels in a figure of eight fashion, thus occluding the vessels during contraction and retraction.

The increase in the size of the uterus is due to hypertrophy & limited hyperplasia of the muscle fibers in the first half of pregnancy, and by stretching because of the growing fetus and amniotic fluid beyond 20 weeks.

The decidua (endometrium of pregnancy): In pregnancy, the endometrial stromal cells enlarge to form polygonal or round decidual cells with round and vesicular nuclei, and clear and slightly basophilic cytoplasm. In early pregnancy, the decidua attains a depth of 5–10 mm that reduces later in pregnancy due to fetal growth and increase in amniotic fluid.

The decidua basalis, underlying the placental site is the most prominent portion. The decidua capsularis surrounding the remainder of the blastocyst consists of flattened epithelial cells without traces of glands. The uterine cavity is lined by the decidua parietalis.

The decidua basalis and capsularis can be divided into a compact surface zone (zona compacta), a spongy middle layer (zona spongiosa) and a basal zone (zona basalis). The upper two layers form the zona functionalis that is shed after delivery. The zona basalis gives rise to endometrium after delivery. The decidual reaction is most prominent in the upper segment while it is poorly developed in the lower uterine segment.

Blood supply of the uterus[13,14,15]

(Fig. 4.6)

The uterine artery is the predominant vessel supplying the uterus. There are two uterine arteries, one arising on either side as a branch of the anterior division of the internal iliac artery. It runs medially towards the cervix, crosses the ureter above the lateral vaginal fornix and 2 cm lateral to cervix, ascends upwards along the lateral uterine wall between the two leaves of the broad ligament and then underneath the fallopian tube anastomoses with the ovarian artery. The uterine vessels anastomose with each other extensively. Each uterine artery gives rise to anterior and posterior arcuate branches along the length of the uterus. These pass transversely into the uterine myometrium giving off radial branches before anastomosing with their counterpart. The radial branches, before reaching the endometrium, supply a basal branch to the basal zone of decidua and enter into the decidua as the tortuous spiral arteries. There is marked spiraling of the uterine arteries that reaches its maximum at 20 weeks. Later, they become straight and engorged, with the blood flow increasing from 50 ml/min to 450-650 ml/min.

The uterine veins, which too become engorged during pregnancy, run along with the arteries and drain in to the internal iliac veins.

The ovarian artery arises from the abdominal aorta just below the renal artery. It descends along the retroperitoneal space along the posterior abdominal wall, crossing the ureter near its origin from the renal pelvis, and enters the suspensory ligament of the ovary. It courses underneath the fallopian tube before anastomosing with the uterine artery.

The ovarian vein, arising from the pampiniform plexus at the ovarian hilum, courses along with the ovarian arteries and drains into the inferior vena cava on the right side and in to the left renal vein on the left side.

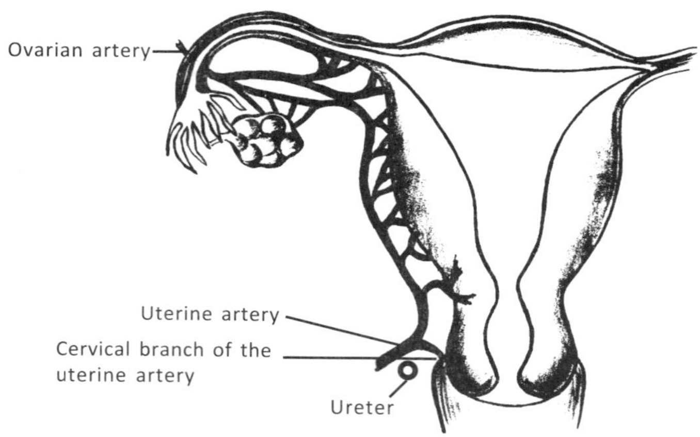

Fig. 4.6 The blood supply of the uterus and its adnexa

THE VAGINA [13,14]

The vagina is a fibromuscular tube lined by non–keratinised stratified squamous epithelium communicating with the cervix superiorly and opening externally at the vaginal introitus. It lies in front of the rectum, anal canal and perineal body, and behind the bladder and urethra. The upper end of the vagina is slightly expanded and receives the uterine cervix which projects into it forming around the margin of the cervix, a circular groove or vaginal fornix. This is subdivided into anterior, posterior and lateral fornices. The posterior fornix is covered by the peritoneum of the front of the rectouterine pouch; this is the only part of the vagina to have a peritoneal covering. The anterior and posterior walls of the vagina are about 8 and 10 cm long respectively in the non-pregnant state and increase in length during pregnancy. This is due to hypertrophy of the smooth muscle along with increased vascularity and hyperemia, with the papillae undergoing hypertrophy to show a hobnailed appearance.

The vagina is supplied by the vaginal artery arising as a descending branch of the uterine or directly from the internal iliac artery. The veins drain into the internal iliac veins.

THE OVARIES[13,15,16]

The ovaries are a pair of ovoid grayish white structures, about 3 x 1.5 x 1.5 cm in size. Each ovary lies in the ovarian fossa on the lateral pelvic wall at the angle between the internal and external iliac vessels and is attached to the uterus by the ovarian ligament. It projects into the pelvic cavity, attached to the posterior leaf of the peritoneum, the mesoovarium. It is in close contact with the fimbrial end of the fallopian tube. The ovary in its normal position can be reached through the vagina by the tip of the examining finger.

The surface appears puckered and uneven due to scarring of previous corpora lutea. A degenerated pale corpus albicans may be noted late in pregnancy – a remnant of the corpus luteum, which loses its function by the twelfth week. Patchy areas of decidual change may occasionally be noted as the surface of the ovary.

THE FALLOPIAN TUBES[13,16]

The fallopian tubes are tortuous ducts lying on either side of the uterus. They are about 10 cm long. Each fallopian tube consists of the following parts:

1) The infundibulum is the fimbriated free lateral end opening into the peritoneal cavity. The abdominal ostium is 3 mm in diameter. This open end lies behind the broad ligament adjacent to the lateral pelvic wall and ovary.
2) The ampulla is about 6–7 cm long and arches over the upper pole of the ovary. Its lumen is 4 mm in diameter. The ciliated columnar epithelium is thrown in 6–12 primary and more complex secondary and tertiary folds.
3) The isthmus is about 2–3 long with a luminal diameter of 2 mm. Its mucosal lining shows 3 - 6 primary folds.
4) The interstitial or intramural portion is the proximal 1 cm of the tube that is embedded in the uterine wall. The tube opens at an angle into the uterine cavity through the narrow ostium, which is about 0.5–1 mm in diameter.

The fallopian tubes receive varying degrees of blood supply from the ovarian and uterine arteries with drainage into the corresponding veins.

THE INTERNAL ILIAC ARTERIES[14,15,17] (Fig. 4.7)

The internal iliac artery is the largest artery in the true pelvis and about 1-½ inches in diameter. It arises as the terminal branch of the common iliac artery on the medial border of the psoas muscle at the level of the upper border of sacrum. It is crossed by the ureter from lateral to medial just beyond its origin. It ends near the upper border of the greater sciatic notch where it divides into anterior and posterior divisions.

The posterior division immediately divides into three branches:

1. The iliolumbar artery
2. The lateral sacral artery
3. The superior gluteal artery

The anterior division gives rise to nine branches:

1) The obturator artery
2) The internal pudendal artery
3) The inferior gluteal artery
4) The middle hemorrhoidal artery
5) The inferior vesical artery
6) The uterine artery
7) The vaginal artery
8) The superior vesical artery
9) The umbilical artery

The branches of the internal iliac artery enter into an extensive collateral anastomosis both with their counterparts as well as with branches from the aorta, external iliac artery and femoral artery. The pathways are:

1) Lumbar branches of aorta with the iliolumbar arteries (internal iliac).
2) Middle sacral artery (aorta) with lateral sacral arteries (internal iliac).
3) Superior rectal arteries (inferior mesenteric) with the middle rectal (internal iliac) and inferior rectal (internal pudendal) arteries.
4) Ovarian arteries (aorta) with the uterine and vaginal arteries (internal iliac).
5) Inferior epigastric artery (external iliac) and medial circumflex artery (femoral) with the obturator artery (internal iliac).
6) Deep circumflex iliac artery (external iliac) and lateral circumflex femoral artery (femoral) with the superior gluteal and iliac branch of iliolumbar arteries (internal iliac).
7) Lateral and medial circumflex femoral arteries (femoral) with the inferior gluteal artery (internal iliac).
8) Superficial and deep external pudendal arteries (femoral) with the internal pudendal artery (internal iliac).

Howard Kelly first described the procedure of internal iliac artery ligation in 1884. The procedure reduces the distal pulse pressure by 77% (unilateral ligation) or 85% (bilateral ligation), blood flow by 49% and mean pressure by 22-24%. This converts the distal circulation from arterial to venous by abolishing the "trip hammer" effect of arterial pulsatile blood flow

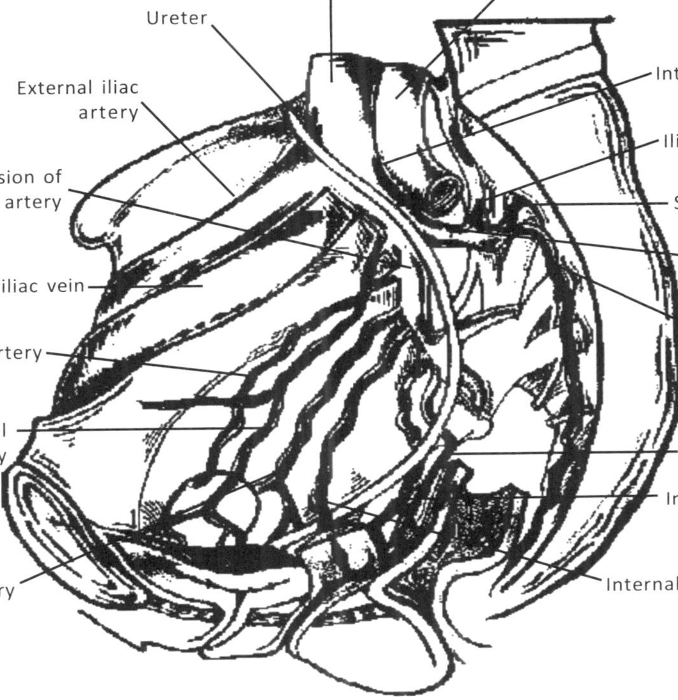

Fig. 4.7 The blood supply of the pelvis

and allowing a stable clot to form at the point of bleeding. Ischemic damage does not occur due to opening up of the pelvic collateral circulation[18].

THE URINARY BLADDER[13, 14, 15, 19]

The urinary bladder is a hollow muscular organ acting as a reservoir for urine. The distended bladder is globular while the empty bladder is flattened from above downwards. It has a superior surface, two inferolateral surfaces and a base, which is in close relationship with the cervix and upper part of the anterior vaginal wall.

The cavity of the urinary bladder is lined by 2–3 layers of transitional epithelium, which on emptying is thrown into rugosities. The detrusor muscle of the bladder is composed of three layers–the outer longitudinal, middle circular and inner longitudinal. There is, however, frequent interchange of fibers so that the muscle contracts as a single syncitial mass.

The trigone is a triangular area at the base of the bladder with its apex near the internal urethral meatus and the ureteric orifices at each end of its base. In the empty bladder the two ureteric orifices are 2.5 cms apart but when distended, as during cystoscopy they may be 5 cms apart. A transverse ridge, the interureteric bar, connects the ureteric orifices. Although the deep trigonal muscle is similar to the detrusor, the superficial muscle is thin with small muscle bundles.

The bladder neck, the junction of the urinary bladder with the urethra, is composed of largely oblique or horizontal muscle fibers with little or no sphincter control in the female, unlike the male, where there is a well-defined preprostatic sphincter.

The female urethra is 3-5 cm in length and is composed of the urethral smooth muscle, the periurethral and urethral striated muscles and the extrinsic periurethral muscle.

The urethral mucosa is made up of non–keratinised, stratified squamous epithelium distally and transitional epithelium proximally.

Parasympathetic nerve supply: They provide the main motor innervation of the bladder and reach the bladder via the pelvic splanchnic nerves. These arise by several rootlets from the anterior surfaces of S2 and S3. They pass forward into the inferior hypogastric plexuses where they mix with the sympathetic nerves and are distributed to pelvic viscera. Sympathetic nerve supply: These come from the T_{10}-L_2 segments of the cord via the superior hypogastric and pelvic plexuses. They inhibit the excitatory parasympathetic supply within the ganglia of the pelvic plexus thus interfering with detrusor contractions.

The sympathetic innervation of the bladder transmits sensory impulses during the fillings and storage phases.

THE URETER[13,14,15,19] (Fig. 4.7 and 4.8)

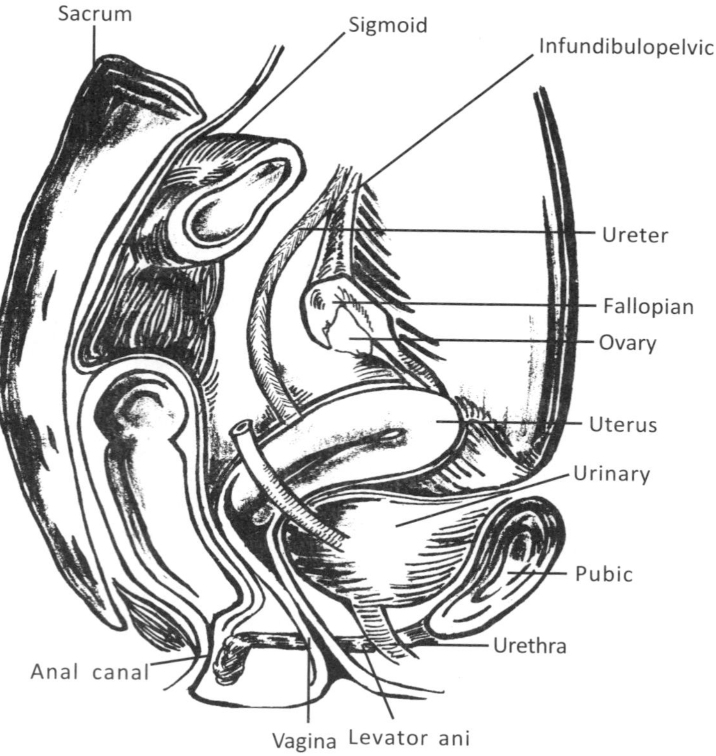

Fig. 4.8 The pelvic organs and their relationships

The ureters are a pair of long muscular tubes one on each side of the abdomen and pelvis connecting the renal pelvis to the urinary bladder. The ureter is 25-30 cm long. It has an abdominal and a pelvic portion each about 12-15 long.

The abdominal ureter

The ureter passes along the anterior surface of the psoas muscle up to the pelvic inlet. The right ureter is located close to the lower portion of the vena cava where the vessel rests on the medial border of the psoas muscle.

The ureter enters the pelvis by coursing over the iliac vessels at the point of bifurcation of the common iliac artery into the external and internal iliac arteries.

The pelvic ureter

The pelvic portion of the ureter forms about half of its length. It passes along the posterolateral pelvic wall adjacent to the anterior border of the sciatic notch and slightly anterior to the hypogastric artery until it reaches deep into the pelvis at the level of the ischial spines. In this area, the ureter lies medial to the branches of the anterior division of the internal iliac artery and lateral to the pouch of Douglas and the uterosacral ligaments.

Deep in the pelvis, the ureter courses along the lateral side of the uterosacral ligaments to enter the base of the broad ligament. The ureter passes beneath the uterine artery about 1.5 cm lateral to the cervix at the level of the internal os. At its distal portions, the ureter passes medially over the lateral vaginal fornix enclosed in a sheath of pelvic fascia called the ureteric tunnel before entering the bladder. This angulation where the ureter passes beneath the uterine vessels to join the bladder is known as the knee of the ureter.

The ureter has three anatomical layers: viz. the innermost layer of transitional epithelium, the middle smooth muscle layer (consisting of inner longitudinal, outer circular and intermediate spiral fibers) and the outer adventitial layer.

The blood supply to the ureter is from the following vessels :

a) Abdominal ureter:

   Superior segment: Renal and ovarian arteries.

   Middle segment: Aorta and common iliac arteries.

b) Pelvic Ureter: uterine, vaginal, middle hemorrhoidal and vesical arteries.

The blood supply of the upper and middle part is from the medial aspect. Hence dissection of this portion of the ureter is from the lateral side. The pelvic ureter derives its blood supply from the lateral side. Thus, its dissection is from the medial aspect.

The ureteral vessels freely anastomose with each other in the surrounding adventitia also known as the fascia of Waldeyer. Trauma to this layer leads to ischemic damage to that segment of the ureter, followed by necrosis and rupture fibrosis or stenosis and hydroureter.

The ureter, through its peristalsis, forms a pseudoperiureteral sheath due to condensation of surrounding tissue. This pseudosheath blends with the Waldeyer's fascia and encloses its lower end just above the bladder.

During pregnancy, the gravid uterus compresses the ureter at the pelvic brim. The resulting dilatation is more pronounced on the right side probably due to cushioning of the left ureter by the sigmoid colon and dextro-rotation of the uterus. The right ovarian vessels overlying the ureter may provide additional compression. Increased levels of progesterone during pregnancy may play a further role in reducing ureteric peristalsis and causing a physiologic hydroureter.

Elongation of the ureter during pregnancy is accompanied by kinks and curves along its course. The ureter also undergoes lateral displacement by pressure of the enlarged uterus and lies as close as 0.9 cm close to the cervix especially on the right side.

SUTURE MATERIALS

Suture materials are required to keep the wound together until they hold sufficiently well by themselves by natural fibre (collagen) to form a strong scar.

Lebas, a French surgeon was the first to close the uterine incision in 1769. Till then, no one thought it conceivable to close the uterus with suture; however, the abdominal incision was closed with a few crude stitches and sticking plaster.

Max Sanger in 1882 described deep sutures of silver wire, which penetrated the peritoneal and muscular layers excluding the decidua to close the uterine incision. Then superficial sutures of silk were inserted at short intervals, thus securing the turned in peritoneum and keeping its serous surfaces in contact.

With the progress in the techniques of the cesarean section, various types of suture materials were introduced for uterine closure varying from silver wire to silk to chromic catgut to polyglactin 910. The research still continues.

Sutures are classified as either absorbable or non-absorbable.

Absorbable sutures

Absorbable sutures lose most of their tensile strength before 60 days when implanted in body tissues. They are further classified into natural and synthetic sutures.

Natural absorbable sutures

The surgical catgut is prepared from the sub-mucosa of the first one third of the small intestine of sheep. Excised intestine is mechanically cleared and subjected to a stripping process, which removes the muscle from one side and the mucous membrane from the other. Casings of 16-18 meter diameter are transported to the suture factory in ice where they are split longitudinally in to 2 or 3 ribbons. Further mechanical cleaning ensures that the final ribbon is purely submucosal collagen. The ribbons are then chromed by treating with 20% chromium salt solution with 5 parts of glycerin for 1 to 96 hours. They are then twisted together, slowly dried under tension, polished and sorted for size. It is sterilized by gamma irradiation or ethylene oxide and packed in fluid containing 70% alcohol with glycerol and water to maintain flexibility. Plain catgut lasts for 10-40 days. It is graded according to thickness and strength from 4/0 to 4. Sutures progressively larger than number 0 are numbered in increasing numeric order (no. 1, 2), sizes progressively smaller than 0-0 are indicated by an increasing number of zeros (i.e. 0,00,000). (The smaller the suture the more the number of zeroes).

Catgut is absorbed through cellular and tissue proteases. Plain catgut is absorbed within 7 days while chromic catgut resists body enzymes and prolongs the absorption time to 4 to 6 weeks. It also causes less tissue reaction and is less irritating than plain catgut during the early stages of wound healing. It is easy to handle and a 2 + 1 knot configuration is very secure.

The aim of uterine suturing is only hemostasis; hence catgut though it does not have much of tensile strength is preferred for uterine incision closure with continuous interlocking sutures.

It maintains more than half of its tensile strength at 7 to 10 days with some measurable strength up to day 21. It loses strength rapidly in infected tissue due to proteolytic enzymes released by inflammatory cells. Since, it is absorbed early, it causes less fibrosis and tissue reaction at the uterine incision. Also it has better knotting properties than polygalactin 910. Studies have shown that the incidence of scar dehiscence in future pregnancies is higher with polygalactin 910 than with chromic catgut.

Number 0.CCG is commonly used for approximation of peritoneum (visceral and parietal), as well as the subcutaneous tissue. These tissues do not require tensile strength or tight suturing but just approximation. It is also recommended by some for B-lynch suturing of the uterus in cases of postpartum hemorrhage.

Synthetic absorbable sutures

Polyglycolic acid and polygalactin 910

These are stronger, longer lasting, less reactive than plain catgut. Polyglycolic acid (Dexon) is a copolymer of glycolic acid, while polygalactin 910 (Vicryl) is a copolymer of lactic and glycolic acid. Breakdown of the two sutures is by hydrolysis.

The polygalactin 910 copolymer is extruded and braided into strands varying in size from 9-0 to 3. It is dyed violet to enhance visibility in tissues. The combination of lactic acid and glycolic acid results in a molecular structure, which maintains 50-60% of tensile strength after 14 days and 20-30% after 21 days. There is no loss in tensile strength in the first 7–10 days after implantation. Absorption is completed by the 60th to 90th day. It is not affected by infection because its degradation is by hydrolysis and not inflammatory cell enzymatic degradation. The handling quality is not as good as catgut sutures; hence various surface coatings have been tried. There is also an increasing tendency for the knots to slip hence a 2 + 1 + 1 + 1 knot configuration is secure.

Polygalactin 910 is the suture material of choice for fascial suturing in patients at low risk for fascial dehiscence. Fascial incisions regain their strength slowly achieving about 10%, 25%, 30% and 40% of original strength by postoperative week 1, 2, 3 and 4 respectively. Facial dehiscence occurs mostly between 2 to 12 days after surgery, with the majority occuring at or around day 7 or 8. Dehiscence rarely occurs after postoperative day 12 but has been reported upto day 18.

Polyglycolic acid (Dexon) is a synthetic, absorbable, braided suture, which is a homopolymer of glycolic acid. The filaments are dyed green to enhance visibility in tissues. The rate of absorption is slower than polyglactin, absorption being maximum after 60-90 days; hence it is preferred for fascial closure. One disadvantage of Dexon is its inferior knot security; hence it is not used for fascial closure in patients who are at high risk for fascial dehiscence.

Polydioxanone (PDS)

PDS is a synthetic, monofilament, and absorbable suture material. It is prepared from polyester. At 14 days after implantation, 70 % of tensile strength is retained, at 28 days 50% of the tensile strength is retained and at 56 days 14% is retained. Absorption is minimal till the 90th day and complete within 6 months. The monofilaments lack interstices that could serve as a nidus for bacterial infection. As a result, chronic inflammation is rarely seen. The disadvantage of being monofilament is that, care must be taken to ensure that the strand is not inadvertently damaged by instruments, needles or other sharp edged material. Such damage can weaken the monofilament suture and may result in suture line disruption after surgery, especially when a continuous suture line is used. The disadvantages are that knots are not so secure and it is known to cause erythema and reaction during absorption.

Poliglecaprone 25 (Monocryl)

It is a synthetic equivalent of surgical gut. The absorption is similar to chromic catgut but is by hydrolysis and hence does not induce the inflammatory response of catgut. It is not recommended for fascial closure because of its low tensile strength. It is used for superficial suturing for more cosmetic healing.

Polygalactin 910 (vicryl rapide)

It is a polyglactin 910 with a low molecular weight. The performance is similar to plain catgut. 70% of tensile strength is lost in first 7 days. Because of its rapid absorption and minimal inflammatory response, it is used for skin suturing with less scarring.

Non-absorbable sutures

Though non-absorbable sutures are resistant to the action of living tissue, they are not completely resistant to absorption. Though, they maintain tensile strength for long periods of time, over time they eventually lose their tensile strength. The disadvantages of non-absorbable sutures include the potential for suture related pain, palpable sutures and occasionally formation of suture sinuses.

<u>Natural non-absorbable sutures</u>

Surgical silk

Though, it is not very relevant to cesarean section, its properties will be reviewed in brief. It is a polyfilament protein thread, which is braided together to form a suture strand. It is then treated to render it non-capillary and dyed with a vegetable dye usually black for enhancing its visibility in tissues. Though, it is referred to as non-absorbable, it is found to lose most or all of its tensile strength in one year and usually cannot be found in tissues after 2 years. It tends to lose tensile strength when exposed to moisture, and hence it is used dry. A 2 + 1 knot configuration is secure. It is available in sizes from 9-0 to 5. Its low tensile strength is its main disadvantage, the other being the inflammatory response that it initiates.

Surgical cotton

It is the weakest of the non-absorbable sutures. It loses half of its original tensile strength within 6 months of implantation, but still retains 30-40% tensile strength at the end of 2 years. Wet cotton is 10% stronger and easier to handle than dry cotton.

Linen

Linen suture is made from long staple flax fibers, which are twisted in to a strand. The tensile strength is lower than that of other non-absorbable suture materials.

Synthetic non-absorbable sutures

Nylon

Nylon is a synthetic polyamide polymer available both as braided polyfilament suture (Surgilon) and as monofilament suture (ethilon). Nylon undergoes slow hydrolysis losing about 15% tensile strength per year. Advantages of Nylon are low reactivity, minimal tissue trauma, elasticity, good tensile strength and ease of handling. Knots of monofilament Nylon are not secure and 2 + 1 + 1 + 1 + 1 knot configuration is required to prevent knot slippage. Nylon is the suture material of choice for fascial suturing in patients at high risk for fascial dehiscence, especially when vertical incisions are made.

Polypropelene suture (prolene)

Polypropylene is a monofilament suture composed of a linear hydrocarbon polymer. It has the least tissue reactivity of all non-absorbable sutures and a high tensile strength. It has a greater knot security than is possible with other monofilament sutures. The knot flattens out and locks against itself. It is unaffected by tissue fluids and can be used in the presence of infection. It is used for fascial closure in patients at high risk for fascial dehiscence.

Metal sutures

Metal suture has the highest tensile strength. It is non reactive but is difficult to handle. It is almost obsolete in Gynecologic surgery, though suturing of the uterus started with silver wire.

ANATOMY AND PHYSIOLOGY OF WOUND HEALING[20,21]

The commonly encountered complications of cesarean section include infections, dehiscence and evisceration as well as incisional hernias and wound sinus formation, which are all a sequelae of improper healing of the tissues. It is worthwhile to know the physiology of the wound healing in order to prevent the complications related to it.

Wound healing is a combination of events that occur in a careful synchronous order. The steps that occur are initiated by a variety of cell-secreted factors such as cytokines, which direct the function of other cells.

Healing of cesarean section wounds is by Primary union (first intention healing) or rarely by secondary union (secondary intention healing).

Wound healing is usually divided into three phases

1) Inflammatory Phase
2) Proliferative Phase
3) Remodeling Phase

Inflammatory phase

Injury leads to disruption of blood vessels with extravasation of red blood cells and other constituents of the intravascular space. The platelets are stimulated by locally generated thrombin and exposed fibrillar collagen. The platelets undergo activation, adhesion and aggregation. Upon activation, the platelets release mediators such as adenosine diphosphate, alphagranules, thromboxane A2, 5HT, fibrinogen, thrombospondin and Von Willebrand's factor VIII, which helps in platelet aggregation and adhesion to fibrillary collagen. ADP and thrombin recruit additional platelets to the site of injury. These events result in formation of a platelet plug.

Coagulation results from the amplification cascade provided by the constituents of the intravascular space. Thrombin is formed by activation of intrinsic and extrinsic pathway. Thrombin converts fibrinogen into fibrin and activates fibrin and platelets. Together fibrinogen and platelet surface receptors bind and polymerize to form a fibrin matrix thus creating a thrombus. The thrombus along with fibronectin allows the formation of a provisional matrix for the migration of monocytes, fibroblasts, and kertinocytes into the wound environment.

Leukocytes: Neutrophils and monocytes migrate to the wound area because of the chemotactic factors produced by the coagulation cascade. The presence of wound contamination prolongs the neutrophilic presence within the wound.

Monocytes and the macrophages become the dominant figures in the inflammatory process after the initial phase.

Tissue macrophages produce various cytokines, which are important in inducing cell migration and proliferation as well as matrix production. Macrophages release biologically active oxygen intermediates and enzymatic proteins, which help in digestion, phagocytosis, killing of pathogenic organisms, scavenging tissue debris and destroying any remaining neutrophils. These processes allow the induction of angiogenesis and the formation of granulation tissue.

Proliferative phase

Reepithelialization: The epidermis reacts to the defect caused by the injury within 24 hrs. The keratinocytes initially respond to the presence of an epidermal defect by migration from the free edge of the wound. It also occurs from the skin appendages including the hair follicle. Approximately 12 hrs after wounding, the cell become flattened and develop pseudopods like projections. The tight binding between these epidermal cells and the basement membrane and the underlying dermis is lost. Fibronectin allows the continual migration of these cells and early provisional matrix is formed of fibronectin, fibrin and type5 collagen. The provisional matrix enables keratinocytes to migrate and dissect under eschar and debris covering the wound bed. TGF beta stimulates keratinocyte production of fibronectin and its deposition in the extracellular matrix.

Angiogenesis: New capillary buds arising from the blood vessels adjacent to the wound extend into the wound. The endothelial cells migrate but do not proliferate. Chemotactic factors, low oxygen tension, lactic acid and biogenic amines potentiate angiogenesis. FGF secreted by the fibroblasts and macrophages are potent stimuli for angiogenesis. Endothelial cells help in the formation of new vessels providing transport of oxygen and nutrients into the wound and secreting biologically active substances.

Fibroplasia: Granulation tissue that forms during healing consists of the new vessels, fibroblast and ground substances. Fibroblast is the most important cell in the formation of dermal matrix. Fibroblasts migrate into the wound between 48 to 72 hrs. Macrophages release the fibroblast chemotactic factors. Fibroblasts migrate by pulling themselves along a fibronectin matrix. This migration occurs by contraction of intracellular microfilaments. The fibronectin enhances fibroblast migration and provides a scaffold for collagen fibrils and mediates wound contraction.

Wound contraction: wound contraction is a result of actin rich myofibroblasts, which align along the line of contraction. Fibronectin also participates in it.

Remodeling phase

It consists of deposition of matrix materials and their subsequent change over time. The total amount of collagen increases early in the repair process reaching maximum between 2-3 weeks after injury. Collagen changes from type 3 to type 1. Bacterial Collagenase, lysosomal proteases and tissue collagenase are then able to restore the post injury tissue towards normalcy and wound repair is considered complete.

By the second week, the basic structure of the scar is established and steady increase in the tensile strength is underway.

The acquisition of the tensile strength follows a sigmoid curve. From the fifth day onwards, the proliferative phase begins, and the skin starts gaining the tensile strength up to day 100, during which 70% to 90% of the strength of unwounded skin is achieved, followed by a plateau. Carefully sutured wounds have approximately 70% of the strength of the normal skin immediately following surgery.

Healing by secondary union (Secondary intention)

It is a more prolonged process because of the need to remove all dead tissue and necrotic debris and to fill in the tissue defect with vital cells. Hence there is ingrowth of granulation tissue with a severe inflammatory reaction and wound contraction.

Few aberrations may occur in wound healing such as accumulation of excessive amounts of collagen may give rise to a protruding, tumorous scar known as keloid. It suggests a genetic tendency, however the mechanisms involved in keloid formation are still unclear.

Healing of Rectus Sheath

The basic healing process of the sheath remains the same as the skin. The predominant collagen is Type-1 collagen, which has 2 types of a chains, both of which are low in hydroxylysine. Initially it is the type-3 collagen, which is the embryonic collagen, is laden down which is gradually replaced by Type-1.

Regeneration of the uterine tissue

The uterine myometrium is made up of smooth muscle cells, which are stable cells. These cells retain the capacity to regenerate but under normal circumstances do not actively replicate because they have a survival time equal to the life of the individual. Thus any injury to the myometrium stimulates the smooth muscle replication. Since it has a low rate of turnover, it takes weeks to months to regain the original strength, which may never be achieved. Repair of the destroyed cells involves some connective tissue proliferation with the formation of a fibrous scar, thus diminishing the reserve of the myometrium.

Schwartz and Pollock (1923) showed that healing is first by fibrous tissue, which is invaded by muscle cells later. They experimented by repairing each horn of pregnant uterus of guinea pig. They repaired and examined from the first day to the end of 10 weeks[22]. Whitridge Williams in the same year proposed new theory that the uterine muscles healed together by the regeneration of muscle fibres from the beginning itself[23]. Current views are however, in agreement with the views of Schwartz and Pollock.

Other factors such as the suture material used, single or double-layered suture, exclusion of the decidua, general factors such as the health and nutrition of the woman, and local factors such as the infection do influence the strength of the uterine scar in the next pregnancy.

CONCLUSION

The value of anatomy in the evolution of the technique of cesarean section, safety, and management and prevention of complication cannot be understated. Each step of cesarean delivery requires awareness of the role of suturing, apposition of tissues and hemostasis in tissue healing and recovery.

Discovery of anatomy is part of the story of medicine and the stirring history of women's age-long struggle against suffering and death due to childbirth. This adventure has lifted the age of ignorance to an era, which allows a woman the benefits, and safety of modern obstetrics.

REFERENCES

1. Snell Richard. Clinical Anatomy for Medical Students. 6th edition, 137-190.
2. Dr Thorek PJ. The Abdomen, Anatomy in Surgery.;J.B.Lipincott company 22(4): 363-397;1951.
3. John Delancey, John Rock, Thompson John D. Surgical Anatomy of female pelvis in Telinde's Operative Gynaecology 6(2),63-93 by Lipincott-Raven,1997.
4. Romanes GJ. The anterior abdominal wall in Cunninham's Manual of Practical Anatomy, Vol.2, 91-104,1986.
5. Last RJ. The Abdomen in Anatomy- Regional and Applied, 256-264,1986.
6. Myerscough PR. Caesarean Section: Sterilization: Hysterectomy Munro Kerr's operative Obstetrics 5(22) 295 320, 2000.
7. Duff DM, DiZerega GS. Is peritoneal closure necessary ? Obstet Gynecol Surv 1994;49:817-22.
8. Elkins TE, Stovall TG, Warren J, Ling FW, Meyer NL. A histologic evaluation of peritoneal injury and repair: implications for adhesion formation and repair :implications for adhesion formation.Obstet Gynecol 1987;70 225-8.
9. Mc Donald MN, Elkins TE, Wortham GF, Stovall TG,Ling FW, Mc Neeley SG. Adhesion formation and prevention after peritoneal injury and repair in the rabbit: J Reprod Med 1988; 33:436-9.
10. Gallup Donald. Incisions for Gynaecologic Surgery John Rock,John Thompson's, Telinde's Operative Gynaecology ,285-321, by Lippincott Raven.
11. Das S. Introduction to Abdominal Surgery in a practical guide to Operative Surgery :21 :206-218.
12. Bhattacharjee et al. Misgav Ladach technique of cesarean section for fetomaternal emergencies . J.of obst. And gynaec. Of India Vol-51, Number-1, 54-56 ,Jan-Feb 2001.
13. Cunningham FG, MacDonald PC, Cant NF et al. Anatomy of the reproductive tract. In Cunningham FG, MacDonald PG, Gant NF et al (eds): William S Obstetrics (20th ed) Prentice – Hall Int Ltd. 3 (I): 37-68, 1997.
14. Cunningham PG, MacDonald PC, Gant NF et al. Maternal adaptation to pregnancy. In Cunningham FG, MacDonald PC, Gant NF (eds): Williams Obstetrics (10th ed) Prentice – Hall Int Ltd. 8 (II): 191- 226.
15. Thorek PJ. The pelvic viscera. In Thorek PJ: Anatomy in surgery. JB Lipincott Company. 31(5): 562- 621, 1951.
16. Williams PL, Warwick R, Dyson M, Bannister LH. The reproductive organs of the female.In Williams PL, Warwick R, Dyson M, Bannister LH (eds): Gray's Anatomy (37th ed) Churchill Livingstone. 8: 1453-1449, 1989.
17. Williams PL, Warwick R, Dyson M, Bannister LH. The arteries of the trunk .In Williams PL, Warwick R, Dyson M, Bannister LH (eds): Gray's Anatomy (37th ed) Churchill Livingstone. 6: 764-780, 1989.
18. Thompson JD, Rock WA Jr. Control of pelvic hemorrhage. In Rock JA, Thompson JD (ed): Te Linde's operative Gynecology (8th ed). Lippincott–Raven. 11(II) 197-232, 1997.
19. Williams PL, Warwick R, Dyson M, Bannister LH.The urinary organs. In Williams PL, Warwick R, Dyson M, Bannister LH (eds): Williams Obstetrics. Churchill Livingstone. 8: 1397-1415, 1989.
20. Robbins Stanley, Kumar Vinay. Inflammation and Repair in Basic Pathology: 28-61 ,W.B.Saunders Company.

21. Kennedy CTC. Reactions to Mechanical and Thermal Injury in Rook, Wilkinson, Ebling's Textbook of Dermatology Vol.2,777-832,1992

22. Schwartz RM and Goldber H. Obst and Gyn 1959:14:773.

23. Chassar Moir J. Cesarean section, sterilization and hysterectomy. In: Chassar Moir J. Munro Kerr's Operative Obstetrics (6th ed). Balliere, Tindall and Cox; 22: 539-607, 1956.

5 | CHAPTER

Indications For Cesarean Delivery

Nagendra Sardeshpande

FRAMEWORK

- Introduction
- Indications for cesarean delivery
- Patterns in cesarean delivery
- Previous cesarean delivery
- Breech presentation
- Fetal distress
- Non progress of labor
- Prolonged pregnancy
- Failed induction
- Failed instrumental delivery
- Intrauterine growth retardation
- Preeclampsia
- Antepartum hemorrhage
- Multifetal gestation
- Maternal diabetes
- Maternal heart disease
- Precious pregnancy
- Uterine fibroids
- Previous uterine surgery
- Ovarian tumors
- Mullerian anomalies
- Maternal HIV infection
- Maternal HSV infection
- Maternal HPV infection
- Fetal anomalies
- Cervical cerclage
- Previous gynecological surgery
- Maternal desire
- Classical cesarean delivery

INTRODUCTION

"I do not know that there was ever any law, Christian or civil in which both ordain the martyring and killing the mother to save the child".

Francois Mauriceau (1637-1709) in "The Diseases of women with child and in child bed".

Since the seventeenth century, when the surgical mortality was extremely high and survival restricted to the fortunate few, dramatic advances in knowledge of anatomy, surgery, anesthesia, microbiology and pharmacology have established the cesarean delivery as one of the commonest and most important surgeries of the modern era.

In the last few decades, the incidence of cesarean delivery has increased from 4.5 per 100 deliveries in 1965 to over 20 per 100 deliveries in the nineties (23.5 per 100 deliveries in the United States in 1993) so much so as to assume epidemic proportions[2].

The relative frequencies of various indications for cesarean delivery have also changed over the past century. At the time of its inception, cesarean birth was primarily a desperate and usually futile last ditch attempt to salvage the moribund mother or fetus in an often prolonged, obstructed labor with the pelvic tissues already compromised by infection. The above mentioned advances in medicine and surgery have transformed the utility of the operation. Along with its increasing use, newer indications have emerged such as its application in primiparae and possibly, by current evidence, in multigravidae with a breech presentation. But, controversies do exist. Its utilisation in preterm delivery and on maternal request has evoked support as well as criticism.

However, no surgical procedure suffers from a lack of purpose at its inception. It is when it becomes established that aims are lost and replaced by a vague ritual. So, what does explain the increased prevalence of this surgery? Is it because of more aggressive management of obstetrical and medical conditions? Is it because of increased patient awareness and desire to avoid the pain of labor? Or is it the monetary temptation or fear of medicolegal problems on part of the obstetrician?

Over the years, many studies and peer reviews have condemned the indiscriminate use of this surgery. In this chapter, an attempt has been made to achieve a critical and unbiased evaluation of the various indications for cesarean section. Inspite of an effort at an exhaustive analysis, some indications may be left untouched and a few questions unsolved.

However, truth suffers from too much analysis. This remarkable operation has stood the test of time and no amount of dissection and criticism can banish it to the mists of the past.

The decision to do a cesarean should be individualized and based on the risk factors associated and the clinical findings at that point of time.

INDICATIONS FOR CESAREAN DELIVERY

Before, evaluating each of them, let us enumerate the indications for which cesarean deliveries are utilized.

There are various ways to classify cesarean deliveries and its indications :

Table - 1. Absolute / relative indications

Absolute	Relative
1. Severe cephalopelvic disproportion	1. Previous uterine scar
2. Major degrees of placenta previa	2. Acute fetal distress
3. Previous H/O of classical cesarean birth	3. Cord accidents
4. Previous H/O of repair for fistula	4. Accidental hemorrhage
5. Advanced carcinoma cervix	5. Prolonged labor
6. Vaginal stenosis / atresia	6. Obstructed labor
7. Transverse lie uncorrected by ECV	7. Failed iduction
8. Brow presentation at term	8. Eclampsia with poor Bishop score
	9. Pregnancy following infertility treatment
	10. Severe heart diseases
	11. IUGR
	12. Genital HPV infection
	13. Fetal macrosomia
	14. Fetal congenital anomalies amenable to correction (e.g. gastroschisis)
	15. Maternal desire

Table - 2. Common / uncommon indications

Common	Uncommon
1. Previous cesarean sections / myomectomy	1. Advanced carcinoma cervix
2. Breech presentation	2. Vaginal atresia / stenosis
3. Fetal distress	3. Previous hysterotomy
4. Cephalopelvic disproportion	4. Maternal HPV infection
5. Antepartum hemorrhage	5. Maternal HSV infection
6. PIH	6. Maternal desire
7. Malpresentation	7. Pelvic tumors
8. Failed induction of labor	8. Medical disorder in pregnancy
9. Precious pregnancy including BOH, infertility conception & elderly primigravida	9. Congenital anomalies in the fetus
10. Maternal HIV infection	
11. IUGR	
12. Preterm labor	
13. Failure to progress	

Table - 3. Fetal / Maternal indications

Fetal	Maternal	Maternal-Fetal
1. Nonreassuring FHR	1. Obstructive benign and malignant tumors	1. Cephalopelvic disproportion
2. Breech	2. Large vulvar condyloma	2. Failure to progress
3. Prematurity	3. Abdominal cervical cerclage	3. Placental abruption
4. IUGR	4. Vaginal stenosis / atresia	4. Placenta praevia
5. Herpes simplex virus		
6. ITP		
7. Congenital anomalies		
8. Maternal HIV infection		

TRENDS IN CESAREAN DELIVERY

Despite relaxed guidelines issued by various obstetrical and gynecological bodies to promote trial of labor for various conditions the cesarean delivery rate has gone up steadily from 4.5% in 1965 to 17.9% in 1981, 18.5% in 1982, 20.3% in 1983, 24% in 1986 and 23.5% in 1993[2, 3]. The probable reasons for this trend are summarized below:

1) ***Labor Factors :***
   - Repeat cesarean sections
   - Electronic fetal monitoring
   - Macrosomia / cephalopelvic disproportion
   - Reduced use of forceps / vacuum
   - Liberal diagnosis of nonprogress / failed induction

2) ***Maternal factors :***
   - Older age of conception
   - Maternal risk factors like HT, PIH, diabetes, etc
   - Patient's desire

3) ***Fetal factors :***
   - Breech presentation
   - IUGR / prematurity
   - Cesarean delivery for a precious pregnancy e.g. infertility conception, previous bad obstetric history
   - Prolonged pregnancy
   - HIV
   - Active genital herpes or HPV infection
   - Multifetal gestation

4) ***Obstetrician factors :***

- Fear of litigation
- Convenience
- ? Monetary gain

Marcoux and Fabia noted a near doubling of cesarean deliveries between 1973 (7.9%) and 1979 (13.6%). Repeat cesarean deliveries accounted for 40.4% of this increase, while primary cesarean deliveries for dystocia, breech presentation and fetal distress explain respectively 21.1%, 21.1% and 21.3% of the rise. Prolonged labor, prolonged rupture of membranes, general anesthesia and preterm repeat cesarean deliveries were observed less frequently in 1979 while the Apgar scores were higher in 1979 than in 1973[4].

In a study of 19,419 deliveries by Gilstrap III at the Wilford Hall USAF medical Centre (9.5% primary cesarean deliveries and 4% repeat operations), from the period of 1970 to 1973 through 1974 to 1977, the primary rate increased from 5.6% to 12.8% ($P < 0.0001$). A significant increase in operations for dystocia, breech presentation and fetal distress was also noted. However, from 1978 to 1981, the primary cesarean rate dropped to 9.6%, principally due to decreased rates for dystocia and fetal distress.[5]

Saudi Arabia too witnessed a tripling of cesarean births from 1979 (3.9%) to 1984 (9.9%), the increase being attributed mainly to repeat sections (37.2%) and fetal distress (28.5%). The increase in diagnosis of fetal distress was related to the introduction of electronic fetal monitoring[6].

A study from the Louis–Mourier Hospital in France concluded that although there was an increase in cesarean birth rates from 1971-75 (5.3%) to 1976-1979 (15.4%), the number of sections for breech presentations was the same. Even though the cesarean rates for previous cesareans, fetal distress, dystocia and toxemia were increased, it was primarily the improvements in fetal monitoring and neonatal resuscitation that accounted for the improvement in neonatal status at birth. It was suggested that the optimum level for cesarean deliveries is 15% with 9% being first cesareans and 6% repeat cesareans[7].

Cesarean section rates vary from country to country and from region to region (Table 4)[8]. Hence, the desired rate in each institution varies according to multiple factors. It may be sensible to define a range for each indication, e.g. cephalopelvic disproportion (2-4%), repeat cesarean delivery (2-6%), breech & other malpresentations (3.5-6.3%), nonreassuring fetal heart rate (1.5-3%) and third trimester bleeding (1%)[9].

Table - 4. Contribution of various indications for cesarean delivery to overall cesarean section rate (no/1000 deliveries)[8]

Indication	Previous cesarean section	Breech	Dystocia	Fetal distress	Others	Overall cesarean rate
Norway						
1980	1.7	1.3	3.1	0.7	2.5	8.4
1985	1.0	1.8	3.6	1.9	3.3	11.6
1990	1.3	2.1	3.6	2.0	3.7	12.8
Scotland						
1980	1.8	1.5	3.7	1.3	3.4	11.7
1985	2.8	1.9	3.8	2.0	2.7	14.2
1990	3.1	2.0	4.0	2.4	2.7	14.2
USA						
1980	5.4	2.1	4.9	0.8	3.8	16.9
1985	7.8	2.3	6.5	1.9	4.3	22.7
1990	8.5	2.6	7.1	2.3	3.2	23.4
Sweden						
1980	2.6	2.1	2.3	2.4	1.6	11.0
1985	3.3	2.2	1.9	1.7	2.4	11.5
1990	3.1	1.8	1.7	1.6	2.4	10.7

In an ICMR study in India, the cesarean delivery rate varied from place to place (11.4% in Mumbai to 25.4% in Trivandrum) and from hospital to hospital (10.8% in KEM hospital, Mumbai to 54% in Eden hospital, Kolkata), the main indications being dystocia, fetal distress and repeat cesarean delivery (Table 5-7)[10].

Table - 5. Cesarean delivery rates in India(1993) [10]

Place	Percent
Bombay	11.4
New Delhi	8.1
Madras	20.6
Calcutta	21.6
Lucknow	20.6
Trivandrum	25.4
India : 1993-94	21.8
1998-99	25.4

Table - 6. Changing incidence of cesarean delivery in India[10]

Hospital	1993-94	1998-99
AIIMS, New Delhi	36.5	32.3
Eden Hospital, Kolkata	34.8	54.0
IOG, Calcutta	20.1	35.7
KEM Hospital, Mumbai	10.8	14.9

Table - 7. Indications of cesarean delivery (ICMR data) 1998-99[10]

Indication	Percent (7017 Patients)
Repeat cesarean sections / uterine surgery	29
Dystocia	37.5
Fetal distress	33.9
Malpresentations	14.5
PIH	12.5
Failed induction	6.2
APH	6.3
Medical causes	2.9
Others	19.7

It may be noted that the changes in the trends include an increase in cesarean section for previous cesarean section scars, for fetal heart rate abnormalities due to advances in fetal monitoring and increasing patient and physician preference for operative intervention in breech presentation. With improvements in neonatal care, greater faith has been reposed in cesarean delivery for preterm and IUGR babies to avoid potential intrapartum complications. Medical conditions like PIH, maternal heart disease and diabetes are liberally managed by cesarean section to avoid worsening of maternal or fetal condition and for better control of maternal-fetal hemodynamics and vital parameters.

PREVIOUS CESAREAN DELIVERY

E. B. Craigin's dictum "once a cesarean, always a cesarean" was issued in an era of dominance by the classical operation. Yet today repeat cesareans account for 34-48% of all cesarean births.[11]Rates for vaginal delivery after a previous cesarean vary from 19.5% in the United States to a high of 56.2% in Norway[11].

There are arguably only four absolute contraindications to trial of labor after previous cesarean delivery:

1) Patient refusal following full discussion and disclosure.
2) The rarely encountered entity of absolute cephalopelvic disproportion.

3) Previous extensive reconstructive uterine surgery, large intramural myomectomies and T shaped extensions of lower segment cesarean sections
4) Previous classical cesarean scar in which the incidence of scar rupture can be as high as 4.7%[12].

Previous one cesarean delivery:

The incidence of scar separation following a previous cesarean delivery is 0.45%-6%[13].

In USA, the incidence of repeat cesarean for a previous cesarean section scar has increased from 25.2% in 1970 to 35.9% of all cesarean deliveries in 1990 (Table 8)[12]. Various reasons suggested for this increase include patient desire, less faith in the ability of maternal-fetal monitoring to detect scar rupture, overdiagnosis of impending rupture and wariness regarding medicolegal implications of uterine rupture.

Table - 8. Cesarean birth rates in the USA and the outcome of patients with a previous cesarean section scar[12]

Year	Total (Per 100 Births)	Primary (Per 100 Births)	Repeat Cesarean (Percent)	VBAC (Percent)
1970	5.5	4.2	25.2	2.2
1975	10.4	7.8	27.1	2.0
1980	16.5	12.1	29.9	3.4
1985	22.7	16.3	34.6	6.6
1990	23.5	16.8	35.9	20.4

Various studies have shown that, following trial of labor for a previous cesarean section, vaginal delivery rates of 60-75% can be achieved with a low incidence of scar dehiscence or rupture (table 9)[14]. In properly selected cases with good monitoring, the incidence of scar separation can be reduced to 0.3-0.8% with a cesarean delivery rate of 17-40%.

Table - 9. Delivery outcome following one previous cesarean birth[14]

	Miller	Flamm	McMahon
Total patients	13594	7229	6138
Elective cesarean section	2714 (20%)	2207 (30%)	2889 (47%)
Trial of labor :	10880 (80%)	5022 (70%)	3249 (53%)
- Vaginal Delivery	9063 (83%)	3746 (75%)	1982 (60%)
- Cesarean section	1817 (17%)	1276 (25%)	1287 (40%)
Uterine rupture during labor	63 (0.6%)	39 (0.8%)	10 (0.3%)

It must be remembered that scar integrity is usually breached during uterine contractions. There is a steep rise in uterine activity during the late first and second stage of labor. Prolonged increase in uterine pressure will result in a uterine rupture. Duration of labor, cervical dilatation and gestational age at repeat cesarean delivery are poor predictors of scar dehiscence or rupture. The signs of rupture including maternal-fetal tachycardia, maternal bradycardia, fetal bradycardia or decelerations and blood stained vaginal discharge are vague and occur variably often leading to a delay in diagnosis. Whether a scar separation will always lead to tenderness is debatable.[15] Facilities for a rapid cesarean section, in cases of suspected or obvious rupture, may not be available in all obstetric centres. Along with a uterine rupture comes the morbidity of a cesarean hysterectomy, bladder and ureteral injuries and blood transfusion, and potential for maternal-fetal mortality. When records of the previous scar and surgery are unavailable, conducting a trial of labor assuming a previous lower segment scar without any extensions, which are a common occurrence, would be unwise. For conducting a trial of scar, knowledge of the previous surgery is vital. In the current pregnancy, an estimate of the fetal weight and presence of a favourable presentation is desirable along with a reasonable idea of feto-pelvic proportion. Facilities for blood transfusion, anesthesia, immediate cesarean section, maternal-fetal resuscitation and intensive neonatal care are necessary. In the deficiency of these, an elective surgery would be a wiser option.

Two or more previous cesarean deliveries

The incidence of scar rupture following previous two cesarean births is quoted to be about 2.3% and 2.8% with three or more[16]. Traditionally, a repeat section is warranted.

Few studies have shown the possibility of a trial of labor in patients with multiple previous uterine scars. Chattopadhay et al in their planned vaginal trial of 115 women with two previous cesarean births for nonrecurrent indications achieved vaginal delivery in 103 (89%) women with one scar dehiscence (0.8%)[17].

However, Al Naim and Krimly performed repeat cesarean in 255 women with four or more previous cesarean sections and found a 4/1000 incidence of scar rupture and 5 times higher incidence of placenta previa (2.4% vs. 0.5% in controls)[18].

Most women in modern obstetrics opt for a small family size. To subject them to an attempt at vaginal delivery with potential for serious complications, especially with multiple previous scars, would not be justified without a detailed discussion and her consent.

BREECH PRESENTATION

Traditionally, elective cesarean delivery for a breech presentation has been advised for a contracted pelvis, fetal weight greater than 4 kg, extended fetal head, footling breech, placenta previa, a previous uterine scar and a Zatuchini-Andros score of less than 3.

Vaginal breech delivery is associated with a PNMR of 42.5 per 1000 breech deliveries (corrected PNMR 40.9) and neonatal mortality rate of 19.0 per 1000 births (corrected PNMR 11.9). Breech deliveries accounted for 25.5% of all still births and 25.8% of neonatal deaths[19]. In a review of 24 studies by Chang and Hannah in 1993, a significantly higher perinatal mortality (OR: 3.86; 95%

CI: 2.22-6.69), lower 5 minute Apgar score (OR: 1.95; 95% CI: 1.45-2.61) and increased birth trauma (OR: 3.96; 95% CI: 2.76-5.67) was noted in infants with breech presentation delivered vaginally[20].

Sudden compression / decompression of the unmoulded fetal head during vaginal delivery, stretching & tearing of the intracranial ligaments & vasculature, and fractures of the fetal skull can cause intracranial hemorrhage. Additionally, Guiliani et al noted a higher incidence of serious perinatal morbidity (2.3%) and developmental delay over 57 months (1.9%) than in controls (0.5% each)[21]. Other complications during vaginal delivery include umbilical cord prolapse and compression; fractures of the clavicle, spine femur and ribs; and trauma to the liver, spleen, kidneys, genitals and mouth. In addition, maternal genital trauma is also significantly greater during the maneuvers involved in vaginal breech delivery. These risks may be obviated with a planned cesarean delivery.

A landmark trial "The Term Breech Trial" was conducted by the Term Breech Trial Collaborative Group involving 121 centers from 26 countries. The women were randomized to either elective cesarean delivery (1041 patients) or vaginal trial (1042 women). The patients were followed up to 6 weeks after delivery. The trial was terminated after enrolling a little over 2000 women when it was noted that the perinatal mortality and serious neonatal morbidity (17/1039 or 1.6%) for the cesarean birth group was significantly lower than that of the vaginal breech delivery group (52/1039 or 5%) with a relative risk of 0.33 (95% CI : 0.19-0.56). There were no differences in maternal mortality or serious maternal morbidity between the cesarean (41/1041 or 3.9%) or the vaginal delivery group (33/1042 or 3.2%; RR: 1.24; 95% CI: 0.79-1.95)[22]. In their words, "the results were clearly in favor of planned cesarean section".

Interestingly, the report noted reduced benefit of cesarean delivery in countries with high perinatal mortality rates probably because of higher levels of experience with vaginal breech delivery. Additionally when data such as prolonged labor, induction or augmentation of labor with oxytocin or prostaglandins, epidural analgesia, footling or uncertain presentation or unavailability of skilled and experienced obstetricians at birth was excluded, the results are similar in both groups.

In a follow up study to the Term Breech Trial of 1596 women at 3 months postpartum, women in the planned cesarean group were found to have less likelihood of urinary incontinence (36/798 or 4.8%) than in the vaginal delivery group (58/797 or 7.3%; RR: 0.82; 95% CI 0.41-0.92) with no difference in the incidence of rectal incontinence.[23]

Krebs & Langhoff-Roos in their study of 15,441 primigravidas with breech presentation concluded that elective cesarean delivery was associated with lower rates of puerperal fever and pelvic infections (RR:0.81; 95% CI : 0.70-0.92), hemorrhage and anemia (RR : 0.91; 95% CI : 0.84-0.97) and postoperative wound infection (RR : 0.69, 95% CI : 0.57-0.83)[24].

The SOGC Interim Position Paper on the management of Term Breech states that the neonatal outcome is better in the cesarean delivery group when compared to the planned vaginal delivery group and that physicians should inform all patients with term breech presentation of the results of the interim analysis of the Term Breech Trial Study. It also suggests that individual physicians should address their own expertise and skills in the management of the term breech and decisions about the method of delivery of the term breech should be made on an individual basis after full disclosure of the risks and benefits[19].

In 2001, ACOG recommended that obstetricians continue their effort to reduce breech presentations in singleton gestations through application of external cephalic version wherever possible and that patients with persistent breech presentation at term in a singleton gestation undergo a planned cesarean delivery[25].

The preterm breech

The mode of delivery of a preterm breech remains uncertain. Many authors like Kitchen et al recommend cesarean birth for babies weighing 750-1500 grams. Babies weighing more than 1500 grams may be delivered vaginally in the absence of other complicating factors[26].

In 1986, Bodmer et al concluded that babies < 1000 g or between 25-28 weeks were more likely to benefit from cesarean delivery[27].

Weissman et al have reported that in the weight bands 500-999g, 1000-1499g and 1500-1999g, there was no statistical difference in survival rates or of IVH by mode of delivery but the fetuses delivered by cesarean had significantly lower long-term morbidity[28].

Prior to term, the head circumference of the fetus is greater than the abdominal circumference thus increasing the likelihood of fetal head entrapment in an incompletely dilated cervix during vaginal delivery. Compression of the fetal head compounded with hypoxia and stress of labor may cause rupture of the fragile subependymal blood vessels with fatal intracranial hemorrhage. Managing a moribund baby than a healthy albeit preterm child is associated with greater complications in the best of intensive care setups. These reasons tend to tilt the obstetrician's decision in favor of cesarean delivery for a preterm breech.

FETAL DISTRESS

Electronic fetal monitoring has a high negative predictive value (90%) but a low positive predictive value (30%)[44]. This is because an abnormal CTG is a mixture of equivocal and frankly ominous traces. Depending on its reserves, a fetus with an abnormal trace ("stressed") is not necessarily born depressed.

High risk situations like PIH, maternal diabetes and IUGR improve the positive predictive value. Fetal scalp blood pH estimation too has a modest positive predictive value (45%). FAST and fetal scalp stimulation too show a positive predictive value of around 45-50%[29].

However much we question the predictive value of the currently available methods of fetal monitoring, these are all we have at moment. The cardiotocographic tracing should be interpreted in the light of the presence situation of the mother and fetus and presence of factors likely to cause fetal compromise and perform a cesarean delivery if necessary rather than persist with attempts at a vaginal delivery in the blind hope of having an unaffected fetus, especially if delivery is not imminent.

Fetal distress is commonly diagnosed either during intermittent auscultation or by a CTG monitor. Expeditious delivery by cesarean, unless vaginal delivery is imminent, is necessary for the following[29]:

1) Baseline FHR > 150 bpm with absent variability and/or repetitive late or variable decelerations.
2) Absent baseline variability (< 5 bpm) for > 90 minutes.
3) Complicated variable decelerations (> 60 bpm lasting > 90 seconds)
4) Repetitive late decelerations
5) Prolonged bradycardia (< 80 bpm for > 10 minutes)
6) Sinusoidal pattern with no accelerations.

Newer methods like fetal base deficit, fetal pulse oximetry, fetal blood lactate estimation and near infrared spectroscopy are under evaluation.

Meconium passage, especially thick meconium and presence of fetal heart rate abnormalities, is associated with intrauterine hypoxemia and low levels of fetal pO_2. Meconium aspiration occurs because of fetal hypoxia induced fetal gasping and breathing movements in utero. In addition, meconium can cause umbilical artery spasm and umbilical cord necrosis[30]. These events are linked to the duration of exposure to meconium. Therefore, presence of moderate to thick meconium especially with fetal heart rate abnormalities, is an indication for cesarean delivery.

NONPROGRESS OF LABOR

Nonprogress of labor is determined by plotting the course of labor on a partogram. Nonprogress may be due to fault in the uterine contractions, fetus or the pelvis.

Abnormalities of expulsive forces

Uterine hypotony is usually managed by watchful expectancy, amniotomy or augmentation of labor with oxytocin. Stewart and colleagues from Ottawa claim that many cesarean deliveries with as many as 40% being performed in the latent phase are undertaken for dystocia without an adequate trial of labor (Table 10)[31,32].

Labor abnormalities due to incoordinate uterine action, pathological retraction and constriction rings often require cesarean delivery[32].

Table - 10. Incidence of cesarean section in dysfunctional labor[31,32]

Types of Labour dysfunctin	Cesarean delivery (%)
Prolonged latent phase	40
Protracted active phase	
- Nulliparas	42
- Multiparas	17
Prolonged deceleration phase	
- Nulliparas	16.7
- Multiparas	8.5
Protracted descent	43
Arrest of descent	30.4

Abnormal presentation, postion and development of fetus

Persistent occipitoposterior or occipitotransverse positions occur in 10% of occipitoposterior positions. They are usually managed by manual rotation, forceps / vacuum rotation and extraction unless there is a significant element of associated pelvic contraction. However, forceps and vacuum extractions fail more often in occipitoposterior than in occipitoanterior positions. (24% versus 7%)[33]. If the accoucheur lacks adequate skill and experience at rotational instrumental delivery, if a trial has proceeded for a reasonable amount of time or if there are adverse changes in the fetal heart rate, a rational option would be to proceed with a cesarean delivery rather than attempt a difficult instrumental delivery and land up with a moribund baby and maternal injury.

Persistent mentoanterior positions which fail to rotates spontaneously, brow presentations and transverse lie require delivery by cesarean section.

Fetal macrosomia

Prophylactic cesarean delivery on the basis of ultrasound and clinical evidence of fetal macrosomia (EFW > 4000 grams) has been justified for prevention of shoulder dystocia and reduction in likelihood of permanent brachial plexus injury.

In macrosomic babies, the relative risk of brachial plexus injury with shoulder dystocia is 1.2-2.6 and absolute risk is 6-35%. For infants with birth weight more than 4500 grams born to mothers with diabetes, the risk exceeds 50%[34].

Ultrasound sensitivity and specificity for the detection of fetal macrosomia of a 4000g or 4500g threshold is 60% and 90% respectively. It would require 3,695 cesarean deliveries to prevent one case of brachial plexus injury with a threshold of 4500g and 2,345 surgeries to prevent one case with a threshold of 4000 grams in a nondiabetic patient. For a diabetic patient, the number would be 443 and 489 cesareans at 4500g and 4000g respectively[34].

Although Nasser et al, in their study of 231 women with EFW > 4500 g achieved vaginal delivery in 88.9% of pregnancies (36.9% operative vaginal deliveries), there was a 7.7% incidence of major fetal injuries and 7 cases of shoulder dystocia[35].

Although universal use of cesarean section in suspected fetal Macrosomia is not necessary, each patient should be individualized and treated as deemed suitable. Babies weighing more than 4.5 kg (4 kg would probably be the upper limit in Indian women), estimated fetal weight more than 4 kg in diabetic mothers, failure of cervical dilatation or descent of the presenting part inspite of good uterine activity in the situation of fetal macrosomia and presence of a suspicious cardiotocographic pattern in a macrosomic baby should be dealt with by a cesarean section as these events tend to be a forewarning of shoulder dystocia.

Fetal abnormalities

Although Chervenak and McCullough recommended liberal cesarean delivery for fetal hydrocephalus, reserving cephalocentesis for fetuses with associated severe abnormalities, precise knowledge of the extent of fetal malformation is difficult and the benefit of cesarean in reducing fetal morbidity and mortality is not clear.[36] Pediatric surgery consultation and a detailed discussion with the patient is advised before making a decision regarding mode of delivery.

Large sacrococcygeal teratomas, cystic hygromas, distended bladder, fetal ascites or enlarged fetal liver or kidneys have been occasionally found to obstruct labor necessitating a cesarean delivery[37]. These are anomalies usually diagnosed before labor. Forceful attempts at delivery may cause rupture of the lesion. Cesarean section is advisable as the fetus can be salvaged in most cases.

Pelvic contraction

Most cases of pelvic contraction are borderline and a trial of labor is justified. Cesarean delivery is reserved for patients with severe pelvic contraction, pathologically distorted pelves (tumors, rachitic pelvis or kyphoscoliosis) or with associated unfavorable conditions (previous cesarean scars, heart disease, suspected macrosomia, etc.). If progress in cervical dilatation or fetal descent is poor in the presence of fetopelvic disproportion, a cesarean section is preferred over a potentially traumatic instrumental delivery in most cases.

PROLONGED PREGNANCY

Prolonged pregnancy implies a pregnancy which has already gone beyond 42 weeks of gestation (294 days). There is a high incidence of antepartum, intrapartum and neonatal deaths due to meconium aspiration, oligohydramnios leading to repetitive cord compression, progressively increasing placental insufficiency leading to fetal hypoxia, large baby leading to prolonged and difficult labor and increased birth trauma due to shoulder dystocia or operative vaginal delivery. A fetal weight of more than 4 kg would be an indication for cesarean delivery. Similarly, an AFI of less than 3, Doppler studies showing absent or reversal of diastolic flow warrant a more liberal approach towards cesarean section. If a vaginal trial is decided upon, the course of labor should be carefully charted. Any suggestion of a prolonged first stage, especially arrest late in the first stage with a loosely applied thickened cervix or a prolonged second stage with a caput, moulding and difficulty in palpating the fetal ear, suggest a difficult vaginal delivery. A cesarean section would decidedly be a more rational or pragmatic approach[38].

FAILED INDUCTION

Since there is no acceptable definition for failed induction, it should be reserved for cases where the cervix fails to dilate beyond 3 cm over a reasonable period of time (8 hours in nullipara and 4 hours in multipara) despite adequate oxytocic stimulation. It is more commonly encountered in nullipara with an unfavourable cervix, and 15-35% cases of oxytocin and 3-5% cases of prostaglandin induction. These cases often end up with a cesarean delivery. Prostaglandins, in spite of their great promise, have reduced the cesarean rate for failed induction by 0-30%[39]. Although repeated attempts at induction can be tried, it is advisable to restrict oneself to 2-3 attempts. The clinical situation should guide decisions. Overzealous efforts at labor induction can result in uterine rupture (spontaneous or scar rupture), fetal distress, and even incoordinate uterine action and atony. The condition of a patient with diseases like PIH, diabetes or heart disease may worsen in the process thus jeopardizing the mother or the fetus. In such patients, an early decision of abdominal delivery is preferred.

FAILED INSTRUMENTAL DELIVERY

A failed forceps is encountered in about 1.4% of all applications while failure of vacuum extraction occurs in 5.4-7.5% of cases[40].

Applying the instrument at a station at or above the ischial spines, nulliparous women, history of previous cesarean section, fetal weight > 4000 grams and fetal head in other than occipitoanterior position are risk factors for a failed instrumental delivery. Sequential use of instrumental delivery carries a significantly higher neonatal morbidity (OR: 4.8; 95% CI: 0.9-19.9)[40].

However, failed instrumental delivery performed in a setting where a cesarean section can follow promptly is not associated with increased morbidity of either mother or baby[41]. In case of a vacuum delivery, judicious use for a limited time of approximately 15 minutes reduces chances of maternal & fetal trauma[42].

In addition, while taking the patients' consent for instrumental delivery, it is advisable to draw her attention to the available alternative mode of delivery, namely, cesarean section.

INTRAUTERINE GROWTH RETAR- DATION

A growth retarded fetus, due to poor oxygen and hepatic glycogen reserves often cannot withstand the stress of labor. Decision regarding delivery should be guided by a Doppler waveform analysis, ultrasound showing the extent of IUGR and oligohydramnios and a cardiotocographic monitoring.

In pregnancies affected by growth restriction, cesarean delivery without a trial of labor, even before 36 weeks, is required in the following conditions[43]:

1) Evidence of fetal hypoxemia and acidemia associated with abnormal venous Doppler waveforms, absent or reversed umbilical artery flow associated with cephalization of flow.
2) Anhydramnios beyond 28-30 weeks gestation.
3) Repetitive late decelerations or a Biophysical Profile score < 6.
4) Doppler studies showing fetal cardiovascular decompensation.

PREGNANCY INDUCED HYPERTENSION

The hypertensive disorders of pregnancy complicate 7-10% of all pregnancies while the incidence of eclampsia varies from 1 in 100 to 1600 pregnancies[44].

Cesarean section is reserved for adverse and deteriorating maternal and fetal conditions or in a preterm gestation with an unripe cervix. Although cesarean delivery in an eclamptic patient is usually recommended on obstetrical issues, provided the patient's condition is not deteriorating, the cesarean rate varies from 11-57%[45]. Cesarean delivery rates in HELLP syndrome are high, especially with a pregnancy below 34 weeks where it varies between 68% at 30-34 weeks and 87% below 30 weeks. It is undertaken on basis of a deteriorating maternal -fetal condition, abnormal fetal presentation or failure to progress during an attempted vaginal delivery[46].

Sibai recommends performing a cesarean section in mothers with an unripe cervix and less than 32 weeks gestation because of high incidence of intrapartum complications[44].

Cesarean delivery is ideal for all deeply unconscious patients with PIH. These patients have probably developed intracranial thrombosis or hemorrhage. Severe edema in severe PIH may cause an altered sensorium. They are at risk for aspiration pneumonitis, deep vein thrombosis, and fetal distress and death. Their condition can be better managed after a rapid cesarean delivery following which maternal hemodynamics can be better controlled, drugs potentially harmful to the fetus such as diuretics can be liberally administered and the blood pressure is likely to reduce spontaneously after delivery.

The very occurrence of an eclamptic convulsion suggests a grave maternal & fetal prognosis. Prolonged labor or induction of labor can cause spikes of high blood pressure during contractions which may precipitate intracranial hemorrhage. The longer the pregnancy continues, greater the chance that the convulsions will recur. Prolonged administration of anticonvulsants may lead to respiratory depression, aspiration, altered sensorium and cardiotoxicity. Hence, if the delivery is not anticipated within 6-8 hours of a seizure, cesarean section should be performed. As has often been noted, the maternal condition rapidly improves following delivery.

ANTEPARTUM HEMORRHAGE

Placental abruption affects 0.49-1.8% of pregnancies with a perinatal mortality rate of 4.4-67% and a maternal mortality of approximately 1%[47]. The outlook for the fetus is poor not only in terms of immediate survival but also in long term survival as 15.4% of live born infants do not survive[48].

Okenofua and Olatubosum noted a perinatal mortality of 52% with vaginal delivery and 16% with cesarean birth in patients with severe abruption[49].

Hurd et al, too, found a clear advantage of cesarean (15% perinatal mortality) over vaginal delivery (20% perinatal mortality)[50]. When abruption is severe, cesarean delivery must be considered in all cases where the fetus is alive, particularly if there is evidence of fetal distress, and that, indecision and delay in delivery worsens fetal prognosis. Even with the advent of excellent modern neonatal intensive care, management and prognosis of an infant delivered without any complications is better than that of a hypoxic baby who has suffered from the stress of labor, trauma and blood loss.

In mild to moderate abruption, the mode of delivery is determined by the condition of the baby, state of the cervix and presentation, cesarean delivery being usually required for abnormal fetal heart rate patterns.

Placenta previa accounts for 31% of cases of antepartum hemorrhage.[47] In general, the diagnosis of placenta previa indicates delivery by cesarean section. In cases of grade I/II anterior previa with an engaged fetal head, elective induction of labor may be considered at 37-38 weeks as emergency delivery has an adverse effect on perinatal outcome. Cesarean section should be performed on all patients in whom the placenta covers the internal os at the time of delivery.

Vasa previa is one of the rare and lethal conditions in pregnancy with fetal exsanguination and death occurring in 75% of cases. In rare cases, it may be accidentally diagnosed on Doppler ultrasound, in which case an elective cesarean delivery at 37-38 weeks is warranted[51]. In most cases, emergency cesarean delivery is undertaken on the bases of severe variable decelerations (sinusoidal pattern) with the presumptive diagnosis of placental abruption.

PRETERM DELIVERY

The optimal route of delivery for a preterm infant remains controversial. The difficulty in assessing accurately the impact of mode of delivery on meaningful fetal outcomes is due to inability to eliminate treatment bias, high cost and inherent difficulty in performing comprehensive long-term follow-up studies of infants, performance of cesarean section for multiple indications (breech presentation, abruptio placentae, etc.), heterogeneous population of patients and major variations in neonatal management in various centers (Table 11 and 12)[52].

Kigawa and colleagues reported that cesarean delivery significantly improved neonatal survival in infants weighing 750-1499 grams[53]. However, an analysis of 1765 newborns weighing less than 1500 grams at birth showed no protective effect of cesarean birth related to mortality or IVH[54].

In a prospective study of 230 infants weighing less than 1750 grams, early intracranial hemorrhage was less common following cesarean section than after vaginal delivery. The incidence of grade 3 or 4 hemorrhage was higher following cesarean delivery performed in the active phase of labor[55].

Vaginal delivery may be attempted when the presentation is cephalic, labor is progressing normally and the fetal heart rate is normal. A preterm fetus withstands acidosis and stress poorly. Compression of the fragile head during the second stage of labor may precipitate intraventricular bleeding. Cesarean delivery must be considered when there are abnormal Doppler studies or fetal heart rate abnormalities.

MULTIFETAL GESTATION

Cesarean delivery in twins is usually required for twin-to-twin transfusion, IUGR, fetal distress, monoamniotic twins. Breech-vertex or breech-breech presentations occur in 15-20% of all twin pregnancies. These are managed by cesarean section because of concern over interlocking of twins and the irreversible fetal loss which will occur following this complication.

Almost all studies show a higher perinatal mortality rate for the second twin with a PNMR of 57.1 per 1000 for the first born and 74.6 for the second[56]. However, if the delay in delivery between the two is reduced, the difference is negligible. This should not be used as a justification for cesarean delivery, which already has reached 27-80% in some centers[57].

A study by Salomon et al found increased evidence of periventricular leukomalacia following vaginal delivery than by cesarean section (OR: 4.7; 95% CI: 1.0-25.15). They recommend routine cesarean delivery for twin infants weighing less than 1500 grams[58].

Breech presentation of the second twin should be managed as that of a singleton pregnancy with vaginal delivery being offered to fetuses weighing between 1500-3500 grams. The number of studies of second breech twin weighing less than 1500 grams is insufficient to draw any conclusion.

A transverse lie in the second twin may be managed by external version or by cesarean delivery depending on the operator's expertise. External or internal version of the second twin should not be carried out in the absence of operator expertise, blood transfusion facilities, availability of anesthesia and resuscitation and a neonatal care setup. Cesarean section would be preferred to risking iatrogenic fetal trauma.

Although case reports of successful vaginal delivery of higher order multiple gestations exist, most authorities recommend cesarean delivery in view of practical difficulties in intrapartum monitoring, although no prospective series exist proving the benefit of vaginal or cesarean birth.

MATERNAL DIABETES

During the first 70 years of the century, experts advocated cesarean section for almost every diabetic pregnancy. This was partly because of attempts of early delivery with an unripe cervix to avoid fetal macrosomia or for prevention and management of other complications like PIH and IUGR.

However, even with excellent glycemic control and an increasingly liberal approach of allowing the fetus to go close to term, the cesarean delivery rates vary between 19-83%[59].

Although diabetes per se is not an indication for cesarean delivery, the cesarean delivery rate is increased in diabetic (OR: 6.2, 95% CI: 4.47-8.61) and gestational diabetic patients (OR: 1.72, 95% CI: 1.41-2.07) unrelated to complicating factors like IUGR, fetal macrosomia or fetal distress[60]. Probably, practice patterns and physician referral to high risk centres may play a role. Certain complications like intrauterine fetal asphyxia and uncontrolled hypertension do increase the likelihood of cesarean delivery.

Planned cesarean delivery is appropriate for a diabetic mother with a previous cesarean scar. Most diabetic women never plan for a large family and the risk of a repeat cesarean is not excessive when compared to the potential morbidity of an uterine rupture in a diabetic patient.

It has been noted that 31% of neonates of diabetic mothers with estimated fetal weight of 4 kg or more experience shoulder dystocia[61]. Cesarean delivery should be recommended for a pregnancy with estimated fetal weight more than 4 kg and clinical suspicion of cephalopelvic disproportion.

Similarly, unstable and breech presentations should be delivered by cesarean section as the diabetic state would impose additional risk of macrosomia and fetal asphyxia on the preexisting risk.

Women with moderate to severe vasculopathy (proliferative retinopathy) should be delivered abdominally due to the risk of retinal hemorrhage and detachment during labor.

Cesarean section is preferred for delay in progress in the late first stage and second stage of labor, fetal distress or brittle diabetes with poor control. As the baby is likely to be of considerable size, a difficult instrumental delivery should be avoided. The incidence of fetal distress in diabetics is 25% and is the commonest reason for cesarean delivery[62]. Due to fetal hyperinsulinemia which is associated with an increased oxygen demand, the fetus is likely to be hypoxic and acidotic prior to onset of labor and is more prone to intrapartum distress[63].

MATERNAL HEART DISEASE

In general, cesarean section should be performed in a case of heart disease only for obstetric indications. However, labor is associated with repetitive expulsion of large amounts of maternal blood from the uterine circulation during contractions. This may place an unacceptable load on an already compromised heart. The pain associated with labor and hypotension due to venous compression may induce tachycardia and precipitate cardiac failure. Most patients of class I and class II heart disease tolerate vaginal delivery without difficulty. In women with functional class III and class IV disease, cesarean delivery may be safer as it avoids the repetitive hemodynamic changes associated with uterine contractions. In addition to being a planned procedure, it can be performed in a short period of time with good control over maternal ventilation and hemodynamics. As with vaginal delivery, cesarean section should be carried out in a setting with adequate intensive cardiac care facilities. This approach also is ideal for patients with pulmonary edema secondary to cardiac disease where, in addition to better management of the mother following delivery, the fetus can also be salvaged as the risk of fetal demise due to hypoxia is very high in this situation[64].

Recommendations for management of a patient with mitral stenosis involves shortening the second stage of labor with a midforceps application. In case of severe disease, cesarean delivery under epidural analgesia has been advocated as the mode of delivery least likely to result in hemodynamic instability[65].

Some authorities strongly recommend premature delivery by cesarean section and sterilization in cases of severe VSD with reversal of shunt. Avila and his associated studied 13 women with Eisenmenger's syndrome, of which seven patients reached term and were delivered by cesarean section. One patient died a month after delivery and all but one baby survived[66].

Although Marfan's syndrome is not an indication for cesarean section, cesarean delivery under epidural analgesia is advised for evidence of aortic root involvement (aortic root diameter more than 40 mm)[67]. Grafting of the aortic root at the same time has been described[68].

PRECIOUS PREGNANCY

Women who have a pregnancy reaching the period of viability after multiple previous pregnancy losses, infertility treatment or have conceived at a late age are considered to have a precious pregnancy. These women are known to have an increased risk of IUGR, preterm labor and perinatal death[69].

Many women may request an elective cesarean section and the obstetrician may consider this or elective induction of labor at term to be appropriate for psychological reasons.

Kozinsky et al, in their study of 284 singleton, 75 twin and 17 triplet pregnancies after ovulation induction, CVI and IVF, noted similar incidences of IUGR (6.3% vs. 4.2%) and preterm births (13.0% vs. 9.0%) as compared to controls. There was, however, an insignificant trend towards increased cesarean rates between singleton (41.2% vs. 34.5%) and twin (66.7% vs. 60.0%) assisted reproduction pregnancies[70].

Dhont found worse neonatal outcomes following assisted reproduction pregnancies with higher perinatal mortality (OR : 2.6, 95% CI : 1.4-4.8), preterm births (OR : 3.5, 95% CI : 2.2-5.7) and cesarean delivery rates (OR : 1.4, 95% CI : 1.2-1.7)[71].

Cesarean section rates significantly increase with advancing maternal age (Table 13)[12]. When the pregnancy outcomes were studied in women aged 45 years or more at the time of delivery and matched with controls (age : 25-29 years), at the Princess Badeea Teaching Hospital in North Jordan, a higher incidence of placental abruption, placenta previa and cesarean deliveries were noted in older patients (6.1 vs. 0.8%, 4.4 vs. 1.6% and 32.4 vs. 10.7%, respectively)[72]. The increased prevalence of hypertension and placental complications may contribute to the increased incidence of cesarean delivery in elderly mothers.

Table 13: Cesarean delivery rates according to age of the mother in USA[12]

Age (Years)	1980	1991
< 20	14.5	18.2
20-24	15.8	21.0
25-29	16.7	24.3
30-35	18.0	26.7
> 35	20.6	28.4

Advanced maternal age is often associated with an increased risk of chronic hypertension, PIH, diabetes mellitus, gestational diabetes, macrosomia and IUGR. In addition, the patient herself may opt for a cesarean delivery. These factors probably account for the increased cesarean rates.

UTERINE FIBROIDS

The incidence of leiomyomas in pregnancy varies from 1.4% to 1 in 500. A cervical fibroid or a pedunculated fibroid impacted in the pouch of Douglas may obstruct progress of labor and an intramural myoma may interfere with uterine contractions necessitating cesarean delivery[73].

Hasan and associates found an increased incidence of obstructed labor with fibroids greater than 6 cms[74] while Rice et al noted an association between cesarean delivery and fibroids greater than 3 cms[73].

Jabiry – Zieniewicz and Gajewska noted that complications such as abruption, fetal malpresentation and incoordinate uterine action were seen more often with fibroids, thus warranting a cesarean delivery (88%)[75].

Intramural fibroids are more likely to cause incoordinate uterine activity while subserous and pedunculated fibroids may obstruct descent of the presenting part.

PREVIOUS MYOMECTOMY

After a previous myomectomy, a cesarean section is often always performed for fear of scar rupture. Cesarean is especially advised following a history of entry into the endometrial cavity during myomectomy or after laparoscopic myomectomy, as suturing during laparoscopy is never precise.

Zheng and Yang found a 4.1% incidence of uterine rupture and higher rates of anterior placenta (51.0%), adherent placenta (7.5%), placenta previa (5.7%), placenta percreta (0.9%) and puerperal morbidity (6.6%) in 161 patients with uterine scarring following myomectomy and previous cesarean delivery[76].

A myomectomy scar involves suturing of thick vascular myometrium, which may result is collection of pockets of blood within, thus compromising healing. Suturing during laparoscopic myomectomy may be imprecise and perfect apposition of surfaces might not be achieved. Many of these patients have conceived after prior infertility or pregnancy wastage, in which case every effort should be made to achieve a safe delivery, by cesarean section if necessary.

OVARIAN TUMORS

Koonings and co-workers report finding one ovarian neoplasm for every 197 cesarean deliveries[77]. Ovarian tumors, if undiagnosed, may obstruct vaginal delivery and lead to a cesarean section. Large neoplasms, particularly if impacted in the rectouterine pouch and not amenable to gentle disimpaction, may rupture. They are best managed by removal after a cesarean section.

PREVIOUS HYSTEROTOMY / METROPLASTY

An incision on the upper uterine segment has been associated with a 3-4% scar rupture and is traditionally considered to be an absolute indication for cesarean delivery[78]. These operations involve large incisions on the uterus with suturing of thick surfaces with poor apposition. The integrity of the scar is thus doubtful. A rupture in such a patient, often with previous pregnancy wastage or infertility, would have devastating psychological consequences in addition to the physical morbidity.

Champault reported his experience of 64 uterine ruptures, most of which were due to hysterotomy, and recommended elective cesarean section in such cases[79].

Pozowski analyzed a series of cases of pregnancy after a Strassmann's or Jones' operation and recommended cesarean section as the optimal mode of delivery[80].

However, hysteroscopic metroplasty has nowadays replaced the more invasive Jones' and Tompkin's metroplasty as the procedure of choice for uterine septae and these patients may be offered a vaginal delivery.

Colacurci et al noted a 52% vaginal delivery rate in 46 pregnancies in 40 women who had undergone a hysteroscopic metroplasty for a septate uterus[81].

MULLERIAN ANOMALIES

Mullerian anomalies, especially septate and bicornuate uteri are associated with increased rate of abortions, preterm labor, malpresentations, cesarean delivery and retained placentae.

Stein and March noted a 61% and 11% incidence of breech and transverse lie respectively, 25% preterm deliveries and 8.3% incidence of cesarean sections in 186 pregnancies in 150 women with mullerian duct anomalies[82].

Ravasia et al state that though vaginal delivery (80%) is common in women with mullerian duct anomalies with previous cesarean births, the rates of uterine rupture (8%) and cord prolapse (8%) are higher than in controls (0.61% and 0.45%, respectively)[83].

Vaginal septa and stenosis following surgical correction of an atretic vagina can obstruct labor. Cases of pregnancies following surgical correction of a cloacal dysgenesis requiring extraperitoneal cesarean delivery have been reported[84].

Singh and Devi successfully reconstructed a cervix and vagina in a 15-year old girl with a nonfused mullerian system and absent cervix and vagina. She subsequently menstruated and conceived. The pregnancy was terminated at term by a cesarean section[85].

MATERNAL HIV INFECTION

In 1999 AD, 32% of reported HIV cases and 23% of AIDS cases in the US were among women. The rate of AIDS among women was 9 per 1,00,000. Reported transmission rates from mother to child vary between 14-33% in industrialized nations and 40-50% in developing countries. 70-85% of neonates are infected during the intrapartum and postpartum periods while antenatal transmission accounts for 15-38% of cases[86].

Several studies have demonstrated a link between the duration of rupture of membranes and the transmission of HIV.

The French Perinatal Cohort study discovered transmission rates of 0.8%, 11.4% and 6.6% following elective cesarean section, emergency cesarean section and vaginal delivery, respectively. All women received zidovudine therapy[87].

Read et al in their meta-analysis of 15 prospective cohort studies noted that the rate of perinatal HIV-1 transmission in women undergoing cesarean delivery was 8.2% and 2% in those receiving no antiretrovirals and in those receiving zidovudine, respectively[88].

The ACOG published a Committee Opinion in 1999[89]:

1) Women infected with HIV should be offered scheduled cesarean section to reduce the rate of transmission beyond that which could be achieved with ZDV alone.
2) Data is insufficient to demonstrate a benefit for women with viral loads less than 1000 copies/mL of plasma as in those patients receiving HAART (highly active antiretroviral therapy).
3) A scheduled section should be performed at 38 weeks of gestation and amniocentesis should not be performed to avoid contamination of the amniotic cavity with viral antigen from maternal blood.
4) Prophylactic antibiotics should be used because of concerns of heightened risks of postoperative infectious morbidity.

   Thus, until further advances in retroviral therapy take place, all patients with HIV infection should be offered a cesarean delivery. This is one area where the benefits of cesarean delivery to the neonate have been established beyond doubt.

As regards management of HIV infected pregnant women in India, clear strategies are yet to be defined. There are several clinical trials underway, the results of which are eagerly awaited. The management of HIV infected pregnant women may differ in developing countries because of different variables, the most important being socio-economic structure.

HERPES SIMPLEX INFECTION

Herpes simplex infection has been found among 0.6% of pregnant women[90]. When primary genital herpes occurs in pregnancy, there is a high risk of fetal and neonatal involvement, especially with infection in the third trimester. Transplacental infection of the fetus is rare (5%). Neonatal herpes is acquired from an infected lower maternal genital tract during vaginal delivery (90%), especially during an acute episode of primary genital herpes (40% or higher) with a neonatal mortality of about 50%. The risk is lower among women with recurrent herpes (1-2%)[91]. Because of the severity of neonatal herpes and the lack of satisfactory therapy, the only current means of preventing neonatal infection is by elective cesarean section or cesarean delivery even if the patient is in labor, irrespective of the integrity of membranes. Vaginal delivery is permitted in the absence of visible genital lesions. If lesions are present, cesarean delivery is indicated[92].

In a study from the University of Washington, cesarean delivery significantly reduced the HSV transmission rate to neonates (1-2% of cesarean group and 7.7% of vaginal delivery group; OR: 0.14; 95% CI: 0.02-1.08; P=0.047) while invasive monitoring during labor significantly increased vertical transmission (OR: 5.8; 95% CI: 14-32)[93].

Broeklehurst et al have suggested a reduced need of cesarean delivery after acyclovir suppression of primary or recurrent episodes of genital herpes[94]. The role of acyclovir and newer antivirals like valacyclovir and famciclovir (class B drugs) remains to be elucidated.

Till more date is available, the International Herpes Management Forum (IHMF) has recommended delivery of pregnant women with primary genital herpes by cesarean section between 34th weeks and term[91].

HUMAN PAPILLOMA VIRUS (HPV) INFECTION

Although the occurrence of grossly visible genital warts is infrequent, epidemiologic data suggests that HPV infection is the most prevalent sexually transmitted disease[95].

Cesarean delivery is indicated for very large lesions which may obstruct labor and, being very vascular, may precipitate severe hemorrhage.

Potential transmission of HPV transmission to the fetus may occur in the antepartum or intrapartum period respiratory papillomatosis in the neonate may produce respiratory obstruction and is often recurrent. However, because of its rarity (1 in 1200), cesarean birth is indicated only in the presence of active genital lesions, irrespective of the status of membranes and labor[96].

FETAL ANOMALIES

Cesarean section has been advised for fetal gastroschisis to avoid contamination of the fetal abdomen with maternal secretions during labor[97].

While some authors recommend cesarean section for a fetal omphalocele, it has not been shown to improve neonatal outcome[97].

Although the optimal route of delivery of a fetus with meningomyelocele is uncertain, studies have suggested that elective cesarean delivery prior to labor may improve neurological outcome in the neonate at two years of age[98]. The probability of trauma to a large meningomyelocoele and contamination of the meninges by the vaginal flora is a real threat to be considered before attempting vaginal delivery.

CERVICAL CIRCLAGE AND OTHER CERVICAL SURGERY

Most patients with a transvaginal circlage dilate spontaneously or following induction after removal of the suture. Treadwell and colleagues reported a 31.8% cesarean section rate following circlage with 11.9% of patients with Shirodkar's circlage and 2.6% with McDonald's circlage requiring cesarean delivery for cervical dystocia[99].

Although an abdominal circlage suture can be removed through a posterior colpotomy, access during late pregnancy is difficult and severe bleeding can occur. A cesarean delivery is always a prudent option.

The occasional patient who conceives following a conization or Fothergill's repair may experience dystocia due to cervical fibrosis and require cesarean delivery. Primary cervical dystocia is a rare condition. In most cases, an abdominal delivery is preferred to a Duhrssen's incision.

PREVIOUS PROLAPSE REPAIR

Most cases of corrected prolapse are counseled for a cesarean delivery for fear of recurrence of the prolapse. A patient with a Shirodkar's sling can be given the option of delivering vaginally since the uterus has been elevated with an artificial suture material. Cases of Purandare's cervicopexy or Shirodkar's uterosacral advancement may benefit from a cesarean delivery, as the fascial supports used to hitch up the uterus and the cervix may give way during cervical dilatation. Following an anterior colporrhaphy or posterior colpoperineorrhaphy, vaginal delivery may lead to recurrence of the prolapse due to tearing of the fascia and denervation injury or vaginal lacerations due to stretching of fibrosed tissues.

PREVIOUS SURGERY FOR RECTAL OR URINARY INCONTINENCE

All patients with corrective surgery for fecal or urinary incontinence should be advised cesarean delivery. An attempt at vaginal delivery can undo a previous repair. A high incidence of internal and external anal sphincter defects has been noted clinically or sonographically, after vaginal delivery. An episiotomy does not offer much benefit in this regard[100].

PREVIOUS VESICOVAGINAL, RECTOVAGINAL FISTULA OR THIRD DEGREE PERINEAL TEAR REPAIR

A cesarean delivery is preferred to avoid recurrence of a fistula after corrective surgery. If a vaginal delivery is to be attempted, it is only if the fistula has been caused by a non-recurring indication (eg. obstructed labor due to malpresentation or surgery), an interposition graft is in place and expert supervision of delivery is available[101].

Vaginal delivery is to be avoided in the presence of an unrepaired fistula or a third degree perineal tear to avoid further trauma. Even following a third degree perineal tear, vaginal delivery may cause trauma to the fibrotic tissues.

Such patients should be offered the option of cesarean section[102].

MATERNAL DESIRE FOR CESAREAN DELIVERY AND PROPHYLACTIC CESAREAN SECTION

In 1985, the New England Journal of Medicine published an article advocating elective cesarean delivery[103]. With improvements in surgery, anesthesia, infection control and blood banking, this issue has been revitalized. Many patients, due to fear of child birth, demand an elective cesarean delivery.

However, the International Federation of Gynecology and Obstetric states "performing cesarean deliveries for non-medical reasons is ethically unjustified" and "the physicians have the responsibility to inform and counsel women in the matter"[104].

Reasons proposed for performing elective cesarean delivery include a probable reduction in stress urinary incontinence & prolapse. The lifetime risk of prolapse and incontinence surgery for a woman is 11:1. Rortvent et al, in their analysis suggested that prophylactic cesarean delivery might reduce a woman's risk of moderate or severe incontinence from 10% to 5%[105].

Other reasons suggested are reduced mother-to-child transmission of infections agents in the peripartum period and reduced risk of intracranial injury due to instrumental vaginal delivery and reduced rates of birth injuries such as fractures and nerve palsies. A study has shown that although cesarean delivery after failed labor carries a lower risk than a failed instrumental delivery, it still carries a higher risk than cesarean delivery without labor[40].

Finally it is suggested that every woman morally has the right to decide regarding subjecting her body to surgery and opt for a cesarean delivery if she desires so.

However, there are many arguments against these suggestions. A large, population-based study in South Australia has shown that disorders of pelvic floor are strongly associated with aging and instrumental vaginal delivery. Cesarean delivery has not been associated with a significant reduction in pelvic floor disorders[106].

Except for HIV and grossly-visible lesion in HPV and HSV infection, there is no benefit of cesarean in reducing vertical transmission in cases of asymptomatic HSV and HPV, hepatitis B, hepatitis C and other infectious agents.

The number of cesarean deliveries required to prevent a single case of birth trauma is scandalous and though mortality due to cesarean delivery has reduced, it was still twice that of vaginal delivery in 1999. Additionally, cesarean delivery is associated with higher morbidity (OR: 1.29, 95% CI: 1.03-1.51) due to wound infection, uterine infection and hemorrhage[107]. Women with a prior cesarean delivery are at risk of long term complications like scar rupture (0.45-6%), placenta previa, placenta accreta, abruption, sterility and adhesion formation[107].

Yamazaki et al demonstrated a higher incidence of respiratory distress and transient tachypnoea of newborn in babies delivered by cesarean section[108].

Finally, Johnson and Slade have proved that emergency cesarean delivery is associated with previous cesarean birth, parity, age and medical risk factors but not with fear of childbirth or anxiety[109]. Adequate counseling will go a long way towards dissuading a woman from an unnecessary surgery. Although available literature may not provide precise estimates of risks and benefits, a qualitative and quantitative assessment must be attempted.

On current evidence, prophylactic or elective cesarean for maternal or physician convenience is not a valid procedure.

CLASSICAL CESAREAN DELIVERY

Most of the early surgeons such as Levret (1770) suggested a longitudinal incision on the uterus. Lauverjat (1788) was the first to recommend a high transverse incision on the uterus[110]. With time and evolution of the lower segment operation, the upper segment or classical cesarean delivery has become less and less acceptable.

Specific indications for a vertical upper segments incision are[111]:

1) Inaccessibility of the lower uterine segment as in fibroids, dense adhesions or placenta percreta
2) Underdeveloped lower uterine segment as in a premature gestation or
3) Advanced cervical cancer, wherein a lower segment approach may invite torrential bleeding.
4) Although a severely contracted pelvis hindering approach to the lower uterine segment has become an unusual obstetric curiosity although in some of the underdeveloped rural areas, it may occasionally be encountered and warrant an upper segment cesarean section.
5) Some authors still recommend upper segment entry for a placenta previa to avoid placental injury and fetal blood loss. This is cumbersome and unnecessary.
6) Postmortem cesarean section

A review of literature for the classical section consists of mostly anecdotal reports.

Bethune and Permezel from the Royal Women's Hospital in Melbourne reported a 20% classical cesarean birth rate when performed at 24 weeks gestation, 5% at 30 weeks and less than 1% at 34 weeks (overall 1%). The majority of the women requiring the classical uterine incision had either a transverse lie or a major degree of placenta previa[112].

In women with cervical cancer and pregnancy advanced beyond 20 weeks of gestation, the current recommendation is classical cesarean delivery after confirming fetal viability followed by a radical hysterectomy (Grade I-IIA) or radiotherapy (Grade IIB-IIIB, or if desired for the lower grades I-IIA). Isolated case reports are available[113].

CONCLUSION

Cesarean section was a surgery primarily conceived as a desperate measure to rescue an often moribund mother or baby in cases of obstructed labor. Today it has broadened its horizons to include a wide array of indications, some elective and at times as an emergency. since judgment teeters on the brink of error, the liberal employment of the surgery in some situations has invited criticism. Knowledge is a game on the edge of uncertainty. Indications for any surgery evolve with time. To give a blanket list of indications and criteria for cesarean delivery is unjustified. The best solution would be to treat every patient as an individual and make decisions with the wellbeing of the mother and the fetus in mind.

KEY POINTS

- Cesarean section is the commonest obstetrical operation with an incidence of 8-25% of all deliveries.
- Dystocia, previous cesarean delivery, fetal distress and malpresentations are the common indication.
- Previous cesarean delivery, in the absence of contraindicating factors, does not warrant a cesarean delivery. However, in the absence of facilities for emergency and intensive maternal and neonatal care, a trial of scar is not indicated. In view of higher risk of rupture, patients with two or more previous cesareans, classical scars, and previous hysterotomy or myomectomy are, in current practice, offered cesarean delivery.
- A breech pregnancy should be managed by informing the patients regarding the findings of the term breech trial, which suggests a better neonatal outcome with cesarean section.
- Cesarean for fetal distress should be considered after evaluating the fetal heart tracing, presence of meconium, high risk factors and, if available, other parameters like fetal scalp pH.
- Failure to progress should be managed according to etiology e. g. uterine hypotony (oxytocin), fetal macrosomia or pelvic contraction (cesarean section).
- Postdatism per se does not warrant a cesarean but the risk is high due to a large baby, IUGR, meconium stained amniotic fluid and fetal distress.
- Newer prostaglandins may reduce the cesarean rate for failed induction.
- Placenta previa and abruption with a live fetus usually necessitate cesarean delivery for fetal salvage.

- Multiple pregnancies, uterine fibroids, PIH, diabetes, maternal heart disease, older maternal age and an infertility conception, per se, do not justify cesarean delivery except for obstetric indications or if labor is likely to jeopardize the wellbeing of the mother or the fetus.
- As per current recommendations, maternal HIV infection, and gross maternal genital HSV or HPV lesions in pregnancy warrant a cesarean delivery.
- Patients with transvaginal cerclage, conization or Fothergill's repair may require a cesarean section due to cervical dystocia while abdominal delivery is a wiser option following an abdominal circlage.
- Cesarean delivery is usually adocated following a prolapse repair except after a Shirodkar's sling.
- Patents with previous incontinence, genital fistula or third degree perineal tear repairs should be advised a cesarean delivery as to avoid trauma and recurrence following a vaginal delivery.
- In cases of the patient demanding a cesarean section, patient counselling will go a long way in allaying fears and doubts regarding vaginal delivery.
- Except for specific indications, classical cesarean section has a limited role to play in modern obstetrics.

REFERENCES

1. Young JH. The History of Cesarean Sections, London, HK Lewis, 1944.
2. National Center for Health Statistics. Rates of Cesarean delivery – United States, 1991. MMWR 42: 285, 1993.
3. Placek PJ. Commentary: Cesarean rate still rising. Stat Bull Metrop Insur Co. 67: 9-10, 1982.
4. Marcoux S, Fabia J. Incidence of and indications for cesarean sections in the Quebec, Canada region 1973 and 1979. Rev Epidemiol Sante Publique. 31 (4): 459-68, 1983.
5. Gilstrap LC 3rd, Hauth JC, Toussaint S. Cesarean section: changing incidence and indications. Am J Obstet Gynecol. 135 (4) : 437-41, Oct 1979.
6. Chattopadhyay SK, Sengupta PB, Edrees YB, Lambourne A. Cesarean section: Changing patterns in Saudi Arabia. Int J Obstet Gynecol. 25(5): 387-94, 1987.
7. Cirau – Vigneron N, Nguyen Tan Lung R, Elnaik S, Barrier J. Evolution of the indication for cesareans-comparison of 1971-1976 and 1976-1979 at the Maternity Center of the Louis-Mourier Hosptial. Review of the literature. J Gynecol Obstet Biol Reprod (Paris) 14(3): 375-84, 1985.
8. Notzon FC, Placek PJ, Taffel SM. Comparison of national cesarean section rates. N Eng J Med. 316: 386-89, 1981.
9. Quilligan EJ. Making inroads against the C-section rate. Contemp Obstet Gynecol. 221, Jan 1983.
10. Kambo I, Bedi N, Dhillon BS, Saxena NC. A clinical appraisal of cesarean section rates at teaching hospitals in India. Int J Gynecol Obstet. 79: 151- 8, 2002.
11. Notzon FC, Cnattingus S, Bergsjo P, Cotes et al. Cesarean section delivery in the 1980s: International comparison by indication. Am J Obstet Gynecol. 139:902-9, 1981.
12. Depp R. Cesarean delivery. In Gabbe SG, Neibyl JR, Simpson JL (eds): Obstetrics- normal and abnormal pregnancies (3rd ed), Churchill Livingstone. 19: 561- 642.
13. Fedorkow DM, Nimrod CA, Taylor PJ. Ruptured uterus in pregnancy : a Canadian Hospital's experience, Can Med Assoc J. 137:27, 1987.
14. Dickinson JE. Previous cesarean section. In James DK, Steer PJ, Weiner CP, Gonik B (eds): High risk pregnancy- management options (2nd ed), W. B. Saunders. 67: 1205- 16, 1999.
15. Arulkumaran S, Chua S, Ratnam SS. Symptoms and signs of scar rupture- value of uterine activity measurements. Aust NZ J Obstet Gynaecol. 32 (3): 208-12, 1992.
16. Lueng AS, Lueng EK, Paul RH. Uterine rupture after previous cesarean delivery – maternal and fetal consequences. Am J Obstet Gynecol. 169: 945-50, 1993.
17. Chattopadhay SK, Sherbeeni MM, Anokute CC. Planned vaginal delivery after 2 previous cesarean sections. Br J Obstet Gynaecol. 101:498-500, 1994.
18. A Mesleh Madawi Al Naim, Krimly R. Pregnancy outcome of patients with previous four or more cesarean sections. J Obstet Gynaecol. 21(4) : 355-57, 2001.
19. Alberta Reproductive Health. Pregnancy Outcomes, Alberta Health and Wellness, 2001.

20. Cheng M, Hannah M. Breech delivery at term: a critical review of literature. Obstet Gynecol. 82(4): 605-18, 1993.

21. Guiliani A, Scholl WM, Basuer A, Tamussino KF: Mode of delivery and outcome of 699 term singleton breech deliveries at a single center. Am J Obstet Gynecol. 187(6) : 1694-98, 2002.

22. Hannah ME, Hannah WE, Hewson SA, et al. Planned cesarean section versus planned vaginal delivery for breech presentation at term: a randomized multicentric trial. Term Breech Trial Collaborative Group. Lancet 356 (9239) : 1375-83, 2000.

23. Hannah ME, Hannah WJ, Ellen D. Outcomes of 3 months after planned cesarean versus planned vaginal delivery for breech presentation at term. The International Randomized Term Breech Trial. JAMA – 287: 1822-31, 2002.

24. Krebs L, Langhoff - Roos J. Elective cesarean delivery for term breech. Obstet Gynecol. 101(4) : 690-96, 2003.

25. Committee on Obstetric Practice. ACOG Committee opinion: mode of term singleton breech delivery. ACOG 265, 2001.

26. Kitchen W et al. Cesarean section or vaginal delivery of 24-28 weeks gestation: comparison of survival, and neonatal and two-year morbidity. Obstet Gynecol. 66: 149, 1985.

27. Bodmer B, Benjamin A, Mclean FH, Usher RH. Has the use of cesarean section reduced the risks of delivery in the preterm breech presentation? Am J Obstet Gynecol. 154 : 244-50, 1986.

28. Weissman A, Blazer S, Zimmar EZ, Jakobi P, Paladi E. Low birth weight breech infants: Short term and long term outcomes by method of delivery: Am J Perinatol. 5(3) : 289-92, 1988.

29. Biswas A, Anandkumar C. Intrapartum fetal monitoring. In Anilkumaran S, Ratnam SS, Bhaskar Rao K: The Management of Labour. Orient Longman Ltd. 4:57-69, 1996.

30. Altshuler G, Arizawa M, Molnar-Nadasdy G. Meconium induced umbilical cord necrosis and ulceration: a potential link between the placenta and poor pregnancy outcome. Obstet Gynecol. 79 (5): 760-5, 1992.

31. Stewart PJ, Dulberg C, Arnill AC, et al. Diagnosis of dystocia and management with cesarean section among primiparous women in Ottawa – Carleton. Can Med Assoc J. 142: 459, 1992.

32. Arias F. Abnormal labor and delivery. In Arias F: Practical guide to high risk pregnancy and delivery (2nd ed), Mosby- Year Book. 19 (5): 385- 412, 1993.

33. Johanson RB, Rice C, Doyle M, et al. A randomized prospective study comparing the new vacuum extractor policy with forceps delivery. Br J Obstet Gynaecol. 100:524, 1993.

34. Rouse DJ, Owen J. Sonography, suspected macrosomia and prophylactic cesarean: a limited partnership. Clin Obstet Gynecol. 43(2) : 326-334, 2000.

35. Nassar AH, Usta IM, Khalil AM, etal. Fetal macrosomia (> or = 4500g): perinatal outcome of 231 cases according to the mode of delivery. J Perinatol. 23(2) : 136-41, Mar 2003.

36. Chua S, Arulkumaran S. prolonged pregnancy. In: Jamees DK, Steer PJ, Weiner CP, Gonik B: High Risk Pregnancy- Management Options (2nd ed). WB Saunders Company. 60: 1057-69, 1999.

37. Chervenak FA, McCullough LB. Ethical analysis of the intrapartum management of pregnancy complicated by fetal hydrocephalus with macrocephaly. Obstet Gynecol. 68:720, 1986.

38. Clark S, DeVore GR, Platt LD. The role of ultrasound in the aggressive management of obstructed labor secondary to fetal malformations. Am J Obstet Gynecol. 152:1042,1985.

39. MacKenzie CZ. Labor induction including pregnancy termination for fetal anomaly in James DK, Steer PJ, Weiner CP, Gonik C (ed): High Risk Pregnancy–Management Options (2nd ed). WB Saunders. 62:1079-1011, 1999.

40. Al-Kadri H, Sabry, Al-Saif S, et al. Failed individual and sequential instrumental vaginal delivery: contributing risk factors and maternal – neonatal complications. Acta Obstet Gynecol Scand. 82(7): 642-8, Jul 2003

41. Revah A, Ezra Y, Farine D, Ritchie K: Failed trial of vacuum or forceps – maternal and fetal outcome. Am J Obstet Gynecol. 176 (1 pt 1) : 200-4, Jan 1997.

42. Greis JB, Bieniarz J, Scommegna A. Comparison of maternal and fetal effects of vacuum extraction with forceps or cesarean deliveries. Obstet Gynecol. 57(5) : 571-7, May 1981.

43. Weiner CP, Baschat AA. Fetal growth restriction: evaluation and management. In James DK, Steer PJ, Weiner CP, Gonik B. High Risk Pregnancy: Management Options (2nd ed). WB Saunders. 18:291-308, 1999.

44. Sibai BM. Preeclampsia – eclampsia. Current problems in Obstetrics, Gynecology and Fertility. 13:1-45, 1990.

45. Dildy GA, Cotton DB, Phelan JP. Complications of pregnancy – induced hypertension. In Clark SL, Cotton DB, Hankins GDV, Phelan JP (eds). Critical cane Obstetrics, 2nd edn, 251-288, Oxford : Blackwell Science Publications, 1991.

46. Magann EF, Martin JN Jr. Twelve steps to optional management of HELLP syndrome. Clin Obstet Gynecol. 42(3) : 532-550, 1999.

47. Green JR. Placental abnormalities: Placenta previa and abruptio placentae. In Greasy RK, Resnik R (eds). Maternal Fetal Medicine: Principles and Practice. Philadelphia: W. B. Saunders, 1999.

48. Abdella TN, Sibai BM, Hays JM, Anderson GD. Relationship of hypertensive diseases to abruptio placentae. Obst Gynecol. 63:365-70, 1984.

49. Okonofua FE, Olatubosun DA. Cesarean versus vaginal delivery in abruptio placentae associated with live fetuses. Int J Obstet Gynaecol. 23:471-474, 1985.

50. Hurd WW, Miodovik M, Lavin JP. Selective management of abruptio placentae: a prospective study. Obst Gynecol. 61 : 467-73, 1983

51. Hata K, Hata T, Fujiwake R, et al. An accurate antenatal diagnosis of vasa previa with transvaginal color Doppler ultrasound. Am J Obstet Gynecol. 171: 265, 1994.

52. Chao CR. Factors affecting optimal mode of delivery. In Witter FR, Keith LG: Textbook of prematurity-antecedents, treatment and outcome (1st ed): Little, Brown and Company. 12: 203- 222, 1993.

53. Kigawa J, et al. Studies on the mode of delivery and the outcome of small preterm infants with less than 32 weeks of gestation. Acta Obstet Gynecol Jpn (Tokyo). 36:2629, 1984.

54. Malloy MH, Oustad L, Wright E. The effect of cesarean delivery on birth outcome in very-low-birth weight infants. Obstet Gynecol. 77:498, 1991.

55. Shaver DC, Bada MS, Korones SB, et al. Early and late intraventricular hemorrhage: The role of obstetric factors. Obstet Gynecol. 80:831, 1992.

56. Wyshak G, White C. Birth hazard of the second twin. J Am Med Ass. 186:869-70, 1963.

57. Bryan EM. Twin Delivery. In Bryan EM: Twins and Higher Multiple Births. Edward Arnold 5 : 73-82, 1992.

58. Salomon LJ, Duyme M et al. Periventricular leukomalacia and mode of delivery in twins under 1500 g. J Matern Fetal Neonatal Med. 13(4) : 224-9, Apr 2003.

59. Siffen Sl, Wapner RJ, Gabbe SA. Maternal outcome in class H diabetes mellitus. Obstet Gynecol. 55: 749, 1980.

60. Remsberg KE, McKeown RE, McFarland KF, Irwin CS. Diabetes in pregnancy and cesarean delivery. Diabetes care. 22 (9): 1561-67, 1999.

61. Acker DB, Sach BP, Freidman EA. Risk factors for shoulder dystocia. Obstet Gynecol. 66 (6): 762-8, 1985.

62. Brundenell M. Delivering the baby of a diabetic mother - proceedings of the Royal Society of Medicine. 71: 207-11, 1978.

63. MacFarlane CM, Tsakalakos N. Relative fetal hypoxia as a contributing factor to fetal Macrosomia in diabetic pregnancy. Med Hypothesis. 11: 365-74, 1983.

64. Ferraris G, Gambotti G. Cesarean section as the method of choice for patients with cardiac decompensation. Minerva Ginecol. 14: 198, 1962.

65. Ueland K, Hansen J, Eng M, et al. Maternal cardiovascular dynamics vs section under thiopental, nitrous oxide and succinylcholine anesthesia. Am S Obstet Gynecol. 108:615, 1970.

66. Avila WS, Grinberg M, Snitcowsky R, et al. Maternal and fetal outcome in pregnant patients with Eisenmenger's syndrome. Eur Heart J 16:460, 1995.

67. Elkayam V, Ostrzega E, Shotan A, Mehra A. Cardiovascular problems in pregnant women with Marfan syndrome. Ann Intern Med. 123:117, 1995.

68. Pinosky ML, Hopkins Ra, Pinckert Tl, Suyderhoud JP. Anesthesia for simultaneous cesarean section and acute aortic dissection repair in a patient with Marfan's Syndrome. J Cardiothorac Vasc Anesth. 8 : 451, 1994.

69. Reginald PW, Beard RW, Chapple, et al. Outcome of pregnancies progressing beyond 28 weeks gestation in women with a history of recurrent miscarriage. Br J Obstet Gynaecol. 94:643-48, 1987.

70. Kozinszky Z, Zadon J, Orvos H, Katona M, Pal A, Kovacs L. Obstetric and neonatal risk of pregnancies after assisted reproductive technology: a matched control study. Acta Obstet Gynecol Scand. 82(9): 850-6, Sep 2003.

71. Dhont M, DeSutter P, Ruyssink G, Marterns G, Bekaert A. Perinatal outcome of pregnancies after assisted reproduction: a case – control study. Am J Obstet Gynecol. 181(3) : 688-95, Sep 1999.

72. Abu-Heija AT, Jallad MF, Abukteish F. Maternal and perinatal outcome of pregnancies after the age of 45. J Obstet Gynaecol Res. 26(1) : 27-30, Feb 2000.

73. Rice JP, Kay HH, Mahomy BS. The clinical significance of uterine leiomyomas in pregnancy. Am J Obstet Gynecol. 160:1212, 1989.

74. Hasan F, Arumugam K, Sivanesaratnam V. Uterine leiomyomata in pregnancy. Int J Gynaecol Obstet. 34:45, 1990.

75. Jabiry- Zieniewicz Z, Gajewska M. The pregnancy and delivery course with pregnant women with uterine myomas. Ginekol Pol. 73(4) : 271-5, Apr 2002.

76. Zheng YY, Yang ZR. On pregnancies with previous uterine scar. Zhonghua Fu Chan Ke Za Zhi. 24(2): 73-5, 123, Mar 1989.

77. Koonings PP, Platt LD, Wallace R. Incidental adnexal neoplasms at cesarean section. Obstet Gynecol. 72:767,1988.

78. Ritchie EH. Pregnancy after rupture of the pregnant uterus. J Obst. Gynaecol Br Commonwealth. 78: 642-48, 1971.

79. Champault G. Uterine ruptures. The experience of 64 cases in Africa. J Gynecol Obstet Biol Reprod (Paris). 71(4) : 844-60, 1978.

80. Pozowski J, Poreba R, Buchacz P. Pregnancy and labor after uterine operations. Ginekol Pol 74(2): 98-101, Feb 2003.

81. Colacurci N, De Placido G, Mollo A, et al. Reproductive outcome after hysteroscopic metroplasty. Eur J Obstet Gynecol Reprod Biol. 66(2) : 147-150, Jun 1996.

82. Stein AL, March CM. Pregnancy outcome in women with mullerian duct anomalies. J Reprod Med. 35(4) : 411-4, Apr 1990.

83. Ravasia DJ, Brain PH, Pollard JK. Incidence of uterine rupture among women with mullerian duct anomalies who attempt vaginal birth after cesarean delivery. Am J Obstet Gynecol. 181(4) : 877-81, Oct 1999.

84. Waters EG. Cloacal dysgenesis: related anomalies and pregnancies. Obstet Gynecol. 59(3) : 398-402, Mar 1982.

85. Singh J, Devi YL. Pregnancy following surgical correction of nonfused mullerian bulbs and absent vagina. Obstet Gynecol. 61(2) : 267-9, Feb 1983.

86. Andieh L. Pregnancy and Infection with Human Immunodeficiency virus. Clin Obst Gynecol. 44(2): 154-166, 2001.

87. Mandelbrot L, Le Chenadec J, Berrebi A, et al. Perinatal HIV-1 transmission: interaction between zidovudine prophylaxis and mode of delivery in the French Perinatal cohort. JAMA. 280 : 55-60, 1998.

88. The International Perinatal HIV group. The mode of delivery and the risk of vertical transmission of human immunodeficiency virus type 1: A meta-analysis of 15 prospective cohort studies. N Engl J Med. 340 : 977-98, 1999.

89. ACOG committee on Obstetric Practice. Scheduled cesarean delivery and the prevention of vertical transmission of HIV infection. Committee opinion. 219, 1999.

90. Kulhanjian JA, Soroush V, Au DS et al. Identification of women at unsuspected risk of primary infection with herpes simplex virus type 2 during pregnancy. N Engl J Med. 326 : 916, 1992.

91. Brkic S, Jovanovic J. Genital herpes with special emphasis on perinatal herpes simplex virus infection. Med Preg 1. 51 (1-2) : 45-9, 1998.

92. American College of Obstetricians and Gynecologists (ACOG). Perinatal herpes simplex infections. Technical bulletin No. 122, 1988.

93. Brown ZA, Wald A, Morrow RA, et al. Effect of serologic status and cesarean delivery on transmission rates of herpes simplex virus from mother to infant. JAMA, 289 (2) : 203-9, Jan 2003.

94. Broecklehurst P, Kinghorn G, Carney O, et al. A randomized placebo-controlled trial of suppressive acyclovir in late pregnancy in women with recurrent genital herpes infection. Br J Obstet Gynecol. 105 : 275-80, 1998.

95. Osborne NG, Adelson MD. Herpes simplex and human papillomavirus genital infections: Controversy over obstetric management. Clin Obstet Gynecol. 33(4) : 801-11, Dec 1990.

96. Shah K, Ashima H, Polk BF, et al. Rarity of Cesarean delivery in cases of juvenile-onset respiratory papillomatosis. Obstet Gynecol. 68 : 795, 1986.

97. Moretti M, Khoury A, Rodriguez J, et al. The effect of mode of delivery on the perinatal outcome in fetuses with abdominal wall defects. Am J Obstet Gynecol. 163: 833- 38, 1990.

98. Luthy PA, Wardinsky T, Shurtlaff DB, et al. Cesarean section before the onset of labor and subsequent motor function in infants with meningomyelocele diagnosed antenatally. N Engl J Med. 324: 662-66, 1991.

99. Treadwell MC, Bronsteen RA, Bottoms SF. Prognostic factors and complications rates for cervical circlage: a review of 482 cases. Am J Obstet Gynecol. 165: 555, 1991.

100. Cutner A, Cardozo LD, Wise BG. The effects of pregnancy on previous incontinence surgery. Am J Obstet Gynecol. 98: 1181-83, 1991.

101. Kelly J. Vesicovaginal fistulae. Br J Urology. 51: 201-10, 1979.

102. Sultan AH, Karim MA, Hudson CN, Bertram CI. Third degree obstetric anal sphincter tears: risk factors and outcome of primary repair. Br Med J. 308: 887-91, 1994.

103. Feldman GB, Freiman JA. Prophylactic cesarean at term? N Engl J Med. 312 : 1264-67, 1985.

104. Schenker JG, Cain JM. FIGO committee report: FIGO committee for the Ethical Aspects of Human Reproduction and Women's Health. Int J Gynecol Obstet. 64 : 317-22, 1999.

105. Rortveit G, Daitveit AK, Hannestad YS, etal. Urinary incontinence after vaginal delivery or cesarean section. N Engl J Med. 348 : 400-407, 2003.

106. MacLennan AH, Taylor AW, Wilson DH, Wilson D. The prevalence of pelvic floor disorders and their relationship to gender, age, parity and mode of delivery. Br J Obstet Gynecol. 107 : 1460-70, 2000.

107. Bewley S, Cockburn J. The infants of 'request' cesarean section. Br J Obstet Gynecol. 107 : 597-605, 2002.

108. Yamazaki H, Torigoe K, Numata O, et al. Neonatal clinical outcome after elective cesarean section before the onset of labor at the 37th and 38th week of gestation. Pediatr Int. 45(4) : 379-82, Aug 2003.

109. Johnson R, Slade P. Does fear of childbirth during pregnancy predict emergency cesarean section? Br J Obstet Gynecol. 109(11) : 1213-21, Nov 2002.

110. Gabert HA. History and development of cesarean operation. In Plauche' WC (ed): Cesarean section. Obst Gynec Clin NA. 15(4) : 591-605, Dec 1988.

111. Driffen F. Technique of cesarean section. Trop Doct. 17:30, 1987.

112. Bethune M, Permezel M. The relationship between gestational age and the incidence of classical cesarean section. Aust NZ J Obstet Gynecol. 37(2) :153-5, May 1997.

113. Liro M, Blsewski J, Kobieski J, Emerich J, Lukaszuk K. An advanced cervical carcinoma coexisting with pregnancy in 19-years old primipara a case report and review of current literature. Ginekol Pol. 73(4) : 325-30, Apr 2002.

6 | CHAPTER

Surgical Techniques for Cesarean Delivery

Ranjit Akolekar

FRAMEWORK

INTRODUCTION

Cesarean delivery is one of the most commonly performed major surgical procedure worldwide[1]. Even in developing countries, especially India, cesarean delivery is a frequently performed surgical procedure. This is especially true since current recommendations necessitate the first referral units to have facilities for cesarean section. It is in this particular background that cesarean delivery should be made as much free of morbidity as possible so that childbirth is fraught with fewer concerns than it is now.

One of the main factors which has contributed to the increase in rate of cesarean delivery is the safety of cesarean birth as a mode of childbirth. Over the past few decades, safety of anesthetic techniques, effective antibiotic prophylaxis, facilities of blood transfusion, and improved surgical techniques have contributed vastly in making cesarean delivery both safe and popular. This popularity of cesarean birth as an effective mode of delivery has not limited itself to the esoteric obstetric populace but has also influenced the lay public[2]. Still, cesarean delivery is not without morbidity.

Over the past few decades, there has been a constant endeavor on part of the obstetric fraternity to decrease these attendant risks. A considerable decrease in the associated morbidity can be achieved with improvement in surgical techniques. Various studies on the techniques of performing a cesarean delivery have focused on reducing the operating time, blood loss, wound infection, and postoperative morbidity. More recently, there are several aspects of the operative technique, which have been studied in randomized controlled trials. It would be unwise to practice modern medicine without keeping abreast of evidence-based knowledge.

This chapter attempts to review surgical steps of cesarean delivery with special reference to the recent evidence based information. It is imperative to emphasize at this juncture that both trainers and trainees follow the best practice of performing a surgical procedure. For the same reason, it is advisable to be aware of the current and recent advances made in this regard so that older techniques can be revised and newer techniques imbibed. While surgical techniques do vary from surgeon to surgeon, good adherence to basic surgical principles and an awareness of recognized methods of performing cesarean delivery will minimize morbidity.

SUMMARY

- Cesarean section is one of the most commonly performed major surgical procedures in developed and developing countries.
- Cesarean delivery has become safer over the years due to better anesthetic techniques, better antibiotics, availability of blood transfusion and improved surgical techniques.
- Constant effort to improve Cesarean delivery techniques should be made both by trainers and trainees and the best practice should be followed.

PREOPERATIVE ASSESSMENT AND PLANNING

It is a well-known fact that the morbidity of an emergency cesarean birth is more than a planned/

elective cesarean delivery. This is true for various reasons. But, incorporating as much planning as possible in the performance of an emergency delivery will certainly minimize the potential complications and make the cesarean birth more comfortable, both for the surgeon and the patient.

The operating surgeon should plan the cesarean birth, so he/she has full knowledge of the patient's history, especially in relation to any high risk factors and previous operative details. It is very important to make a note of the high risk factors and any other details and highlight them in the history sheet. This will ensure that these important points are not only prioritized in the mind of the operating surgeon, but also the assistants, anesthetists and the surgical paramedical staff who view those history sheets.

A brief history, even in emergency situations, should include certain basic minimum necessary information, which would have an immediate bearing on the performance of the cesarean delivery. These brief points to be kept in mind are mentioned below :

- Presenting complaints
- Medical high risk factors e.g. heart disease, diabetes, hypertension
- Obstetric history
- Accurate gestational age assessment
- Review of antenatal records
- Hemoglobin level and blood group type
- History of known drug sensitivities / reactions
- Details of previous surgery / surgeries

A religious adherence to these details will definitely highlight certain facts about the patient's history, which would have been otherwise missed.

One of the most important points in the above checklist is the history of any known drug reactions or drug sensitivities. Drug allergies are rare; but when a patient has a known sensitivity to a particular drug, its administration can have devastating consequences.

Although it might be tempting in certain situations to make a clinical estimate of the patient's hemoglobin level, the practice should be refrained from. It is necessary to document and ascertain a recent and satisfactory preoperative hemoglobin level. The blood group should also similarly be documented and checked. It is recommended that availability of the same blood type should be checked with the blood bank prior to the surgery.

During history taking, an estimate should be made about the patient's level of intelligence regarding provision of a proper history. This is important in situations where at times patients are not forthcoming with the necessary information. This may be because at times they do not think it necessary or sometimes it slips their mind! It is very important in such a situation to ask direct questions (e.g. a patient who has undergone a repair for atrial septal defect in childhood may not volunteer this information very readily).

A quick review of the previous operative records is necessary as knowledge of intraoperative/ postoperative complications in previous surgeries would help the surgeon to make informed decisions during the course of the present surgery.

A preoperative examination is most valuable as it provides information, which makes planning the surgical procedure easier. The gestational age assessment, number of fetuses, the lie & presentation of the fetus, maternal health & presence of certain high risk factors (which mandate certain modifications in the anesthetic and surgical technique) and lastly the degree of urgency in question, are important factors, which are necessary for planning the current cesarean birth. Although surgical technique is broadly speaking the same, but the above determining factors do mandate a minor modification in the technique e.g. while performing a cesarean delivery for a preterm fetus, the surgeon should anticipate that the lower segment would not be properly formed and therefore make the necessary modification in making the uterine incision.

Anticipation and proper planning are the keys to avoid potential complications.

Planning also involves a good dialogue and understanding amongst the operative team. Although each person in the operative team has a defined job but sharing of the necessary patient information between the surgeon & the assistants, between the surgeon & the anesthetist and between the surgeon & the paramedical staff only increases the level of efficiency and makes patient management more risk free.

It is extremely worthwhile, especially for trainee doctors, to mentally rehearse the surgical steps prior to the surgery. The surgeon should anticipate complications and make a plan of dealing with them intra-operatively. Preoperative rehearsal of the surgical steps in this way would result in the intraoperative decision-making based more on planning than on instinctive judgment.

SUMMARY

- Plan a Cesarean delivery, even an emergency one!
- Elicit proper history e.g. high risk factors, previous operative details, drug sensitivities and highlight them in history sheet.
- Make a note of necessary investigations.
- Appropriate preoperative examination
- Good dialogue between the surgeon, assistants, anesthetist and the paramedical staff
- Rehearse the surgical steps prior to surgery and anticipate complications and ways to deal with them.

MAKING THE SKIN INCISION

Skin incisions have their own unique importance in cesarean delivery. Traditionally, skin incisions for cesarean delivery were vertical incisions. These incisions were initially planned in line with conventional surgical principles i.e. proper and adequate exposure of the operative field. At that time, vertical incisions were used and preferred because of their less vascular rapid entry.

As the rates of cesarean delivery increased paralleled by their increasing safety, there was a concomitant rise in cosmetic considerations. There were an increasing number of women with vertically scarred abdomens who found the vertical scar on the abdomen cosmetically unsightly. This realization was not only on the part of the patients but even obstetricians, who realized the cosmetic benefits of transverse abdominal incisions. As more and more transverse incisions began to be used for cesarean deliveries, other benefits were also apparent viz. the benefits of early ambulation, and a lower incidence of wound disruption[3]. For a lot of years, advocates of vertical skin incisions reported increased intraoperative bleeding and increased incision to delivery time (I-D interval) associated with transverse abdominal incisions. But recently, there have been several studies, which have refuted this claim[4, 5]. Nevertheless, vertical skin incisions do have their own advantages and should be preferred in certain situations, which warrant their use.

The choice of a particular skin incision should be based on relative simplicity and speed of various incisions, the desired exposure, the estimated fetal weight, the anticipated cosmetic results, and the risk factors for infection and dehiscence.

Vertical skin incisions

The vertical incisions used in cesarean deliveries are the low midline vertical incision and the paramedian incision. In present day parlance, vertical incisions are used when there is a sense of extreme urgency involved, in cases of massive hemorrhage, in patients with bleeding tendencies, or in cases when an upper abdominal exploration is required. One of the strongest arguments in favor of performing a low midline vertical incision is when an upper abdominal exploration is warranted. Paramedian incisions are rarely used nowadays for cesarean delivery, as they do not serve the purpose of performing a vertical skin incision.

Vertical incisions allow more rapid access to the lower uterine segment, have less blood loss, provide for greater feasibility for incisional extension around umbilicus, and allow easier examination of the upper abdomen. In pregnancy, the speed of entry through a midline vertical incision is facilitated by the common occurrence of diastasis of the rectus muscles.

It is of particular importance to note here that care should be exercised in making the vertical skin incision. In extremely thin and asthenically built patients, the rectus muscle and sheath are thin and already divaricated; to this is added the virtual absence of subcutaneous tissue in the midline. In an emergency setting, when there is a haste to reach the lower uterine segment, undue pressure on the scalpel may at times cut through the skin and the underlying linea alba with remarkable ease, with the incision extending to the superficial layers of the uterus.

Transverse incisions

There has been an overt bias in the use of transverse abdominal incisions compared to vertical incisions. There are many types of transverse abdominal incisions viz., the Pfannensteil, the Joel-Cohen, Modified Joel-Cohen, Maylard's and Cherney's. Of all these types the commonly employed incisions are Pfannensteil incision, the Joel-Cohen incision and sometimes the Maylard's incision.

Transverse skin incisions are preferred cosmetically. They are generally less painful, allow early postoperative ambulation, are associated with a lower risk of subsequent herniation[3], and yet provide equal, if not better, visualization of the pelvis. Some surgeon's argue that there is also a decreased risk of postoperative pulmonary complications when a transverse incision is used[6]. Although transverse incisions are somewhat more time consuming, the difference in time of entry between the two incision types may be only 30 to 60 seconds in the hands of an experienced surgeon[7]. An important drawback associated with transverse incisions is limitation of view of the upper abdomen.

The Pfannensteil incision is a curvilinear transverse incision about 15 cms long made at the pubic crease. The incision has a gentle curve with the concavity upwards. It is generally made at a point approximately 3 to 4 cms above the symphysis pubis at the level of the pubic hairline. The determination of the lateral extent of the incision should be a function of the estimated fetal size but it is generally extended to the lateral border of the rectus muscles[7]. The Pfannensteil incision involves sharp dissection of the subcutaneous tissue layer and the anterior rectus sheath, which at times may extend upto the external oblique muscles. It is in these situations that chances of nerve entrapment are high and the iilioinguinal and iliohypogastric nerves may be injured[8].

The Maylard incision was originally described for use in radical pelvic surgeries. But it is a commonly used transverse skin incision for cesarean delivery in some obstetric centers. The Maylard incision involves cutting the anterior rectus sheath and the rectus muscles bilaterally either with knife or with cautery. The superficial inferior epigastric vessels, which are present at the lateral edge of the incision, may be individually ligated[9]. After separation of the rectus muscles, the fascia and the peritoneum are then incised transversely, as opposed to the Pfannensteil incision in which they are incised vertically. In most cesarean deliveries, pelvic exposure is sufficient if only the medial two thirds of the muscles are divided. This avoids the necessity to separate surgically the deep inferior epigastric vessels, as is the case with radical pelvic surgery[7]. Maylard's incision is recommended and is considered when certain risk factors are present e.g. macrosomia or twins needing maximal exposure. But as more tissue dissection is required, postoperative discomfort is likely to be more and is comparable to vertical incisions in terms of complications and outcome[10].

The Joel-Cohen incision was originally introduced for abdominal hysterectomies in the mid-fifties and since then has been widely used by obstetricians for performing cesarean delivery[11]. The Joel Cohen incision is a straight incision as compared to the curvilinear Pfannensteil incision. It is placed at a slightly higher level than the conventional Pfannensteil incision i.e. about 3 cm below an imaginary line drawn between anterior-superior iliac spines or about two fingerbreadths above the usual Pfannensteil incision. The subcutaneous tissues are not sharply dissected but separated by blunt dissection. The rectus sheath is extended with fingers after a small incision is made in the anterior rectus sheath; the rectus muscles are also not separated from the overlying sheath. The Joel-Cohen incision is positioned where the fascia is not firmly attached and moves freely over the muscle, therefore there is no need to separate the fascia from the muscle for want of adequate exposure. In a study conducted by Stark and Finkel, a comparison was made between the Pfannensteil and Joel-Cohen incision, the operating time was less by 1.6 minutes in the Joel-Cohen group and so

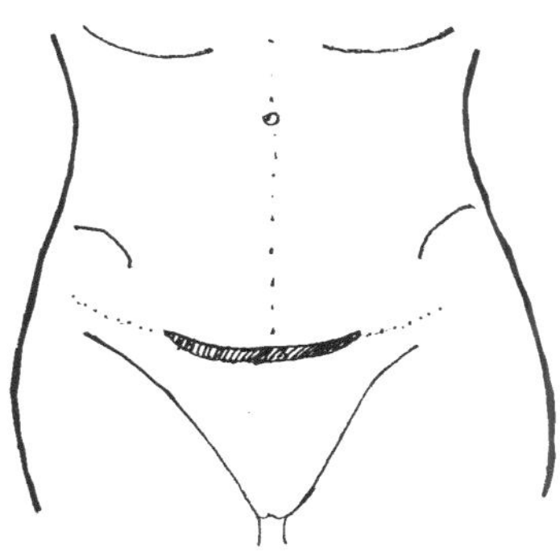

A. Pfannensteil incision

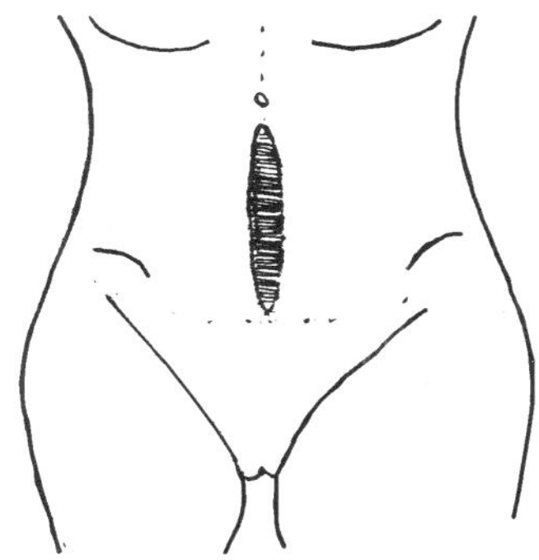

B. Vertical midline infraumbilical incision

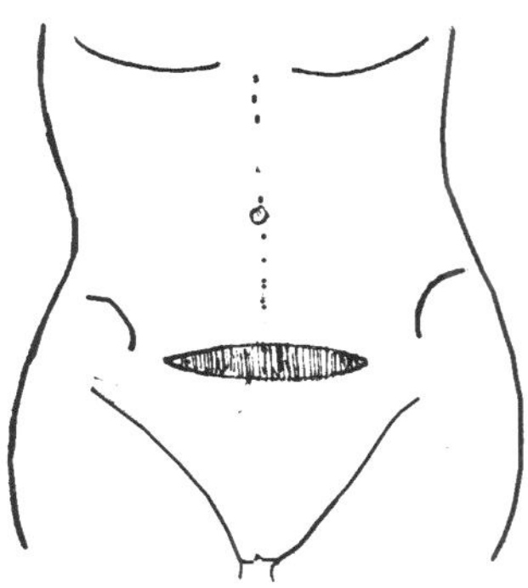

C. Joel Cohen incision during Misgav Ladach method for cesarean section

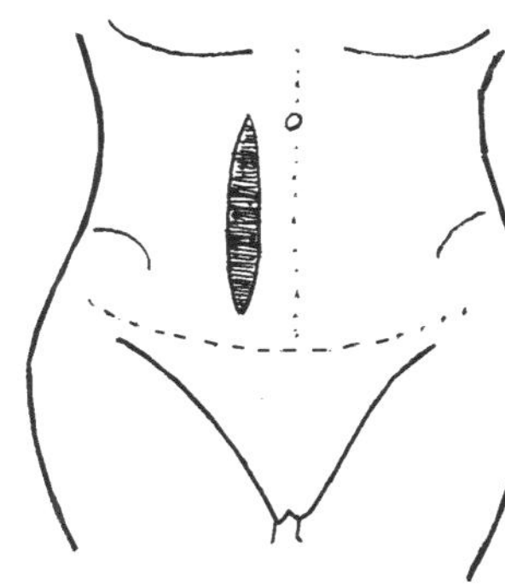

D. Vertical paramedian incision

Fig. 6.1 Various types of abdominal incisions during cesarean section

was the postoperative morbidity[11].

The standard Joel-Cohen incision has been modified and is being used by obstetricians for performing cesarean deliveries. In this modification, the technique of performing the incision remains the same but the placement of the incision differs. In this modified technique, the incision is made 3 cms above the pubic symphysis and all the subsequent layers are bluntly dissected as in the standard technique[12]. The modified Joel-Cohen incision has been studied in various randomized controlled trials. Darj and Nordstrom compared the modified Joel-Cohen incision with the Pfannensteil incision and reported that the former was associated with lesser operating time, blood loss and a decreased analgesic requirement in the postoperative period[13].

As intraoperative bleeding is one of the factors associated with standard transverse incision, the Joel-Cohen incision became more popular because it was associated with a lesser degree of hemorrhage. As the Joel-Cohen incision does not involve sharp dissection of the subcutaneous tissue, it avoids the attendant intraoperative bleeding, which occurs due to the same. Also, as the Joel-Cohen technique does not recommend the separation of rectus muscle from the overlying rectus sheath, it avoids whatever little bleeding, which occurs from the inadvertent dissection of the perforating vessels, which travel between the rectus sheath and rectus muscles.

Additional considerations

Regardless of the type of the incision chosen, there are certain surgical principles that should be borne in mind. While making the skin incision, the surgeon and the assistant should apply traction at right angles to the intended incision site in a symmetric manner so that the incision develops with a uniform length and depth.

The 'Allis' test may be used to determine if the abdominal incision will be adequate enough for performance of the cesarean delivery. If an Allis forceps fits between the retractors placed at the ends of the incision, little difficulty will be encountered in delivering the fetus[14].

In performing cesarean delivery for a patient with a previous abdominal scar, it should be borne in mind that excision of the previous scar will improve wound healing and give better cosmetic results.

Also, in making the abdominal incision, one firm and brisk stroke of the scalpel may be cosmetically better than multiple strokes of the scalpel, which may lead to poor healing and infection.

The obese patient is at a significant risk for postoperative wound complications[15]. In such patients, it is best to use an incision that does not involve the underside of the panniculus as this area is heavily colonized with bacteria, difficult to surgically prepare and is difficult to inspect in the post operative period. The choice in such cases is between a midline vertical incision, which is developed periumbilically both above and below the umbilicus and a transverse incision closer to the umbilicus.

SUMMARY

- The choice of incision is based on indication for cesarean delivery, desired exposure, anticipated cosmetic result and risk factors for infection and dehiscence.
- Incision to delivery interval is same in vertical and transverse incisions, especially Joel-Cohen and modified Joel-Cohen incisions.

- Transverse skin incisions are preferred cosmetically, are generally less painful, allow early postoperative ambulation, have been associated with a lower risk of subsequent herniation, and provide a good visualization of the pelvis.
- Joel-Cohen and Modified Joel-Cohen incisions are associated with a lesser operating time, a decreased blood loss and a decreased postoperative morbidity compared to Pfannensteil incisions.

REACHING THE LOWER UTERINE SEGMENT

After making the skin incision, there are several layers of the abdominal wall, which have tobe negotiated before the operating surgeon reaches the desired destination – i.e. lower uterine segment. There are five basic structures that need to be dissected prior to making the uterine incision. They are:

- Subcutaneous tissue
- Rectus sheath
- Rectus muscle
- Parietal peritoneum
- Visceral peritoneum

The subcutaneous tissue in the lower abdominal wall is made up of the superficial Camper's fascia and the deeper Scarpa's fascia. During the making of a bold abdominal skin incision, especially in non-obese patients, the Camper's fascia is inadvertently dissected for the most part. It is only the tough Scarpa's fascia that needs to be dealt with for further access to the abdomen.

The standard technique of cesarean delivery using the Pfannensteil incision advocates sharp dissection of this fascia. As the Scarpa's fascia forms the plane for vascular travel in subcutaneous tissues, the blood vessels are also inadvertently cut with resultant hemorrhage from these vessels. This bleeding can at times be troublesome, which increases the operative effort and operative time.

In the Joel-Cohen technique as well as in its modified version, this unnecessary surgical effort and investment of operative time is avoided[12]. In this technique, a 2.5 to 3 cms long nick is made in the midline in Scarpa's fascia, which is extended on both sides by fingers traction. This technique causes considerably less bleeding as the vessels curve behind the advancing edge of the finger and are not cut. Blood vessels and nerve fibers have a certain amount of elasticity and on stretching they get pushed behind the finger and are not torn or severed[12]. The only vessels that bleed when this technique is employed are thin walled vessels; the resultant bleeding is little and is temporary as spontaneous thrombosis in a very short time occludes these vessels. So, the operating surgeon should bear in mind that while employing this technique, effort should not wasted in achieving hemostasis as most of these vessels stop bleeding by themselves in a short time. It should be noted that Scarpa's and Camper's fascia are not encountered when a vertical midline incision is employed for cesarean delivery.

The anterior rectus sheath is the next layer of abdominal wall that meets the surgeon. When transverse incisions are employed for cesarean delivery, the posterior layer of rectus sheath is not encountered, as it is deficient below the arcuate line.

In the conventional technique of cesarean delivery using the Pfannensteil incision, the anterior rectus sheath is incised and the incision is extended on both sides by sharp dissection with tissue cutting scissors. After an adequate incision has been made, the next surgical step entails separation of the underlying rectus muscle from the rectus sheath. The rectus sheath is densely attached to the underlying rectus muscle in the midline and this is attachment is sharply dissected with the aim to achieve a better surgical exposure. On both sides of the midline, the muscle is bluntly separated from the rectus sheath. However, also in this plane are perforating vessels, which traverse between the rectus sheath and the rectus muscle, which are also inadvertently dissected. These vessels are notorious in that they retract quickly and cause bleeding. So, dissection in this plane should be done carefully, taking care not to injure the obvious vessels.

In the Joel-Cohen technique, a 2.5 to 3 cms long transverse incision is made in the midline, which is extended on both sides by finger traction. No effort is made to separate the rectus sheath from the underlying rectus muscle, as the placement of the incision is such that the fascia is not firmly adherent but freely mobile over the muscle[12]. Therefore, there is a significant decrease in intraoperative bleeding as well as a decrease in operative time.

In vertical midline incisions, the dissection is at the linea alba, which is incised and the incision advanced cephalad and caudad as is required.

The rectus muscle lies below the plane of the anterior rectus sheath. While doing routine cesarean deliveries in those patients who have not had a prior surgical procedure, sharp dissection of the rectus muscle is rarely required. In transverse abdominal incisions, the muscle bellies of the rectus muscle are split and not sharply cut. The rectus muscle can be split by the operating surgeon and the assistant in two ways viz. vertically and transversely. It is the latter, which should be avoided. A good surgical exposure can be achieved by splitting the bellies of the rectus muscle while the traction is applied in a vertical plane. When transverse stretching of the rectus muscle is done, there is a potential risk of damage to the inferior epigastric vessels which lie on the underside of the muscle bellies; these vessels are wide bore vessels and damage to them can cause significant bleeding. In those patients who have had a prior surgical procedure/childbirth, the rectus muscle can be fibrosed to a variable degree, which may require the use of sharp dissection by the operating surgeon to achieve a necessary exposure.

The parietal peritoneum follows the rectus muscle as the next and the last layer of the abdominal wall. Incision and extension of the peritoneum is an important step in the technique of cesarean delivery as improper techniques can lead to a variety of complications.

In the conventional technique of cesarean delivery with a transverse Pfannensteil incision, the peritoneum is incised as high as possible in between two artery clamps after ascertaining that the parietal peritoneum is free from the underlying bowel. The incision is then extended vertically on either side and access to the abdominal cavity is gained. In the Joel-Cohen technique, the peritoneum is opened bluntly with fingers as high as possible and the incision is extended on either side with finger traction by the surgeon and the assistant[12].

It is worthwhile to note at this juncture that inadvertent bladder injuries can occur during extension of the peritoneal incision. This is primarily because of the fact that the bladder is advanced on the parietal peritoneum in advanced gestation, especially the dome of the bladder. In some patients it may be unusually high, so particular care should be taken.

Alternatively, the peritoneum can also be opened transversely with sharp dissection, as doing so not only avoids inadvertent bladder injury but also gives adequate exposure. This transverse opening of the parietal peritoneum is not what is achieved with conventional and Joel-Cohen techniques; the peritoneum is vertically opened in the conventional technique while in Joel-Cohen technique, as the traction is applied transversely, the shearing force develops in a direction perpendicular to it, which is vertical.

Additional considerations

Following opening of the layers of the abdominal wall, access is gained to the abdominal cavity. Before attempting to open the vesico-uterine space to gain access to the lower uterine segment, there is an important anatomical relationship to note. In quite a few patients, the uterus is dextro-rotated, thus bringing the left round ligament closer to the midline than the right. The surgical importance of this fact is that, while making the uterine incision, extension of the incision without this knowledge may lead to an unplanned tear on one of the angles of the uterine incision. Sometimes, the dextro-rotation is severe enough to warrant correction of the rotation prior to entry into the vesico-uterine space.

After all the above necessary considerations, the vesico-uterine fold is identified and a small incision is made in the center in the loose part just over the desired site of uterine incision. A retroperitoneal space is created bluntly with the scissors, tenting the peritoneum on either sides of the incision. The incision is extended on both sides with sharp dissecting scissors and then the bladder flap is developed. Development of the bladder flap needs the loose vesico-uterine fascia to be separated from the lower uterine segment. This can be done by blunt dissection with fingers or by sharp dissection of the flimsy tissue with scissors. Some surgeons also use a sponge on a holder to separate and dissect the vesico-uterine fold from the lower uterine segment. The latter practice however, is not common. The vesico-uterine fascia in a patient undergoing a primary cesarean delivery is very flimsy and can usually be separated from the lower uterine segment with one or two 'sweeps' of the finger/s and should be preferred. Use of sharp dissecting scissors is however recommended if there are dense adhesions between the lower uterine segment and the vesico-uterine fascia, as is the case in some patients undergoing repeat cesarean birth. Care should be taken while using the dissecting scissors as at times the dense adhesions are accompanied by blood vessels. The dissection of the vesico-uterine fascia should be done mainly in the center and too much of lateral dissection should be avoided to prevent injury to the vascular plexus that lie laterally. The bladder flap is then retracted with the use of a bladder retractor. The bladder retractor keeps the bladder away from the surgical field but it should be remembered that undue pressure on the retractor should be avoided as it might cause minor mucosal bladder injury at times.

SUMMARY

- Blunt dissection of the Camper's and Scarpa's fascia is advisable, as it is associated with a decreased intraoperative bleeding, and less operative time.
- During dissection of the anterior rectus sheath from the underlying muscle, care should be taken as perforating vessels might get cut and subsequently bleed. Such a bleeding is not a part of the modified Joel-Cohen technique, as it does not require the said dissection.
- Rectus muscle should be split vertically and not transversely. Care should be taken to avoid injury to the vessels on the underside of the muscle bellies.
- Peritoneum should be opened as high as possible. It can be cut transversely to avoid inadvertent injury to the bladder. If opened in any other way, care should be taken to avoid bladder injury.
- Dextro-rotation of uterus should be noted prior to opening the vesico-uterine space.
- Development of the bladder flap should entail dissection in the midline and not laterally to avoid vessel injury.

UTERINE INCISION

Making the uterine incision is a very important surgical step in the cesarean delivery. As far as possible, the incision should be planned preoperatively as aforementioned, to avoid potential complications associated with extended and misdirected uterine incisions. Uterine incisions may be of several types:

- Lower segment transverse (Kerr incision)
- Lower segment vertical (Krönig incision)
- Classical incision
- Variations of transverse incisions e.g. J–shaped incision, U-shaped or trap door incision, and the T-shaped incision.

Lower segment transverse incision:

By far, the lower segment transverse incision is the most commonly employed incision for cesarean birth and will be focused on in greater detail.

For making a lower segment transverse incision, a small incision is made in the center, about 2-3 cms long, with the scalpel, until the membranes are reached. Considerable caution should be exercised in making this incision, as in times of emergency cesarean deliveries; haste and undue enthusiasm may result in undue pressure on the scalpel. This results in the incision being made on the uterus as well as the baby.

After the initial small incision being made on the uterus, the incision can be extended in two ways: either with the use of sharp dissection or with blunt, finger dissection[16]. Sharp dissection can be done with dissecting scissors on both sides and the incision advanced. Alternatively, blunt finger dissection and traction on both ends of the incision can also extend the incision. These two techniques of extension of the uterine incision have been compared in randomized clinical trials[16, 17] and it has been noticed that there is no difference in both the techniques as far as the ease of delivery, blood loss, unintended extension or post-operative endometritis is concerned. In a prospective, randomized controlled trial Rodriguez AI et al showed that blunt and sharp dissection of the uterine incision are equivalent in ease and safety and that there was no difference in the incidence of unintended extension, postoperative endometritis, duration of surgery or unintended blood loss[17]. However, in another randomized clinical trial conducted by Magann EF et al, it was studied whether blunt vs. sharp dissection of uterine incision affected the incidence of intra-operative hemorrhage. They concluded that sharp dissection of the uterine incision significantly increases intra-operative blood loss and the need for a subsequent transfusion[16].

Usually, a surgeon uses only one of these techniques as his/her experience might dictate but it is advisable to be abreast with both these techniques as they can be used in different surgical situations. Blunt splitting with fingers is preferable when the lower uterine segment is thin and effaced while sharp dissections is more recommended if the lower uterine segment is not fully effaced. Therefore a surgeon should use a particular technique depending on the effacement of the lower uterine segment. However, the choice of a particular technique usually depends on the surgeon's level of comfort and ease with a particular method.

One point of importance to note here is that when the uterus is dextro-rotated, the force used on the left side should be less than that on the right side to avoid hemorrhage and extension of the left uterine angle. While using fingers to extend the uterine incision, it is important to curve the incision upward (cephalad), so that the incisional length that develops is maximum without the inadvertent extension of the uterine angles. Splitting the uterine incision with fingers is more unpredictable as it results in a variable degree of shearing force; this technique therefore needs more experience to be effectively used.

Another technique has been tried to decrease the amount of blood loss, which occurs during the making of the uterine incision. In this technique, a stapling device was used. After the making of the small uterine incision in the center, the stapling device is introduced between the amniotic membrane and the uterine wall. As the stapler is closed, a cutting device is activated and a double row of staples seals blood vessels and secures uterine layers just before the blade cuts the uterine wall[18]. This technique causes less bleeding from the cut edges of the uterine incision but results in an increased operating time and the time needed to deliver the baby. In a systematic Cochrane review, Wilkinson and Enkins analyzed four trials, which studied the use of absorbable staples at cesarean section. They concluded that there was no difference in the total operating time but the time needed to deliver the baby was prolonged[19]. The device is expensive and at present there is not enough evidence to justify its routine use but it may be useful in patients with vascular lower segment e.g. placenta praevia.

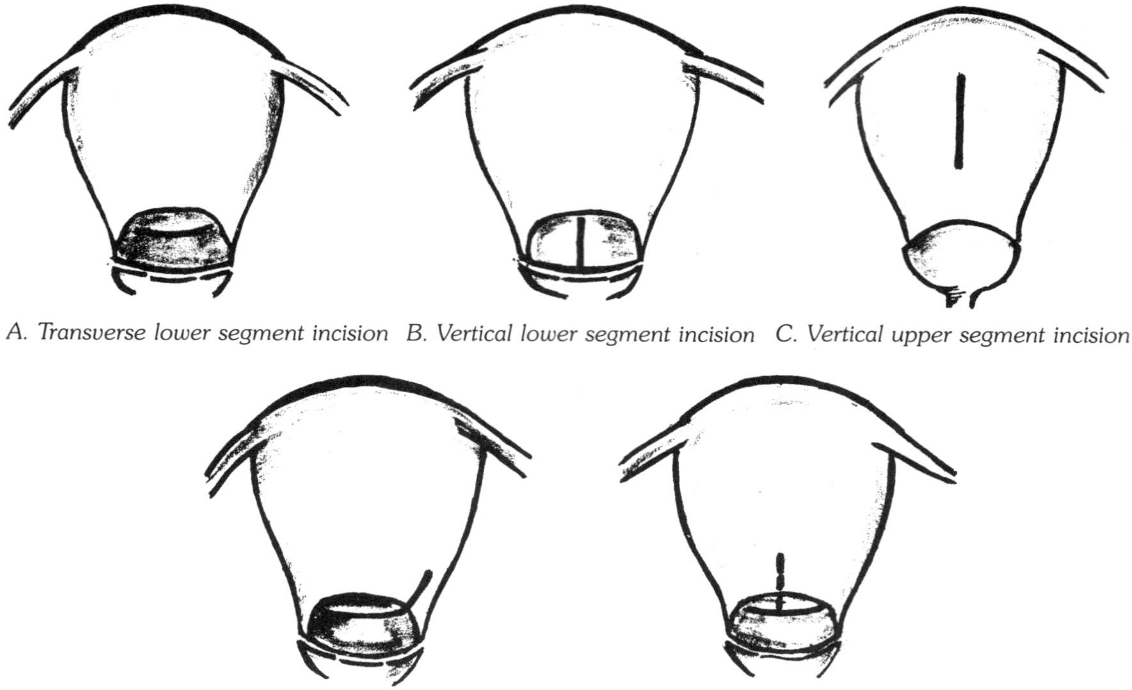

A. Transverse lower segment incision B. Vertical lower segment incision C. Vertical upper segment incision

D. J shaped incision E. Inverted T shaped incision

Fig. 6.2 Various types of uterine incisions employed during cesarean section

Some other uncommonly used methods are also described for limiting the amount of bleeding that occurs during making of the uterine incision. In patients with thin and effaced uteri, the chances of extension of uterine angles and resultant hemorrhage are relatively higher. Some surgeons recommend taking stay sutures at two predetermined sites at lateral angles of the uterus prior to making and extending the incision. This limits the lateral extension of the uterine incision upto the stay sutures and thus does not cause inadvertent extension of uterine angles. This technique however, increases the amount of operative time and also the time needed to deliver the baby. This technique has not been studied in randomized trials and is not recommended for routine use during cesarean birth.

It is worthwhile to note that intraoperative bleeding can be decreased and inadvertent extensions can be prevented even when routine techniques are used (i.e. sharp or blunt dissection), provided preoperative planning is done and correct technique is used.

Lower segment vertical incision

Preterm patients, in whom lower uterine segment is not well developed, and in fetuses presenting with a transverse lie, the lower segment vertical incision can be used[7]. After the lower uterine segment is exposed, the bladder is displaced downwards to expose more of the lower uterine segment. This downward displacement of bladder is more inferior than that usually done for lower segment transverse incision. This downward displacement of the bladder is necessary to ensure that the low vertical incision does not extend into the upper segment. This is a very important step in the making of the low vertical incision. If the downward displacement of the bladder is not enough, it is very likely that the incision may extend either upwards or downwards; upward extension will involve the upper segment and downward extension can either extend into the bladder or rarely the vagina. Once the bladder is displaced downwards, an incision is made at the lowest margin of the incision and extended cephalad with either the scalpel or the tissue cutting scissors.

The low vertical incision evolved with the aim of avoiding an incision in the upper segment, which has a higher risk of scar dehiscence in subsequent pregnancy. Although the incision is made in the lower segment; in practice, a true lower uterine vertical incision that does not extend into the contractile portion of uterus is actually uncommon[7]. The clinical implication of making a vertical incision in the lower segment is that it poses a lesser risk in a subsequent gestation than an upper segment vertical incision. The risk of scar dehiscence following a lower segment vertical and a lower segment transverse incision was compared in some trials[20, 21, 22]. One of the earlier studies (1983) conducted by Schutterman EB and Grimes DA compared the safety of lower uterine transverse and vertical incision in cesarean deliveries conducted for fetuses with breech presentation. They found that the incidences of an Apgar score of 6 or lower, extension of the uterine incision, a decrease in hematocrit by 6 points or more, blood transfusion, and maternal fever were not significantly different in both these groups. They concluded that since both these types of incisions appear to have comparable safety, the possibility of a vaginal delivery with later pregnancies suggests that the low transverse uterine incision is preferable to the low vertical incision[20]. In a more recent study (1999), Ship et al studied whether gravidas with a lower vertical incision were at a higher risk for dehiscence during trial of labor in a subsequent gestation. They concluded that gravidas with a prior low vertical uterine incision are not at increased risk for uterine rupture during a trial of labor compared with women with a prior low transverse uterine incision[21]. Martin JN Jr. et al retrieved and reviewed American Obstetric literature from 1981 relating to pregnancy outcome in patients with a prior low transverse incision. They concluded that in the otherwise uncomplicated pregnancy the patient with one previous non-extended lower-segment vertical cesarean incision should be considered a candidate for trial of labor in her current singleton pregnancy[22].

However, because the risks of extension into bladder and upper segment remain higher with the performance of a lower segment vertical incision, a low transverse incision should be used whenever it is possible.

Classical incision

The Classical upper segment vertical incision was the standard uterine incision for cesarean delivery until the lower uterine segment incision was introduced and popularized by Munro Kerr in 1926[23]. In this technique, an initial incision is made with the scalpel 1 to 2 cms above the bladder reflection. After the fetus or the fetal membranes are visualized, the incision is extended upwards with the scalpel or the tissue cutting scissors. The extent of upward extension depends on estimated fetal size[7]. The classical upper segment incision is associated with considerable intraoperative hemorrhage from the cut edges of the uterine incision. There is an increased risk of infection, poor healing contributing to the increased risk of rupture during a subsequent gestation[3]. The performance of 'Classical' cesarean delivery is a rare occurrence in recent times but there are certain clinical situations when its use is warranted. In maternity set ups supported by good neonatal care, performance of cesarean delivery done for extreme prematurity (especially deliveries prior to 28 weeks), warrants the use of classical upper segment incision. This incision is also used when a large cervical fibroid prevents the making of an incision in the lower uterine segment. One might be forced to use a classical incision when severe dense adhesions from previous cesarean delivery make the lower uterine segment inaccessible. Some older texts have quoted placenta praevia, especially with large vessels in the lower segment, as an indication for classical cesarean delivery; but this should be individualized and a lower transverse incision should be taken whenever possible.

Variations

Sometimes, as a desperate measure for baby delivery, few modifications of the above mentioned incisions might be required. These are the J-shaped incision, the U-shaped incision or the trap door incision and the inverted T-incision.

After making the initial uterine incision, when it is realized that there is difficulty in delivering the fetal presenting part, and effort should be made to quickly assess the cause of the difficulty. This is because at times the resistance to baby delivery is due to factors other than inadequacy of the uterine incision (e.g. inadequate skin incision, inadequate fascial incision). Once other factors are ruled out and the reason for entrapment of the fetal presenting part is found to be inadequacy of uterine incision, the incision will need to be extended. The options for further extension of the incision, in these situations, are limited. In such situations, when a further extension of the incision is desired, the only direction in which the incision can be extended is perpendicular to the transverse incision, and towards the upper segment. The uterine incision can be extended into the upper segment either at the uterine angles or in the center. This results in the three variations of the uterine incision as aforementioned. If the incision is extended upwards from only one uterine angle, it results in a J-shaped incision. If this is done at both the uterine angles it results in a U-shaped incision. If, however, the upward extension is done from the center of the upper edge of the incision, it results in the T-shaped incision.

All these incisions are associated with intraoperative complications, poor healing and prolonged hospital stays[25]. As the healing in these incisions is poor, the scar formed is weak and therefore more liable to rupture in subsequent pregnancies. The worst healing, however, is seen with the T-shaped incision and its use should be avoided.

SUMMARY

- Anticipating the intraoperative findings, the uterine incision should be planned as far as possible.
- One should be abreast of blunt as well as sharp expansion of the uterine incision. Sharp dissection leads to a slightly increased intraoperative blood loss compared to blunt dissection.
- Low vertical incision may be preferred in poorly formed lower segment, transverse lie, and preterm patients. Patients who have had a prior birth with an uncomplicated low vertical incision can be given trial of labor in the current pregnancy without increasing risk of dehiscence.
- The classical incision is rarely required but its use may be warranted in extreme prematurity, large fibroid in lower segment, and patients having dense adhesions from previous surgery when access to lower segment is not possible.
- J-shaped, U-shaped and T-shaped incisions are associated with poor healing and increased postoperative morbidity. But when such an incision is warranted due to difficulty in baby delivery, J-shaped incisions heal better than T-shaped incisions.

TECHNIQUES OF BABY DELIVERY

After the uterine incision is made, the next step is to deliver the fetus. This is a very important step in the surgery, as it is the purpose of performing a cesarean delivery. The degree of urgency required while performing a cesarean section is mandated by the indication of the cesarean birth. But on a general principle, induction-delivery intervals of more than 8 minutes under general anesthesia and incision delivery intervals of more than 3 minutes under both general and regional anesthesia are associated with increased incidence of low Apgar scores and neonatal acidosis. This fact should be kept in mind while performing a cesarean section and conducting a baby delivery during the same[26].

After the uterine incision is made, if the membranes have not been inadvertently cut, they should be ruptured and the amniotic fluid suctioned. Techniques for baby delivery differ according to the part of the fetus occupying the lower uterine segment. Fetal presentations may be cephalic, breech or transverse. Cephalic presentations are by far commoner and will be discussed in detail.

Techniques for delivery of the fetal head may also differ depending on whether the head is floating, engaged, deflexed or deeply impacted. Delivery of an uncomplicated cephalic presentation can be comfortably accomplished but certain facts should be borne in mind. After completion of the uterine incision and ascertaining that the membranes are ruptured, a hand is introduced into the uterine cavity to elevate the fetal head, which is then brought out through the incision. It is important to bear in mind that the flexion of fetal head should be maintained all through the delivery, as deflexion might lead to head entrapment. (The importance of the preoperative clinical examination cannot be overemphasized. An adequate knowledge of the fetal lie, presentation, station, degree of flexion and the position of the occiput is of paramount importance). After the delivery of the fetal head, the nose and oropharynx are suctioned and the rest of the delivery accomplished. The rest of the baby delivery should be done carefully and quickly but without haste. The shoulders should be delivered one by one and not at the same time as trying to accomplish delivery at the same time will lead to enlargement of the uterine incision with the shearing force being concentrated either on angles or on the thin lower uterine segment. The rest of the baby is then delivered by a gentle but a firm traction.

If the fetal head is deflexed, then after introduction of the hand into the uterine cavity, the head should gently flexed in the opposite direction prior to delivering the fetal head out of the uterine incision.

While delivering the floating head, some technical considerations are important. After making of the uterine incision, if an attempt is made to immediately deliver the fetal head, the head may slip, as the grip is not firm. This might cause some inadvertent fetal movement and rotation in the uterine cavity with the result that the fetal lie is now changed and may become oblique, especially if the fetus is preterm. This leads to an increase in intraoperative time with prolonged incision to delivery interval[27]. To avoid such a situation, some technical modifications are necessary. After the uterine incision, the membranes are ruptured, the amniotic fluid is suctioned out and the fetal head is allowed to descend till it reaches the incision made in the lower uterine segment. The fetal head can then be delivered by adherence to surgical techniques described above. Some surgeons advocate the use of vacuum or the forceps in a controlled manner for delivering the floating head[28]. Both these instruments can be used for delivering the fetal head. For use during cesarean delivery, short forceps (e.g. Wrigley's or Simpson's) are generally preferred. One can also use only one blade of forceps as a vectis to gently elevate and deliver the fetal head[3]. It should be remembered that forceps should be applied such that the flexion of the fetal head is maintained. This can be accomplished by adhering to the norms of a perfect cephalic application i.e. along occipital-mental diameter and in the biparietal malar plane. When vacuum is used for delivery of the fetal head, normal principles of vacuum applications should be followed e.g. flexing application. More recently, sialistic vacuum cups have been used for delivery of fetal head during cesarean delivery[28]. They are less traumatic and effective for use in cesarean delivery.

The use of instruments during cesarean delivery however, is associated with an increase in operating time which is especially associated with increased interval from uterine incision to delivery (called as the U-D interval to distinguish it from the I-D interval, which is used to assess the time elapsed between skin incision and baby delivery). In most instances, this increase in U-D interval is not associated with significant changes in the Apgar scores and acid base values in umbilical cord blood. However, caution should be exercised when instruments are used to deliver babies during cesarean deliveries[29]. The chances of cup slippage, when vacuum is used during cesarean births, are less compared to vaginal deliveries but when this occurs, no persistence should be shown to deliver babies with instruments and immediate resort to more conventional methods should be made without hesitation.

A more challenging scenario prevails when the head is deeply engaged in the pelvis. Diagnosis of deeply engaged head should preferably be a preoperative diagnosis so that necessary planning can be done for accomplishing the baby delivery. During the cesarean delivery, this can be ascertained when the operating surgeon cannot reach the leading part of the fetal head. Accomplishing the delivery of the deeply engaged fetus without having extensions of the uterine angles is a tight rope walk, and needs considerable surgical expertise. There are certain matters of surgical technique, which are important at this stage. There are two different methods of baby delivery, which are described to deliver deeply engaged heads. One method is the abdomino-vaginal method and can be found mentioned in standard textbooks of obstetrics. In this technique, an extra assistant is kept ready, and after the making of the uterine incision, pushes the fetal head upwards per vaginum. This enables the operating surgeon to reach beyond the leading edge of the fetal presenting part, which is then elevated and brought out of the uterine incision. This should be done as gently as possible, without unnecessary panic and haste, so that no undue force is generated during the elevation and delivering of the fetal head. Attempts at delivery of the head without proper elevation and maintenance of head flexion can lead to undesirable uterine extensions. Landesman and Graber evaluated the use of abdomino-vaginal method in delivery of deeply engaged head and opined that with the decreasing use of rotational and mid-forceps delivery, this technique is very valuable in effecting safe childbirth in difficult labors[30]. Another technique of accomplishing delivery in such situations, which has found mention in literature, is to deliver the fetus as a breech. This is easier said than done and usually is reserved as a last resort when all other efforts fail. Before attempting to deliver as breech, one should always try to deliver by what has been described as the "Patwardhan's Maneuver". In fact, some surgeons use this technique as the first and the preferred method to deliver deeply engaged heads. This technique is difficult to learn and master but once learnt, has minimal complications. In this technique, after an adequate uterine incision is made, one of the fetal upper limbs is delivered and brought out of the incision. If the back is not already anterior, then the arm which is out of the incision is gently pulled so that the fetal back rotates anteriorly and the other fetal arm is now closer to the midline. The other arm is then delivered. Delivery of the fetal upper limb should be done skillfully; the axilla is hooked, the arm is followed down upto the forearm, the hand is held and brought out over the chest thus maintaining flexion all through at all joints. At this instance, both the upper limbs now lie outside the uterine cavity with the back anterior. The operating surgeon, with both the hands, now holds the fetal trunk and applies gentle traction so that successive parts of the fetal trunk, buttocks and the lower limbs are delivered. An important technical detail that should be borne in mind is the holding of the fetal trunk; it should be held firmly yet no compression of the fetal abdomen should be caused. The fetal trunk should be held so that the thumbs of both hands of the operating surgeon are parallel to the fetal spine and gentle traction should be applied downwards which invariably results in delivery of successive fetal parts. After the fetal trunk and lower limbs have been delivered, the head is then pulled out, and suction of nose and oropharynx is done.

Fasubaa et al conducted a randomized controlled trial of two techniques of baby deliveries for impacted head at cesarean section: the push and the pull method. Patients in the push group had statistically significant higher rates of maternal morbidity (longer operation time, more blood loss, extension of uterine incision, endometritis, longer hospital stay and higher hospital bills) than the pull method ($P < 0.05$). Also the fetal morbidity was worse in the push group. They concluded that the 'pull' method of delivery of impacted fetal head at cesarean section for obstruction is safer and faster than the 'push' method[31].

In all the above techniques described, it would be advantageous to use a uterine relaxant for accomplishing baby delivery. Glyceryl trinitrate has been tried for use during cesarean deliveries and has no significant maternal or fetal side effects. Its use was studied in a randomized controlled trial at elective cesarean section, and the authors concluded that although it did not have significant benefit at an elective cesarean section, it might be worth trying in difficult deliveries[32]. Also, as aforementioned, if during the above maneuvers, any further difficulty is encountered, a planned extension of the uterine incision is made in a J-shaped or U-shaped manner to effect delivery. This increases the postoperative morbidity of the surgery but is advantageous than having inadvertent, uncontrolled extensions[25].

Other cephalic presentations at cesarean delivery may be face or brow presentations. Again the same principle described above applies: head flexion, elevation and delivery through the uterine incision. Flexing the head in brow presentations might at times be difficult but should be accomplished before an attempt to deliver the head through the uterine incision is made.

Breech presentation is a common indication for cesarean birth. More recently, after the publications of the results of the Term breech trial, an increasing number of clinicians find themselves more inclined towards cesarean delivery when faced with a breech presentation at term. However, it should be kept in mind that as in vaginal breech delivery, improper conduct of breech delivery at cesarean birth increases the perinatal morbidity with the unfortunate result that the whole purpose of performing a cesarean delivery is defeated. Therefore, even during performance of a cesarean delivery for breech presentation, proper technique should be used. The technique is the same as that for vaginal delivery, using slow and steady traction, and avoiding unwarranted haste and speed. In case of a flexed breech, one or both feet are grasped and gently pulled out of the incision. In case of an extended breech, gentle groin traction can achieve the same. Delivery of shoulders should be conducted one followed by the other, as in vaginal breech delivery. The position of the back should be maintained anterior. The aftercoming head should be delivered with considerable caution, as head entrapment can occur with improper conduct of delivery. The assistant should maintain fundal pressure and the operating surgeon can use one of the two methods: Mauriceau-Smellie-Veit or Burn-Marshall. Alternatively, Piper's or a long Simpson's forceps can also be used for delivery of the aftercoming head. Locksmith et al. published an interesting article on the usefulness of Laufe-Piper forceps during cesarean delivery in breech presenting fetuses. During this study, they also evaluated its value in teaching residents, the use of forceps in after coming head of breech. They concluded that Laufe-Piper forceps can be used for cesarean delivery of breech-presenting infants. This practice also promotes confidence and skill for their use at vaginal delivery[33].

If the fetus presents in a transverse lie, it is advisable to try version prior to making the decision for cesarean delivery[34]. In such cases when version is not possible or when membranes have ruptured or worse, in cases of neglected shoulder presentation, the only recourse is a cesarean delivery. During the cesarean delivery, one of the most important decisions is about making the uterine incision. This depends on the development of lower uterine segment. If the lower segment is narrow and not well formed, a low vertical incision should be considered as it can be extended upwards if necessary. Strong advocates of lower segment cesarean delivery usually advocate the making of a transverse incision, which, if necessary, is then extended on any one side as a J-shaped incision. Shoham et al studied the use of transverse incision for fetuses in transverse position during a cesarean section. They found no significant complications in the mother and fetus during the postoperative period and concluded that transverse uterine incision is safe for cesarean delivery of a transverse lying fetus[35].

A transverse incision is made in the lower segment and extended adequately on both sides. A hand is introduced in the uterine cavity and the lower limb is grasped and delivered out of the incision and the rest of the delivery is accomplished as a breech. It is not uncommon to find the hand closer to the incision than the foot and so a proper identification of the limb should be made prior to taking it out of the incision. If by error, the upper rather than the lower limb is brought out inadvertently, it should be reposited and the lower limb subsequently delivered. In some cases, however, especially with ruptured membranes, this is not possible and the hand invariably comes out and attempts to reposit the hand and deliver the lower limb fail. In these desperate situations, the uterine incision should be extended as a J-shaped incision, the hand brought out, followed by the lower limb of the same side. This should be followed by the a gentle pull on the lower limb already delivered and then the delivery of the second lower limb and the rest of the delivery can then be conducted as in breech. This technique should be reserved for the most desperate situations, which are unfortunately not uncommon in patients presenting with transverse lie.

Administration of a uterine relaxant should be considered in such patients prior to baby delivery as this makes manipulations for delivery easier[32].

SUMMARY

- Induction delivery intervals of more than 8 minutes and incision delivery intervals of more than 3 minutes adversely affect Apgar scores and neonatal outcome.
- Maintain flexion during delivery of fetal head.
- Floating head can be delivered by conventional methods, vacuum or forceps. The latter increase the U-D interval.
- Deeply engaged head can be delivered by abdomino-vaginal method, modified Patwardhan's method or rarely by breech. Patwardhan's maneuver needs expertise but has minimal complications if skillfully performed.
- Fetuses in breech presentation at cesarean delivery should be delivered with the same care and caution as at a vaginal delivery.

PLACENTAL DELIVERY

Following the delivery of the fetus, purpose of performing a cesarean birth is accomplished but the surgery is far from over. The next important step in the surgical childbirth is delivery of the placenta. Placenta can be manually removed or may be allowed to spontaneously expel.

Both these techniques are equally popular but not equally rewarding. There are several studies, which have shown that when the placenta is manually removed at a cesarean birth, there is increase in the amount of blood loss compared to when spontaneous expulsion is allowed[36,37,38]. Also, it was noticed that the incidence of postoperative infections was higher in the manually delivered group compared to the spontaneous delivery group[38]. In a systematic Cochrane review, Wilkinson and Enkins concluded that manual removal of placenta may do more harm than good by increasing maternal blood loss and increasing the risk of infection[39]. This is because manual shearing of placenta does not allow time for retraction of the myometrial fibres and therefore leads to increased blood loss. It is therefore more prudent to allow spontaneous expulsion of the placenta during cesarean birth. While the placenta still expels, the uterine angles can be sutured, thus saving intraoperative time. This will lead to a decrease in the amount of intraoperative hemorrhage and a consequent decrease in operative morbidity.

At a cesarean delivery the mean time required for spontaneous placental delivery is 3-4 minutes. Should it take longer, no hesitation should be shown in attempting manual removal, as one of the causes of delayed separation in such cases can be morbid adherence of placenta.

In a randomized controlled trial, Atkinson and colleagues showed that the incidence of postoperative endometritis is also increased in those patients who undergo manual removal compared to those who experienced spontaneous expulsion[40]. This has been studied in various trials and one of the plausible explanations was that after manual removal, the uterus is not well retracted and contracted, so the chances of bacterial inoculation deep into decidua and myometrium are higher. A policy of glove change after baby delivery was compared with no glove change in a randomized controlled trial and it was realized that change of gloves did not alter the incidence of postoperative endometritis[40].

At this point, it is worth noting that some surgeons use a gauze sponge after placental delivery to explore the uterine cavity to check for retained placental bits. This practice of doing mop curettage has not been adequately studied in trials but an exploration manually with fingers can also accomplish the same.

SUMMARY

- Spontaneous placental delivery should be preferred to manual removal of placenta as the former causes less blood loss and is associated with a decreased incidence of postoperative infections
- Glove change after delivery of the fetus is not associated with a reduced incidence of postoperative endometritis.

EXTERIORIZATION OF UTERUS VERSES IN-SITU REPAIR

Following the delivery of placenta, the actual repair of the uterine incision is begun. There is however, one important technical detail that needs to be considered before actual suturing of the uterine incision is begun. For suturing of the uterine incision, there is an option of where the uterus should be placed i.e. whether it should be brought out of the incision for suturing or it should be sutured in-situ.

The technique of manually bringing the uterus out of the abdominal incision for ease of suturing is called exteriorization. In this technique, the uterus is manually brought out of the abdominal incision, covered with a moistened laparotomy pack and the uterine incision is inspected for any obvious bleeding points. The uterine angles are held with either Green Armytage clamps or with Allis forceps and the suturing of the uterine incision is started. Exteriorization of the uterus through the uterine incision has several advantages[41]. It allows for the manual uterine massage, observation of uterine tone, the Mathew Duncan folds, and allows for routine examination of the adenexa. It also allows for easy performance of tubal ligations if they need to be concurrently performed with a cesarean delivery. At the same time, exteriorization of the uterus allows for better visualization of the bleeding points in the lower segment, especially, when there is an associated extension of the uterine incision. The ease of suturing, manual massage and traction on the uterus have been shown to cause a decrease in the amount of intraoperative bleeding[41]. There are, however certain demerits associated with exteriorization of the uterus. Manual removal of the uterus out of the uterine incision leads to peritoneal irritation resulting in pain, nausea and vomiting[7]. This is especially true when there is an associated inadequate regional anesthesia. Secondly, there was a reported increased incidence of venous air embolism when uterus was exteriorized[42]. The possible explanation for this fact is that when the uterus is exteriorized, it raises the uterus to a level higher than the heart. This coupled with traction, which enlarges the uterine sinuses, increases the hydrostatic gradient, thereby promoting the air embolism[43].

In situ repair of the uterus is technically slightly difficult, especially for trainees, but is without the above demerits. There is no increase in the amount of blood loss, no difficulty in examining the adenexa or in performing tubal ligations; as all that is required to perform the tubal ligation is a gentle tilt of the uterus in situ. At the same time, there is no unnecessary traction on the uterus and no associated peritoneal irritation. It is also less likely that venous air embolism occurs when uterus is repaired in situ[43].

Several studies have compared these two techniques as regards intraoperative blood loss, postoperative wound sepsis, pyrexia, blood transfusion and length of hospital stay. In a recent study, Edi-Osagie et al studied the influence of exteriorization and in-situ repair on cesarean section morbidity. They concluded that there are no clinically significant differences between uterine exteriorization and in situ repair as regards pulse rate, mean arterial pressure, oxygen saturation and hemoglobin concentrations. The also found that the incidence of vomiting and pain was similar[44]. In another randomized controlled trial, Wahab et al studied the surgical and anesthetic benefits and problems associated with exteriorization of uterus at cesarean delivery. They concluded that with effective anesthesia, exteriorization of uterus was not associated with significant problems and is associated with less blood loss[45].

In a systematic Cochrane review, Wilkinson and Enkins evaluated four prospective trials of exteriorization of the uterus to repair the uterine wound and found that, there was insufficient data to permit definite conclusions about exteriorization[46].

It should be remembered strict adherence to a particular technique at all times is not advisable. Modifications in surgical technique exist so that they cause minimal morbidity in different surgical situations and scenarios. The clinical implication is that the surgical procedure and technique should be individualized according to the clinical findings and demands of the surgery. Therefore, surgeons comfortable with in-situ repair should not hesitate to exteriorize the uterus should there be an extension of the uterine incision.

SUMMARY

- Uterine exteriorization at cesarean section allows for ease of suturing, manual uterine massage, observation of uterine tone, and allows for routine examination of the adenexa. It also allows for easy performance of tubal ligations.
- There is a slight increased incidence of vomiting, nausea, peritoneal irritation and in some cases possibly a venous air embolism associated with exteriorization but these adverse effects are not seen with improved anesthetic techniques.
- In-situ repair, in experienced hands, does not cause increased blood loss, and is without any technical complications.

UTERINE CLOSURE

The uterus is a very important tissue for repair during the cesarean birth as it has a bearing not only on the immediate postoperative period but also on subsequent gestations.

Before proceeding with the actual repair of the uterine incision, meticulous attention should be paid to inspecting the margins of the incision. As an initial step, the angles of the uterine incision are identified and held with Allis forceps or Green Armytage clamps. Application of these clamps controls bleeding and identifies the lateral limit of the uterine incision. Beginning at one angle, the upper margin is then followed upto the other angle and in the same way, the lower margin of the incision is followed from one to the other angle. Especially along the lower margin, bleeding points are noted and if needed held with additional clamps. The lower margin of the incision should be carefully inspected as in some situations it might escape notice resulting in faulty repair of the uterine incision. Also, if the lower margin of the incision is not bleeding, it should not be held with more than one clamp as it unnecessarily clusters the operative field with instruments. After such a careful inspection of the uterine incision, it is advisable to proceed with suturing of the incision.

Reapproximation of the uterine incision can be done in either two layers or one layer. Closure in two layers has been the conventional and anachronistic way of suturing the uterine incision. A brief mention of the some historical aspects at this point would highlight certain pertinent facts. Munro Kerr for the first time introduced the lower uterine transverse incision in 1926[23]. Prior to this time, uterine incisions were either upper segment vertical or lower segment vertical. Upto the late 1800s, mortality of the cesarean birth was very high, mainly due to infection and hemorrhage. In

1882, Sanger recommended that all uterine incisions should be sutured immediately after delivery[47]. This procedure immediately reduced the operative mortality of a previously fatal operation. From then on, all upper segment vertical incisions (because they were the only incisions in vogue) were sutured in two layers. The suturing of uterine incisions was done in two layers even after the introduction of the lower segment vertical incision by Krönig in 1912[48]. The lower segment vertical incision frequently extended into the upper segment and indeed required two layers to close. But this was to change after the introduction of lower segment transverse incisions in 1926[23]. The practice of suturing the lower uterine transverse incision in two layers was borrowed directly from the initial vertical incision closure. This two-layered closure continued to be a standard part of surgical technique and was widely used by one and all.

It was for the first time in 1976 that Pritchard and MacDonald noted that satisfactory approximation of the edges of the uterine incision can also be obtained with a single layer closure[49]. Subsequently, the single layered closure was tried by many other surgeons, was found to be satisfactory and thus became popular.

At the same time, vaginal birth after cesarean delivery was also gaining popularity, and in this background, it was suggested that a two-layered closure of the uterine incision is associated with a decrease in the incidence of scar rupture in subsequent gestation. This however, is not entirely accurate. The behavior of a uterine scar in the subsequent gestation depends on many factors viz. the extent of extension of the uterine incision, the myometrial apposition achieved at uterine closure, the suture material used for uterine closure, the occurrence of postoperative infections and wound complications.

The basis for use of a single layered closure in approximation of the uterine incision is that it achieves hemostasis in a lesser operative time. At the same time the amount of foreign material introduced, in form of suture, is lesser[3]. Hauth et al randomized 906 women and compared methods of suturing the uterine incision. They concluded that the outcome of a one-layer closure was similar to that of a two-layer closure except that the operative time was significantly shorter and fewer additional hemostatic sutures were required. They also showed that a double layered closure in no way was superior to single layered closure as regards other outcomes e.g. hemostasis, and post operative endometritis[50]. Animal, histological and hysterographic studies, have demonstrated that a single layered closure provides the best anatomical result and the strongest scar[51]. Single layered closure has also been compared to the double-layered closure as far as risk of scar dehiscence in a subsequent trial of labor is considered. Franchi M et al analyzed the behavior of uterine scar after single and double layered suturing and found that there were no statistically significant differences[52]. In another study, the risk of scar dehiscence was evaluated after a single and double layered suturing, and it was concluded that asymptomatic ruptures were not higher in the single layered group[53]. Chapman et al studied the outcome of subsequent delivery in women with single and double layered suturing and concluded that there were no differences in the two groups in terms of maternal and fetal outcomes[54].

Wilkinson and Enkins in their systematic Cochrane review assessed the effects of a single layer closure of the uterine incision at cesarean section, in contrast to conventional two-layer closure. In one of the trials evaluated, single layer closure was associated with reduced operating time (5.6 minutes). In another trial evaluated, radiographic scar appearance showed fewer scar defects at three months with single layer group. There were no significant differences in the use of extra hemostatic sutures, incidence of endometritis, decrease in postoperative hematocrit or use of blood transfusion. They concluded that there are no advantages or disadvantages of a single layer closure, except a shorter operating time[55].

The uterus can be sutured in a single layer fashion without compromising the scar behavior in subsequent gestation. However, it should be kept in mind that each patient should be individualized and a particular technique should not be strictly adhered to. Should the need arise; the uterus may be sutured in additional layers for want of adequate hemostasis.

While performance of a double-layered technique, the first layer should be sutured with an absorbable suture in a continuous locking or a continuous running fashion. After the first layer is complete, a second continuous layer (Lambert or Cushing) is used to invert the first layer; the inverting stitch may be horizontal or vertical. Thereafter, the incision should be inspected again for bleeding points and hemostasis checked[7]. While a double layered closure is performed, the first layer can be closed in continuous running, continuous locking or interrupted fashion. The continuous running and interrupted stitches are used as some surgeons feel that use of a locking stitch increases the likelihood of tissue ischemia and therefore affecting wound healing. The interrupted stitches have the disadvantage of introducing more suture material into the wound, which elicits a more profound tissue reaction. Additionally, the use of interrupted stitches may not achieve satisfactory hemostasis, therefore requiring more tissue bites and more effort to achieve hemostasis.

A single layered closure is performed like the first layer of a double-layered closure. It is sutured with an absorbable material preferably in a continuous locking fashion. The continuous locking stitch should be used with caution, as it should be only adequately tightened to achieve hemostasis and myometrial apposition. An undue amount of traction on the suture material while taking the continuous locking stitch may actually cause tissue ischemia with resultant poor healing. Also, especially in those patients with an effaced lower segment, too much pull on the suture while taking locking stitches may cause the suture to cut through.

There has been some concern voiced about avoiding the incorporation of the decidua in the uterine suture line, as it might cause development of endometriosis at the scar site. Myometrial apposition is the aim but development of endometriosis at scar site due to incorporation of the decidua is a remote possibility[56].

The suturing of the uterine incision is usually done with chromic catgut but some surgeons also prefer to use delayed absorbable suture material e.g. vicryl for suturing the uterine incision. The latter is a sharp and braided suture material with increased tensile strength; while using it to suture the uterine incision too much traction or pull should not be exerted as it might cause a 'cheese wire' effect. Another important fact that is to be kept in mind while using vicryl for uterine closure is that, being delayed absorbable, it gets absorbed after a longer time compared to chromic catgut. This means that it elicits a prolonged tissue reaction at the scar site, which might have a bearing on the scar behavior in subsequent gestation. In a study conducted by Zuidema and colleagues, the outcome following suturing the uterine wound with either chromic catgut and vicryl was studied. They reviewed subsequent outcomes in 537 women in whom 237 had chromic closure and 302 had vicryl closure. Subsequent scar separation was increased almost four fold in the vicryl group (4.6% vs. 1.2%)[57].

While suturing the uterine incision with chromic catgut, the suture sometimes breaks, especially at the angles, resulting in the need for additional sutures. The breaks in the suture material may not be due to the fault with the chromic material but may be due to two important reasons; if the suture material used is not fresh or if the surgeon uses an unusual amount of force while using chromic catgut. Both these situations should be avoided. The delayed absorbable material meets the surgeon, as a tough suture material. This particular strength of the suture appeals to the surgeon and mentally reinforces his/her strength while uterine suturing. The uterus is sutured, and the hemostasis controlled but the suture stays there for a longer time than it is required, thus eliciting a prolonged tissue reaction and more fibrosis, which might compromise the strength of scar in future pregnancies.

The suturing of the uterine incision is done for achieving hemostasis during the surgery and as the uterus is a muscular tissue, with a good vascular supply, it heals rapidly. Therefore, having a suture material with delayed absorption characteristics, as is required for fascial closure, may not be required. This needs to be evaluated in properly conducted trials.

SUMMARY

- Uterine incision should be meticulously inspected for bleeding points and extensions prior to suturing.
- Only the bleeding points should be held and unnecessary clustering of operative field with instruments should be avoided.
- A double-layered closure is not superior to single layered closure as regards hemostasis & postoperative endometritis and requires more operative time.
- Single layered suturing does not lead to an increased risk of scar dehiscence in a subsequent gestation.
- Individualize each patient and whenever deemed necessary, a second layer may be taken.

PERITONEAL CLOSURE

After the uterine incision is closed, two important structures meet the surgeon: the visceral peritoneum and the parietal peritoneum. Conventionally, these structures were closed with chromic catgut, until recently, when non-closure was advocated and found to be effective and better. There are, however, many surgeons, who remain vehemently against the technique of non-closure.

Non-closure of the peritoneum has been compared with peritoneal closure in numerous trials and the conclusion has unequivocally been in favor of non-closure[58,59,60,61,62,63]. This is because non-closure is associated with decreased operative time[58,60,61,62,63], a decreased postoperative morbidity[62,63,64] and a decreased requirement of postoperative analgesia[59,62,63]. At the same time, there is quicker return of bowel activity after cesarean delivery if the peritoneal surfaces are not closed[59,65]. Also, there is a decreased adhesion formation if the peritoneal surfaces are not closed[65,66,67,68]. The merits of peritoneal non-closure are numerous and it is beneficial to the patient in the immediate and late postoperative period if the peritoneal surfaces are not closed.

For clearly understanding the debate between peritoneal closure and non-closure, an understanding of the basis for closure and non-closure is essential. Ever since, Sanger advocated in 1882 that all uterine incisions should be closed following delivery[47], the practice of suturing all structures incised was a part of surgical practice. Since then, closure of all layers of abdomen, which have been incised, became a part of traditional surgical training. In the early times, when surgical techniques were not as improvised as today, when infections were strife, and when effective antibiotics were not available, the closure of abdominal wall layers provided considerable benefit. As medicine advanced, more effective antibiotics were available and postoperative surgical infections were increasingly less common. At the same time there was an improvement in techniques of surgical practice. All this progress dramatically changed the vista of surgical practice. A lot of surgical techniques were modified and several alternative techniques were suggested. One such technique was peritoneal non-closure. The succeeding paragraphs discuss the scientific basis of peritoneal healing for an insight into logic of peritoneal non-closure.

Peritoneum is a mesothelial tissue. It develops from the celomic epithelium and differs in many ways from the other differentiated tissues. One of the main differences is the pattern of healing. Healing in the epidermal tissue begins from the wound borders and advances gradually towards the center. In contrast, to the epidermal tissue, peritoneum begins healing simultaneously throughout the wound[69]. Healing of the peritoneal surfaces occurs by mesothelialization, in which small islands of mesothelial cells are formed throughout the wound, which grow gradually towards each other and ultimately bridge the gap in the peritoneal structure. This process of reperitonealisation begins to occur in 48-72 hours and is complete in 5 to 6 days[70,71].

Another important fact to be considered in regard to peritoneal healing is the amount of fibrosis and degree of adhesion formation after injury. Healing in any tissue occurs in conjunction with fibroblasts, which lay down fibrous tissue. The degree of fibrosis and adhesion formation in any healing tissue depends on two factors: the activity of fibroblasts and the ability of the healing tissue to lyse excessive fibrin, which is formed as a process of repair. The lysis of excessive fibrin in peritoneal healing is due to release of fibrinolysin from incised peritoneal surfaces. Deperitoniealised surfaces, which have otherwise not been traumatized, heal without permanent adhesion formation[66]. Based on this above information, the closure and non-closure of peritoneum are now reviewed.

Closure of peritoneum with absorbable chromic catgut introduces foreign material into the wound site. Introduction of foreign material into the healing sites promotes fibrosis during wound healing. The normal peritoneal surfaces, which have been further traumatized by suturing, lose their ability to lyse fibrin. Not only do they lose this ability; they also inhibit fibrinolysis by normal tissue, leading to excessive fibrosis and adhesion formation[66]. Closure of the visceral peritoneum also advances the bladder and vesico-uterine fascia on the lower uterine segment. At the same time, closure leads to increase in the repair activity, thus contributing to delayed convalescence in the postoperative period. There is delayed return of bowel activity in those patients who have undergone peritoneal closure.

Non-closure on the other hand is more physiological, allows for a more natural repair, saves operating time, causes decreased postoperative pain, leads to a quicker return of bowel activity and is associated with decreased adhesion formation. And last but not the least, it is cost-effective[72,73].

SUMMARY

- Peritoneal non-closure is associated with a shorter operating time.
- Peritoneal non-closure is associated with a reduced need for a postoperative analgesia.
- Peritoneal non-closure is associated with a decreased postoperative morbidity.
- Peritoneal non-closure is associated with a quicker return of bowel activity.
- Peritoneal non-closure is associated with a decreased adhesion formation.

ABDOMINAL CLOSURE

After discussing the peritoneal closure / non-closure, the other structures which merit a surgeon's attention are the two muscle bellies of the recti, the rectus sheath, the subcutaneous tissue and the skin. All of these structures are important and should be appropriately dealt with during closure of the abdominal wall.

The muscle bellies of the recti should be inspected for any bleeding and any obvious points of bleeding should be ligated/cauterized. A special attention should be given to the undersurface of the muscle bellies, as inferior epigastric vessels situated there can be a source of bleeding. The muscle bellies of the recti may not be approximated during repair of the abdominal wall, as they heal otherwise also[7]. If the muscles are sutured, vigorous tight suturing along the entire length of the incision is not required. The muscle bellies should be gently approximated with one or two sutures to appose them. A very enthusiastic and tightly approximating closure of the rectus muscle bellies should not be done as it might cause tissue ischemia, which might impair and delay healing leading to a slower convalescence in the postoperative period.

The closure of the rectus sheath is the most important step in the closure of the abdominal wall. It is the most important structure of integrity, which protects against wound dehiscence. Proper closure and suturing of the rectus sheath is necessary for preventing abdominal wall dehiscence and it should be done with meticulous detail. A proper selection of the suture material is of paramount importance. The healing of the fascial tissue occurs in about 12 weeks and a return to near normal tensile strength occurs in a matter of 24-26 weeks. Therefore, the approximating suture should be of sufficient strength and should last most of that period. Therefore, it would be extremely improper to use chromic catgut for the repair[7]. If the incision is a vertical, closure of the incision in a monolayer fashion with non-absorbable suture is the correct technique. In transverse incisions, use of non-absorbable sutures provides the strong fascial support needed, however, delayed absorbable sutures can also be used. In those patients undergoing repeat cesarean delivery with transverse incisions, again a non-absorbable suture should be preferred, as the chances of a dehiscence are higher than patients undergoing a primary surgery. The obese patient is also at high risk for fascial dehiscence and suturing of the fascia should be done with meticulous concern.

Another important technical detail is the method chosen for facial repair. As the rectus sheath is the most important structure, which protects against occurrence of dehiscence, a method of suturing which reinforces the strength of the incision along the entire length of the incision should be preferred; therefore, fascial closure should be in interrupted fashion. Alternatively, if the continuous running or locking stitch is used, every third stitch should be reinforced with a cobbler knot. Amongst the running and the locking stitches, the former is preferable. Use of a continuous running or locking stitch without interspersed cobbler knots or interrupted stitches is not advisable as a break at one point can compromise the integrity of the whole fascial tissue.

The technique of facial closure should be accorded equal attention. The angles of the incision should be identified and should be secured individually. The knots should be tied beyond the angles and should be surgical knots. The healing of the rectus sheath is best if the stitches are spaced not more than 1 cm apart from each other and not less than 1 cm from the fascial edge. This is because collagenolysis occurs in the 1 cm zone near the facial edge[74].

A rare but important error, which might complicate the fascial repair, is improper identification of the edges of the rectus sheath. The Scarpa's fascia, which overlies the rectus sheath at times appears similar and might be mistaken for the fascial edge, which is in a deeper plane at slightly higher level. This should be kept in mind and consciously avoided.

There are several factors, which predispose to fascial dehiscence in the post-operative period and the technique of repair should not be one of them.

The subcutaneous tissue in the anterior abdominal wall below the umbilicus is divided into two layers: the superficial fatty layer-Camper's fascia and the deep membranous layer-Scarpa's fascia. The Camper's fascia continues into the thigh while the Scarpa's fascia ends at the inguinal ligament and is continuous with the fascia lata of the thigh. The superficial blood vessels and nerves run in the plane between these two layers of subcutaneous tissue. There have been no systematic studies relating to separate closures of Scarpa's fascia and Camper's fascia. But it seems prudent to suture the Scarpa's fascia, especially in patients at high risk for dehiscence, as it is a membranous fascial sheet, which might contribute to the integrity of the abdominal wall wound. It should be closed with absorbable sutures either in continuous running or in interrupted fashion.

The Camper's fascia is the superficial fatty layer in the subcutaneous tissue containing variable amount of adipose tissue. Closure of this layer has often been debated. Surgeons advocating closure and suturing of the Camper's fascia do so for following reason: closure of the potential dead space created in the subcutaneous tissue, thereby avoiding seroma/hematoma formation and subsequent infection. Formation of seroma/hematoma in the subcutaneous tissue planes along with a coexistent infection compromises wound healing and predisposes to wound dehiscence[3]. But it has been noted that non-closure of this layer, in non-obese patients, does not predispose to wound infection and wound dehiscence[7]. Del Valle et al conducted a randomized controlled trial to study the effect of closure and non-closure of subcutaneous tissue on wound disruption. The concluded that the incidence of would disruption was higher in the non-closure group. But, in their study they made no distinction between obese and non-obese groups[75].

It should be kept in mind that in the modified Joel-Cohen technique of Cesarean delivery, separation of subcutaneous tissue from the underlying fascia is not advocated so there is practically very little dead space created[11]. The superficial fascia is an adequately vascular structure, so healing is good provided no extensive tissue trauma is done. If the closure of the subcutaneous tissue is done, it should be done in interrupted fashion taking care not to tighten the knots so much so as to cause tissue ischemia.

The most important factor responsible for formation of seroma/hematoma is the depth of subcutaneous tissue. In those patients where the depth of subcutaneous tissue is more than 2 cms, closure is advisable as it also improves skin approximation. Cetin A and Cetin M studied the superficial wound disruption after cesarean section in their study and found that in women with a subcutaneous tissue thickness of 2 cms or more, the incidence of infections was higher in the non-closure group[76]. Alternatively, in patients with a thick subcutaneous tissue (2 cms or more), placement of a drain above the rectus sheath with a continuous suction is also advantageous and has been shown to reduce the incidence of wound complications[77]. The use of this drain however, in non-obese patients has no advantage.

Closure of the skin is the last step of the surgical childbirth. This part of the surgery is often not given its due merit with the result that assistants or trainee residents suture the skin more often than not. This does not mean that trainee residents or assistants should not suture the skin but should do so only after they have demonstrated the necessary skill to do so under supervision.

The importance accorded to the skin suturing techniques is due to necessary reasons. Transverse skin incisions are commonly performed in obstetrics and one of the major factors, which make them popular, is cosmesis. So, it should be the duty of the operating surgeon to use the best suturing techniques so that the skin scar formed is cosmetically superior.

There are three basic suturing techniques that can be employed while suturing the skin: the intracutaneous sutures, the percutaneous sutures, and the skin staples. A fourth technique, which strictly speaking is not a suturing technique but is used uncommonly for skin approximation – cyanoacrylate. The two most commonly used techniques are the percutaneous and the intracutaneous techniques (subcuticular stitch). No matter which technique is used, the results are more or less the same if suturing is done with the necessary care and effort. However, minor differences do exist.

In case of vertical incisions, percutaneous sutures give the same benefit as the intracutaneous suture. The width of the skin scar is however, less when intracutaneous sutures are used for suturing vertical skin incisions. Lindholt et al studied the cosmetic outcome of scar formation after cesarean section with percutaneous and intracutaneous sutures. They found that intracutaneous suture after lower midline incision produced scars 40% narrower than with percutaneous sutures, (6.8 versus 11.3 mm)[78]. The vertical skin scar is cosmetically inferior to the transverse incision, as the skin incision is across the lines of Langer.

Transverse incisions are made along the lines of Langer and healing takes place along these embryological segments, providing greater cosmetic benefit. In patients with transverse incisions, percutaneous and intracutaneous suturing techniques can give nearly the same result, especially if proper surgical technique has been used for suturing.

While using subcuticular stitch, there is a choice of suture materials and use of a particular suture type may make a difference in the final appearance of the skin suture. One of the most commonly used suture type for subcuticular suturing is the delayed absorbable variety, which causes good approximation of skin edges and does not require removal. Especially at the time of the discharge from the hospital, the skin suture is healthy, well approximated, dry and has a good cosmetic appeal. The same cosmetic appeal is generated amongst both, the surgeon and the patient, if the skin is sutured with subcuticular non-absorbable sutures. But a non-absorbable suture has to be removed at the first postoperative visit[3]. The non-absorbable suture has a little advantage over the delayed absorbable suture, as it evokes no tissue reaction. The delayed absorbable suture, by virtue of it being absorbable albeit in a delayed fashion, evokes a tissue reaction. The tissue reaction takes some days to phenotypically manifest itself, and a variable degree of induration/hyperpigmentation is visible at the scar site, depending on the patient's tendency for scar formation. This is not seen with non-absorbable sutures as they evoke no tissue reaction and are removed within the first two weeks following the cesarean delivery. The non-absorbable suture serves the purpose of skin approximation in the initial phase of healing, after which it is removed, thus, allowing the skin to heal in the most natural way.

Skin staples have also been tried for skin suturing and have been studied in randomized clinical trials. It has been seen that subcuticular sutures are associated with less pain post operatively and were more cosmetically more attractive to the surgeon and the patient alike[79].

Cyanoacrylate has been used to approximate the skin edges at the cesarean delivery and its use has been compared to nylon and silk in a case controlled study. The authors found that the use of cyanoacrylate on the cesarean wounds closure showed: efficiency, safety and surgical time reduction, the scar aesthetics was improved and costs were reduced[80]. This however needs more evaluation.

Alderdice F et al analyzed the techniques and materials for skin closure in a systematic Cochrane review. They concluded that there is no conclusive evidence about how the skin should be closed after cesarean section. Questions regarding the best closure technique and material and the outcomes associated with each remain unanswered. The appearance and strength of the scar following cesarean section is important to women and the choice of technique and materials should be made by women in consultation with their obstetrician based on the limited information currently available[81].

SUMMARY

- Muscle bellies do not need to be sutured. If they are sutured, gentle apposition should be done and tight suturing should be avoided.
- Most important structure of integrity in abdominal wall is rectus sheath.
- It should always be closed in interrupted stitches. If continuous sutures are used, a cobbler knot should be at every third row.
- Vertical incisions are at best closed with monolayer suturing.
- Chromic catgut should not be used for suturing rectus sheath. Delayed absorbable or at best non-absorbable sutures should be used.
- Rectus sheath should be sutured so that stitches are 1 cms form the edge and 1 cms from each other.
- Non closure of the subcutaneous tissue in non-obese patient does no harm. It should, however be closed in women with a subcutaneous tissue of 2 cms or more in depth.
- Skin closure should be done with meticulous care.
- An effort should be made to hone skills in skin suturing techniques, so as to provide maximum cosmetic benefits to the patient.
- Cosmetic considerations should be kept in mind while suturing the skin incision, whether vertical/ transverse.
- Transverse skin incisions are cosmetically superior to vertical incisions.
- Both subcuticular and percutaneous closure techniques in transverse incisions give good results but subcuticular sutures, especially with non-absorbable sutures, may give an added cosmetic superiority.

REFERENCES

1. Stirrat G. The place of cesarean section. Contemporary Reviews in Obstetrics Gynecology 1998; 10: 177-183.
2. Cotzias C & Fisk N. Patient demand for cesarean section. In. Lieberman BA, Shaw RW, Sutton CI & Thomas EJ (eds) Advances in Obstetrics and Gynecology, pp9-16. Oxford: The Medicine Group. 1999.
3. Hema KR, Johanson R. Techniques of performing cesarean section. In. Drife J, Walker J. Best Practice & Research, Clinical Obstetrics and Gynecology, 2001; 15(1):17-47.
4. Ellis H, Coleridge-Smith PD, Joyce AD: Abdominal incisions – Vertical or transverse? Postgrad Med J 60; 407, 1984.
5. Greenail MJ, Evans M, Pollack AV: Midline or transverse laparotomy? A random controlled clinical trial. Br J Surg 67;188, 1980.

6. Becquemin J-P, Piquet J, Becquemin M-H et al: Pulmonary function after transverse or midline incision in patients with obstructive pulmonary disease. Int Care Med 11:247. 1985.

7. Depp R. Cesarean delivery and other surgical procedures. In. Gabbe SG, Niebyl JR, Simpson JL. (eds) Obstetrics: Normal and Abnormal Pregnancies; pp 635-692. 4th ed. Churchil Livingstone, 2002.

8. Sippo WC, Burghardt A & Gomez AC. Nerve entrapment after Pfannenstiel incision. Am J Obstet Gynecol 1987;157: 420-421.

9. Maylard AE: Direction of abdominal incisions. Br Med J 2:895, 1907.

10. Rayburn WF & Swartz WJ. Refinements in performing Cesarean delivery. Gynecol & Obstet Surg 1996;51: 445-451.

11. Stark M & Finkel A. Comparison between the Joel-Cohen and Pfannenstiel incision in Cesarean section. European Journal of Obstetrics, Gynecology and Reproductive Biology 1994; 53:121-122.

12. Holmgren G, Sjoholm L & Stark M. The Misgav Ladach method for Cesarean section: method description. Acta Obstet Gynecol Scand 1999; 78: 615-621.

13. Darj E & Nordstrom ML. The Misgav Ladach method for Cesarean section compared to Pfannenstiel method. Acta Obstet Gynecol Scand 1999; 78 : 37-41.

14. Finan MA, Mastrogiannis DS & Spellacy WM. The Allis test for Cesarean Delivery. Am J of Obstet Gynecol 1991;164: 772-775.

15. Pitkin RM: Abdominal hysterectomy in obese women. Surg Gynecol Obstet 142: 532. 1976.

16. Magann EF, Chauhan SP, et al. Intraoperative hemorrhage by blunt verses sharp expansion of the uterine incision at cesarean delivery: a randomized clinical trial. Br J of Obstet Gynecol 2002; 109(4):448-452.

17. Rodriguez Al, Porter KB, O'Brien WF. Blunt versus sharp expansion of uterine incision in low-segment transverse cesarean section. Am J of Obstet Gynecol 1994;171(4):1022-1025.

18. Villeneuve MG, Khalife S, Marcoux SA & Blanchet P. Surgical staples in Cesarean section: a randomized controlled trial. Am J of Obstet Gynecol 1990;163: 1646

19. Wilkinson C & Enkins MW. Absorbable staples for uterine incision at cesarean section (Cochrane review). In The Cochrane Library, Issue 2. Oxford: Update Software, 2000.

20. Schutterman EB & Grimes DA. Comparative safety of the low transverse versus the low vertical uterine incision for cesarean delivery of breech infants. Obstet Gynecol. 1983 May;61(5):593-7.

21. Shipp TD, Zelop CM, Repke JT, Cohen A, Caughey AB, Lieberman E. Intrapartum uterine rupture and dehiscence in patients with prior lower uterine segment vertical and transverse incisions. Obstet Gynecol. 1999; 94: 735-40.

22. Martin JN Jr, Perry KG Jr, Roberts WE, Meydrech EF. The case for trial of labor in the patient with a prior low-segment vertical cesarean incision. Am J Obstet Gynecol. 1997 Jul; 177:144-8.

23. Kerr JMM. The technic of cesarean section, with special reference to the lower uterine segment incision. Am J of Obstet Gynecol 1926; 12: 729.

24. Bethune M and Permezel M. The relationship between gestational age and the incidence of classical cesarean section. Aus & New Zea J of Obstet Gynecol 1997; 37: 153-155.

25. Boyle JG & Gabbe SG. T and J vertical extensions in low transverse cesarean births. Obstet Gynecol 1996; 87:238-243.

26. Datta S, Ostheimer GW, Weiss JB et al. Neonatal effect of prolonged anesthetic induction for cesarean section. Obstet Gynecol 1981; 58: 331-335.

27. Warenski JC. A technique to facilitate delivery of the high-floating head at cesarean section. Am J Obstet Gynecol. 1981;139(6):625-627

28. Pelosi MA & Apuzzio.J. Use of the soft, silicone obstetric vacuum cup for delivery of the fetal head at cesarean section. J of Repro Med 1984;29: 289-292.

29. Arad I, Linder N & Bercovici B. Vaccum extraction at cesarean section-neonatal outcome. Perinat Med 1986;14: 137-140.

30. Landesman R, Graber EA. Abdominovaginal delivery: modification of the cesarean section operation to facilitate delivery of the impacted head. Am J Obstet Gynecol. 1984;148(6):707-10.

31. Fasubaa OB, Ezechi OC, Orji EO, Ogunniyi SO, Akindele ST, Loto OM, Okogbo FO. Delivery of the impacted head of the fetus at caesarean section after prolonged obstructed labour: a randomised comparative study of two methods. J Obstet Gynaecol. 2002 ;22(4):375-8.

32. David M, Halle H, Lichenegger W et al. Nitroglycerine to facilitate fetal extraction during cesarean delivery. Obstet Gynecol 1998; 91: 119-124.

33. Locksmith GJ, Gei AF, Rowe TF, Yeomans ER, Hankins GD. Teaching the Laufe-Piper forceps technique at cesarean delivery. J Reprod Med. 2002;47(8):693

34. Pelosi MA, Apuzzio J, Fricchione D, Gowda VV. The "intra-abdominal version technique" for delivery of transverse lie by low-segment cesarean section. Am J Obstet Gynecol. 1979;135(8):1009-11.

35. Shoham Z, Blickstein I, Zosmer A, Katz Z, Borenstein R. Transverse uterine incision for cesarean delivery of the transverse-lying fetus. Eur J Obstet Gynecol Reprod Biol. 1989 Aug;32(2):67-70.

36. McCurdy CM Jr, Magann EF, McCurdy CJ & Saltzman AK. The effect of placental management at Cesarean delivery on operative blood loss. Am J Obstet Gynecol 1992; 167: 1363-1367.

37. Magann EF, Dodson MK, Allbert JR et al. Blood loss at time of Cesarean section by method of placental removal and exteriorization versus in situ repair of the uterine incision. Int J Obstet Gynecol 1993; 43: 35-40.

38. Lasley DS, Eblen A, Yancey MK & Duff P. The effect of placental removal method on the incidence of postcesarean infections. Am J of Obstet Gynecol 1997; 176: 1250-1254.

39. Wilkinson C & Enkins MW. Manual removal of the placenta at cesarean seciton (Cochrane review). In The Cochrane Library, Issue 2. Oxford: Update Software, 2000.

40. Atkinson MW, Owen J, Wren A & Hauth JC. The effect of manual removal of the placenta on postcesarean endometritis. Obstet Gynecol 1996;87:99-102.

41. Hershey DW & Quilligan EJ. Extraabdominal exteriorization at cesarean section. Obstet Gynecol 1978; 52: 189.

42. Handler JS & Bromage PR. Venous air embolism during cesarean delivery. Regional Anesthesia 1990; 15: 170.

43. Lowenwrit IP, Chi DS & Handwerker SM. Nonfatal air embolism during cesarean section: a case report and review of literature. Obstet Gynecol Surv 1994; 49: 72-76.

44. Edi-Osagie ECO, Hopkins RE, Ogbo V et al. Uterine exteriorization at cesarean section: influence on maternal morbidity. Br J Obstet Gynecol 1998; 105: 1070-1078.

45. Wahab MA, Karantizis P, Eccersley PS et al. A randomized controlled study of uterine exteriorization and repair at cesarean section. Br J Obstet Gynecol 1999; 106: 913-916.

46. Wilkinson C & Enkins MW. Uterine extriorization versus intraperitoneal repair at cesarean section. (Cochrane review). In The Cochrane Library, Issue 2. Oxford: Update Software, 2000.

47. Eastman NJ. The role of frontier America in the development of cesarean section. Am J Obstet Gynecol 1932; 24: 919-929.

48. Kronig B. Transperitoneal Cervikaler Kaiserschnitt. In: Doderlein N, Kronig B eds. Operative gynakologie. 3rd ed. Leipzig G. Thieme, 1912; 879.

49. Pritchard JA, MacDonald PC. Cesarean section and Cesarean hysterectomy. In: Pritchard JA, MacDonald PC eds Williams obstetrics 15th ed. New York: Appleton-Century-Crofts, 1976: 903-923.

50. Hauth JC, Owen J & Davis RO. Transverse uterine incision closure: one versus two layers. Am J Obstet Gynecol 1992; 167: 1108-1111.

51. Jelsema R, Wittingen J & Vandenkolk K. Continuous, non locking, single layer repair of the low tranverse uterine incision. J of Repro Med 1993; 38: 393-396.

52. Franchi M, Ghezzi F, Balestreri D et al. A randomized clinical trial of two surgical techniques for cesarean section. Am J Perinat 1998; 15: 589-594.

53. Tucker JM, Hauth JC, Hodgkins P et al. Trial of labor after a one or two layer closure of a low transverse incision. Am J Obstet Gynecol 1993; 168: 545-546.

54. Chapman SJ, Owen J & Hauth JC. One versus two layer closure of a low transverse cesarean: the next pregnancy. Obstet Gynecol 1997; 89: 16-18.

55. Wilkinson C & Enkins MW. Single versus two layer suturing for closing the uterine incision at cesarean section (Cochrane review). In The Cochrane Library, Issue 1. Oxford: Update Software, 2003.

56. Chatterjee SK: Scar endometriosis: a clinocopathologic study of 17 cases. Obstet Gynecol 1980; 56: 81.

57. Zuidema L, Elderkin R, Cook C, Jelsema R: Is vicryl suture closure of uterine wounds associated with more dehiscence. Am J Obstet Gynecol 1996;174: 357.

58. Pietrantoni M, Parsons MT, O'Brien WF et al. Peritoneal closure or non-closure at cesarean. Obstet Gynecol 1991; 77: 293-296.

59. Hull DB & Varner MW. A randomized study of closure of peritoneum at cesarean delivery. Obstet Gynecol 1991.; 77: 818-820.

60. Luzuy F, Irion O & Beguin F. Non-closure of the visceral and parietal layers of peritoneum at cesarean section: a randomized controlled trial. Br J Obstet Gynecol 1996; 103: 690-694.

61. Ho WP, NorAzlin M, Patrick C et al. Peritoneal closure at cesarean section. FIGO 1997. Acta Obstet Gynecol Scand 1997; 76:30.

62. Nagele F, Karas H, Spitzer D & Staudach A. Closure or nonclosure of the visceral peritoneum at cesarean delivery. Am J Obstet Gynecol 1996; 174: 1366-1370.

63. Irion O, Luzuy F & Beguin F. Non-closure of the visceral and parietal peritoneum at cesarean section: a randomized controlled trial. Br J Obstet Gynecol 1996; 103: 690-694.

64. Grundsell HS, Rizk DEE & Kumar RM. Randomized study of non-closure of peritoneum in lower segment cesarean section. Acta Obstet Gynecol Scand 1998;77: 110-115.

65. McNally OM, Curtain AC. Does closure of the peritoneum during caesarean section influence postoperative morbidity and subsequent bladder adhesion formation? J Obstet Gynaecol 1997;17:239–41.

66. Buckman RF Jr, Buckman PD, Hufnagel HV, Gervin AS. A physiological basis for the adhesion-free healing of deperitonealized surfaces. J Surg Res 1976;21:67–76.

67. Stark M, Chavkin Y, Kupfersztain C, Guedj P, Finkel AR. Evaluation of combinations of procedures in cesarean section. Int J Obstet Gynecol 1995;48:273–6.

68. Joura EA, Nather A, Husslein P. Non-closure of peritoneum and adhesions: the repeat cesarean section. Acta Obstet Gynecol Scand 2001;80:286.

69. Duffy DM, diZerega GS. Is peritoneal closure necessary? Obstet Gynecol Surv 1994;49:817–22.

70. Elkins TE, Stovall TG, Warren J, Ling FW, Meyer NL. A histologic evaluation of peritoneal injury and repair: implications for adhesion formation. Obstet Gynecol 1987;70:225–8.

71. Hubbard TB, Khan MZ, Carag VR, Albites VE, Hricko GM. The pathology of peritoneal repair: its relation to the formation of adhesions. Ann Surg 1967;165:908–16.

72. Pietrantoni M, Parsons MT, O'Brien WF, Collins E, Knuppel RA, Spellacy WN. Peritoneal closure or non-closure at cesarean. Obstet Gynecol 1991;77:293–6.

73. Grundsell HS, Rizk DEE, Kumar RM. Randomized study of non-closure of peritoneum in lower segment cesarean section. Acta Obstet Gynecol Scand 1998;77:110–15.

74. Rayburn WF & Schwartz WJ. Refinements in performing a cesarean delivery. Obstet Gynecol Surv 1996; 51: 445-451.

75. Del Valle GO, Combs P, Qualls C & Curet LB. Does closure of camper fascia reduce the incidence of post cesarean superficial wound disruption? Obstet Gynecol 1992; 80: 1013-1016.

76. Cetin A & Cetin M. Superficial wound disruption after Cesarean delivery: effect of the depth and closure of subcutaneous tissue. Int J Obstet Gynecol 1997; 57: 17-21.

77. Ranaboldo CJ & Rowe-Jones DC. Closure of Laparatomy wounds: Skin staples versus sutures. Br J Surg 1992; 79: 1172-1173.

78. Lindholt JS, Moller-Christensen T, Steele RE. The cosmetic outcome of the scar formation after cesarean section: percutaneous or intracutaneous suture? Acta Obstet Gynecol Scand. 1994 Nov;73(10):832-5.

79. Frishman GN, Schwartz T & Hogan JW. Closure of Pfannenstiel skin incisions. Staples vs subcuticular suture. J Repr Med 1997; 42: 627-630.

80. Gorozpe-Calvillo JI, Gonzalez-Villamil J, Santoyo-Haro S & Casteneda-Vivar JJ. Closure of the skin with cyanoacrylate in cesarean section. Ginecol Obstet Mex. 1999 Oct;67:491-496.

Alderdice F, McKenna D, Dornan J Techniques and materials for skin closure in caesarean section (Cochrane Review) In: The Cochrane Library, Issue 3. Oxford: Update Software, 2003.

7 | CHAPTER

Difficulties and Complications During Cesarean Delivery

Reena Wani, Pallavi Naik

FRAMEWORK

- Introduction
- Difficulties in cesarean deliveries
  - Choice of indication
  - Choice of anesthesia
  - Difficult abdominal access
  - Difficulties with uterine incision & closure
  - Difficult baby deliveries
  - Difficult placental deliveries
  - Difficulties in controlling hemorrhage
  - Difficult abdominal closures
  - Difficulties in tubal ligations
- Complications in cesarean deliveries
  - Maternal mortality
  - Maternal morbidity
  - Complications of anesthesia
  - Intraoperative complications
  - Early postoperative complications
  - Late postoperative complications
- Conclusion

INTRODUCTION

"It must be acknowledged that all errors of practice do not proceed from ignorance of the act. Some of them may justly be imputed to our entertaining too much confidence in our own dexterity, or too little dependence on the natural efforts and resources of the constitution..."
-Thomas Denman (1795)

Cesarean section (C.S.) is one of the most commonly performed operations worldwide. Should this undisputed fact be taken as a testament to the safety and acceptability of this procedure? Although it is true that mortality related to Cesarean birth has reduced dramatically over the past decade, to practically negligible numbers, there is still a definite morbidity associated with this surgical procedure. While the world has been facing an epidemic of rising C.S. rates over the past few decades, good clinical practice requires us to exhibit our judgment, based as far as possible on evidence-based medicine to decide when the C.S. operation is necessary.

DIFFICULTIES IN CESAREAN SECTION

CHOICE OF INDICATION

Pregnancy and childbirth are basically physiological process and as obstetricians, our goal is to see that the outcome is a healthy mother and a healthy baby. It has often been said that the journey undertaken by the fetus through the mother's birth canal is probably the most dangerous one it will embark on for a long time. Hence, while it is true that a trial of vaginal birth is sometimes more hazardous than an elective Cesarean, this cannot justify offering Cesarean as a matter of choice without a valid indication.

A review of indications for cesarean delivery in the U.S.A. in 1985 and 1994 found that dystocia was the leading indication for cesarean delivery in both years. While CS for dystocia and breech increased, those attributable to fetal distress did not change significantly, and elective repeat cesarean declined[1].

A Meta analysis of published literature found that active management of labor is associated with a 34% decrease in the rate of CS for dystocia in nullipara[2].

Cesarean section for fetal indications are being performed more commonly such as for breech, selected cases of prematurity, multiple pregnancies and others. Special discretion is required when choosing route of delivery of infants with congenital anomalies. The choice of vaginal versus abdominal delivery must be based on knowledge of the nature of the individual malformation in question, the presence or absence of associated fetal malformation, karyotype abnormalities, fetal presentation and maturity. Clear evidence of benefit to the fetus is not available for many malformations that are considered for CS. However, certain malformations that produce sufficient enlargement of fetal structures are at possible risk of dystocia, such as severe hydrops, severe hydrocephalus or large sacrococcygeal teratoma. These may benefit from abdominal delivery[3].

In some women, childbirth can be a very painful experience, often associated with feelings of being out of control. Most women recover quickly post partum, others appear to have a more difficult time. Reynolds suggests that a variant of post-traumatic stress disorder (PTSD) which he calls "Traumatic birth experience", may occur after childbirth. Seeking of elective CS for psychological reasons exemplifies the avoidance behavior typical of PTSD[4]. Women seeking elective CS for such or other psychological reasons need special evaluation and counseling by the health care provider.

On the other hand, one may find resistance to CS as a mode of delivery particularly for fetal indications, more so in the Indian scenario. This is because some women perceive having an abdominal delivery to be a failure in the natural process of childbirth. Proper counseling and communication is often the key to resolve such situations.

CHOICE OF ANESTHESIA

The success of any endeavor depends on teamwork and this is true for operative deliveries too. Regional anesthesia, appropriate monitoring and risk awareness markedly reduce risks and complications related to anesthesia. More and more patients also question their obstetricians regarding anesthetic options prior to surgery. However, regional anesthesia (spinal or epidural) may not be suitable for all cases, and an absolute contraindication is an unwilling patient who doesn't wish to have regional anesthesia. When general anesthesia is opted for, a rapid anesthetic induction and intubation utilizing continuous cricoid pressure (Sellick's maneuver) is mandatory. However, fear of aspiration should not lead to persistent intubation attempts without intervening mask ventilation during difficult intubations. Regional anesthesia or awake intubation offers an alternative to rapid sequence induction for patients with known or suspected difficult airways[5].

DIFFICULT ABDOMINAL ACCESS

Changing trends in surgical techniques over past few decades have seen a shift from vertical midline incisions to transverse incisions for most gynecological and obstetrics laparotomies. For C.S deliveries, a transverse incision remains the choice for most obstetricians. This could be either

- Pfannensteil incision
- Joel-Cohen incision (modified)
- Maylard type

The choice of incision should be made after considering the need for haste, fetal size and presentations and previous operations. For situations in which rapid delivery and maximum exposure are required, the vertical midline skin incision might be still the best choice[6].

Current literature suggests that the skin incision and entry into the abdominal cavity is best achieved by the modified Joel-Cohen's incision[7].

In emergency situations in which the surgeon has underestimated the need for operative exposure Pfannensteil incision may be converted to the Maylard incision by incising the rectus muscles. In fact if thick scars or dense adhesions are suspected or known to exist, a muscle cutting incision may be a better primary choice if a transverse incision is to be used or else a vertical midline incision to be taken. Meticulous hemostasis is mandatory as subfascial hematomas may follow large amounts of tissue disruption. A subfascial drain may provide some prophylaxis against a hematoma[6].

Personal experience mandates the mention of special situations like severe preeclampsia or eclampsia with unknown coagulation status or HELLP syndrome (hemolysis, elevated liver enzymes and low platelets) where special precaution is required to guard against rectus muscle hematomas.

Another challenging situation is when there are two or more previous abdominal scars, of which one is vertical and the other is transverse. Which should be the chosen route of entry, keeping in mind that most operators prefer to excise the previous abdominal scar while opening the abdomen? The decision should be based on type of previous surgery and suspected adhesions, and need for adnexal evaluation such as for a concomitant tubal ligation. If both prior surgeries have been cesareans, we prefer to take transverse incision as it usually gives adequate exposure, direct access to the lower uterine segment and has a lesser risk of post-operative wound disruption. However, special care is required while entering the peritoneal cavity to avoid bladder or bowel injury. As far as possible, peritoneum should be opened as high up as possible, after confirming by palpation and by three-artery forceps method that there is no underlying viscus.

DIFFICULTIES WITH UTERINE INCISION AND CLOSURE

The primary requirement of the uterine incision is that it should be adequate to deliver the fetus in an atraumatic manner[6]. This is particularly true when the CS is being done for a "fetal" indication in the belief that abdominal delivery offers the fetus benefit over vaginal birth. The lower segment transverse incision has stood the test of time over a period of 75 years and remains the best way to enter the uterus[8]. However variations in technique exists as described below:

1) Incision with scalpel till membranes bulge/rupture and then extension of incision transversely using bandage scissors, curved slightly upwards. The desired length of incision is achieved under direct vision and inadvertent extension downwards or into the uterine vessels is less. However, possibility of fetal injury exists, particularly if amniotic fluid has been depleted, and due to cutting of muscle fibres, blood loss maybe more.
2) Digital tearing of the lower uterine segment after initial incision: There may be a tendency to create a downwardly concave incision[9] on finding the incision inadequate for smooth fetal delivery.
3) Misgav Ladach method: Uterus is opened with an index finger and the hole enlarged between the index finger of one hand and the thumb of the other.

Lower segment vertical incision may be preferable where difficult baby delivery is anticipated. The advantages are that extension into uterine vessel does not occur and the incision can be extended upwards if additional space is needed, particularly in a poorly formed lower uterine segment. The potential disadvantages include possibility of downward extension into bladder and cervix. If the extension of the incision into the corpus is required, it may disqualify the patient from trial of vaginal birth in subsequent pregnancy[9].

However a large study by Shipp et al compared the rate of rupture in 377 women with low vertical incision and 2912 women with low transverse incisions. The rate of rupture was similar in the two groups, 0.8% for low vertical versus 1 % for low transverse incisions[10].

Classical cesarean section, namely a vertical incision on the upper uterine segment may be required in very selected cases of multiple previous surgery, densely adherent bladder, anterior placenta praevia, leiomyomata on lower segment or a cervical carcinoma. The maternal and perinatal morbidity is higher than inverted T cesarean and much higher than low transverse cesarean as found by a recent Meta analysis of 19-year review of perinatal database from 1980-1998[11].

Inverted T incision : Sometimes an operator is faced with a situation where a transverse lower segment incision proves to be inadequate for fetal delivery, and an extension of the incision is needed. In such situations, it has been suggested that a J-shaped extension upwards with scissors might be a better option than converting to an inverted T incision. However, the Meta analysis by Patterson et al[11] of 19,726 deliveries found that the rates of lower transverse cesarean and classic cesareans have remained stable at 98.5% &1.11% respectively. However, the rate of inverted T cesarean rose from 0.2% in 1980 to 0.9% in 1988. They have also found that there is no increase in maternal or perinatal morbidity if an attempted low transverse incision has to be converted into an inverted "T" incision compared to performing a classic cesarean section.

Closure of transverse lower segment uterine incision can be safely done as a single layer without compromising future pregnancy outcomes[6, 8] with further hemostatic sutures taken as required. However both inverted T & classical incision requires meticulous closure usually in 3 layers.

Vaginal entry when planned is known as laproelytrotomy. This usually happens when inadvertently due to placing the incision too low; often following prolonged labor when the cervix is fully dilated. Repair of a vaginal incision and the bleeding that frequently is associated with it must be tackled carefully, since the uterus and bladder are at higher risk than they would be with a properly placed incision[6].

DIFFICULT BABY DELIVERIES

One of the major advantages of CS delivery is the fact that the fetal journey through the birth canal is eliminated and a controlled baby delivery under direct vision is accomplished. This more true when fetal considerations such as abnormal lie or presentation, or dystotic labor are the indications for operative deliveries. Paradoxically, these are the situations in which the delivery of the baby may not be as easy as it seems and a difficult or traumatic abdominal delivery would defeat the very purpose for which the CS was being performed.

The key to avoiding problems is anticipation. One must know when to expect trouble, and plan the anesthesia, abdominal entry and uterine incision keeping all the factors in mind. Certain situations in which such difficulties may arise, and ways to negotiate this has been discussed below:

A) Extracting fetus: Cephalic presentation

As far as possible after an adequate incision, the fetal head is delivered by flexion, maintaining occipito-anterior position. The exact procedure is operator dependent but the possible ways include

- Using a right hand inserted below the head as a "Shoehorn" and levering out the head.

- Using a combination of both hands, disimpact the fetal head from the pelvis. Then with the help of fundal pressure, delivery is accomplished.
- Instrumentation: this is not a very popular approach, however various techniques include:
  1. Murless head extractor
  2. Short obstetric forceps applied through the uterine incision
  3. One forceps blade used to lever out the fetal head.

B) Extracting fetus: Floating head

A high floating head often presents difficulties that may result in extension of the uterine wound or delay in delivering the infant. Any of the above maneuvers described above may be utilized. Other special technical details include:

- Rotation of chin or occiput to the front as possible, and application of forceps.
- Kielland forceps application in the classic fashion was described by Warenski[12] with traction on the fetal head as occipito transverse, then rotation to occipito anterior position and delivery by extension.
- Vacuum extractor has been suggested by certain authors[13]
- Historically certain procedures were mentioned which are now obsolete.
  - Use of Bonney's uterine compressor, and Willets scalp traction forceps.
  - Grasping the foot, performing a version and a breech extraction.

C) Extracting Fetus: deeply impacted head

Attempts to deliver a presenting part that is wedged deeply in the pelvis may result in extension of the incision or, may be difficult unless proper measures have been taken. Possible options include :

- Deepen the plane of anesthesia; achieve uterine relaxation if the presenting part is being gripped tightly.
- Head-low position may help to disimpact the fetal head from the pelvis, along with upward pressure on the fetal shoulder by the operator.
- While the operator's hand is inserted to lever out the head, pressure by an assistant on the fetal shoulder and an attempt to bring the chin anterior can be made. This may be followed by the use of one or both blades of obstetrics forceps to deliver the fetal head.
- An assistant using suitable aseptic precautions may push the fetal head upward from the vagina. If this is planned it may be advisable to drape the patient in a low lithotomy or frog position and prepare the abdomen and perineum, so this "Push" method can be used to elevate the presenting part at the level of uterine incision[6].
- If the arm or shoulder has been extruded from the uterine incision and other methods cannot or have not worked extraction may be achieved by any of the following[14]
  - Patwardhan's maneuver: One arm, opposite arm, trunk, one leg, other leg, and finally the head are delivered in succession.

- Modified Patwardhan's maneuver: One arm, the same side legs, buttock, opposite leg, opposite arm and lastly the head are delivered in succession.

- Low vertical incision may be taken especially if there is a prolonged labor with suspected constriction ring.

Obstructed labor is still a common obstetric complication in rural areas of our country and in parts of the developing world. A study of 108 women with obstructed labor at term with live fetus undergoing CS was conducted in Nigeria[15]. This randomized study compared the morbidity associated with two methods of delivery of the impacted head-the push method and the pull (reverse breech) method. They found that the pull method of delivery was faster and safer than pushing the fetus up from below.

D) Malpresentations: Breech

CS for breech seems to be the rule nowadays, with very few women or obstetricians opting for vaginal breech delivery. However, certain issues need to be considered such as timing of CS to avoid iatrogenic prematurity. Especially with an elective CS, unformed lower uterine segment may be encountered. This is also frequently seen in preterm breech, and in cases with associated prelabor rupture of membranes.

It would be wise to remember that the maneuvers to deliver a breech baby are similar whether vaginal or abdominal birth is chosen. The major difference is, of course, that the options to facilitate delivery such as anesthesia, widening the uterine incision are under the operators control at CS. Yet trapping of the fetal head is possible at CS, particularly in premature breech, or with inadequate uterine or abdominal incisions.

Faulty technique in breech delivery has often led to many breech babies being "done to death"[16]. This includes errors due to excitement or haste, failure to maintain the occiput anterior, pulling the trunk upward or undue pressure on fetal abdomen or pelvis.

Certain authors suggest that there are inherent factors with breech presentations with higher perinatal mortality (such as anomalies, preterm labor etc); hence despite doing CS one cannot eliminate all the other variables[17]. Routine use of CS may in fact be a factor in perpetuating inexperience, and lead to further difficulty when an unanticipated breech delivery is encountered.

The premature breech is more prone to injury, whether vaginally or abdominally delivered. In fact, for fetuses < 1500 gm weight there has been controversy regarding justification of CS routinely being chosen as mode of delivery[18]. The unformed lower segment is thick walled, narrow and retractile. Extraction of the trunk and arms may involve undesirable forcefulness and the after coming head may be trapped by the retracting uterus[19].

E) Malpresentations: Transverse Lie

CS for transverse lie may present difficulties in two situations:

- Preterm labor with or without prelabor rupture of membranes: the lower uterine segment is poorly formed; the fetus is in an unfavorable position. Here it may be prudent to take a lower segment vertical incision, extending it upward if required.

- Neglected transverse lie: although less frequently seen in modern obstetrics, this is a dangerous situation. Possibility of inadvertent extension of the uterine incision exists and probability of atonic PPH is also more. One also has to watch for sepsis. At times an obstetric hysterectomy may be required for such problems. It is wise to advise the patient if CS has been for this indication, that future pregnancies must end in elective CS.

F) Multiple Pregnancies

With assisted reproductive technology, not only twins but high order multiple pregnancies are often being encountered. These may have malpresentations, placenta praevia, preterm labor or PROM associated with them and cesarean birth is often the chosen route of delivery.

Special precautions include:

- Adequate abdominal and uterine incisions
- Knowledge of placental site and location
- Experienced neonatologist at hand
- Double clamping of cord after delivery of first baby to avoid retrograde bleeding from placenta
- Prophylaxis for PPH

Depending on fetal lie and presentation, each baby is delivered as discussed in the section above.

DIFFICULT PLACENTAL DELIVERIES

At cesarean, placental delivery can be accomplished by manual removal of the placenta after creating plane of cleavage, as was often done in the past. However, current opinion suggests that placental delivery should be by controlled cord traction after spontaneous expulsion[8]. This is not only associated with less blood loss, but also with lesser risk of post-cesarean endometritis. A randomized study of 760 women found manual extraction of placenta to be associated with higher risk of endometritis, but that intra-operative glove change did not decrease post-cesarean endometritis[20].

The placenta being normally located on the upper uterine segment, in the days of classic CS, it was encountered in 40% cases. However with lower segment incisions this is fortunately not the case. However a low-lying placenta or previa have certain special problems.

Placenta Praevia has always been associated with higher maternal and fetal morbidity and mortality. This is true till today, in fact, elective CS for placenta previa is not a surgery which can be assigned to less experienced residents, and consultant involvement is advisable.

When the placenta is low lying, the placental bed tends to bleed more as it is located on the less contractile lower uterine segment. More so, the plane of cleavage between placenta and uterine wall may not be well defined and there may be large dilated tortuous vessels present.

Even though known placenta previa may be present, a lower segment uterine incision is still preferred. Special precaution may be required with an anterior placenta previa, in which case the options are taking a low vertical uterine incision, or underrunning large vessels with ligatures before incising. The final decision of course needs to be taken on the operating table. Regarding baby delivery in such situations, the options include:

- Incising or pushing through the placenta: associated with more bleeding, possibility of fetal exsanguination too.
- Slipping the fingers between placenta and uterine wall, rupturing the membranes and delivering the baby. This is often preferable but may take more time and the neonate may have low Apgar if delivery cannot be expedited.

Abnormal placentation such as a succenturiate lobe, or an unusually large placenta should not create any difficulty if the operator ensures the completeness of placenta and membranes on table before uterine closure. Mop curettage of the uterine cavity is also useful to remove remnants of membranes and placental tissue.

Adherent placenta due to abnormal trophoblastic invasion (placenta acreta, increta and percreta) has been increasing in recent years; through stastically it is still a rare complication. The increasing incidence is probably partly due to increasing rates[21] and also due to procedures interfering with normal decidua formation like curettage, myomectomy, and manual removal of placenta[22]. The risk of placenta previa was 0.26% in an unscarred uterus, increasing linearly to 10% in patients with four or more previous cesareans, in a study by Clark[23]. They found the clinical risk of accreta increased with the number of previous cesarean deliveries. If an adherent placenta is suspected in advance, particularly percreta, a multidisciplinary operative team should be kept ready and an adequate operative field exposure, intravenous access and availability of blood products is essential[21, 22].

However, when this is found (as is often the case) as an unexpected problem on table, the options include:

- Suitable uterine incision (low vertical or classical as appropriate) to avoid incising into an anterior placenta percreta.
- Obvious increta/percreta: attempts to remove the placenta should be avoided, uterus can be closed, oxytocics given, after ligating the cord close to placental attachment. Post-operative adjuvant chemotherapy with methotrexate can be given to increase rate of resumption of placental tissue[22].
- Hemorrhage occurring from partially separated placenta: resuscitative measures, bilateral uterine artery ligation, or if required bilateral hypogastric artery ligation may be helpful. However, in some cases expeditiously performing a cesarean hysterectomy may be a better option, sometimes even life saving.

DIFFICULTIES IN CONTROLLING HEMORRHAGE

Hemorrhage with the need for blood transfusion is one of the more common, and potentially serious complications of cesarean section.

Strategies to minimize intraoperative blood loss include:

1) Ensuring that the loose uterovesical peritoneal fold is picked up and incised, rather than the fascia over the uterine serosa (De Lee's fascia) as that leads to unnecessary blood loss[19].

2) Avoiding wide lateral dissection of the bladder to avoid damaging enlarged venous plexuses in the broad ligament.
3) Planning the uterine incision suitably
4) Careful delivery of the fetal head, to avoid extension of the uterine incision, which is often the commonest cause for bleeding at CS[24].
5) Preferring spontaneous expulsion of the placenta-which may reduce blood loss upto 300ml[25].
6) Prophylactic use of oxytocic drugs.
7) Clamping the cut edges of the uterine incision with hemostatic forceps such as four Green Armytage clamps-two for the angles, and two for the most vascular areas anteriorly and posteriorly.
8) Rapid closure of the uterine incision-a single closure is usually adequate, with interrupted hemostatic bites in addition if required. If angle bleeding is profuse, it may be better to take the angles separately[24]. If uterus was exteriorized prior to closure, it is mandatory to confirm hemostasis after repositing it.

Control of Intraoperative bleeding

A) Localized site:

Pressure by a sponge on holder or pack to isolate the bleeding site, and then deep interrupted sutures to ligate the bleeder usually suffice. It may be wiser to use no. 1 or 2 chromic catgut rather than delayed absorbable sutures to prevent cutting through or sawing of the bleeding area.

B) Uterine artery ligation:

Bilateral ligation of the uterine artery along with the veins (O'Leary's stitch) can be very effective in most cases. The surgeon should grasp and elevate the uterus, and pass no. 1 chromic catgut suture on a large atraumatic needle through the myometrium medial to the uterine vessels from anterior to posterior. The suture is then brought forward through the avascular area in the broad ligament, lateral to the artery and vein. The suture is below the level of the transverse uterine incision, bladder mobilization is not required and the ureters are not at risk[6].

C) Internal Iliac (Hypogastric) artery ligation:

This may be required in selected cases, and done bilaterally. It does not provide absolute hemostasis, but reduces pulse pressure in the vessels facilitating hemostasis. The procedure is more technically challenging, carries risk and may not be successful in all cases. Hence, it should be reserved for hemodynamically stable women of low parity who desire future reproductive capability[21, 24].

D) Hysterectomy

It is very occasionally required to control hemorrhage if other measures have failed. Certain clinical situations may mandate a decision to proceed directly with hysterectomy rather than try other measures like hypogastric artery ligation-such as bleeding placenta percreta, upper uterine segment rupture or hemodynamically unstable patient.

Certain technical points need to be kept in mind:

- It is often difficult to decide where the cervix ends and the vagina begins
- The laxity of tissues in pregnancy allows the uterus to be pulled up quite easily; an inadvertently low incision across the vagina may injure the uterus[19].
- The increased vascularity and tissue edema, although making dissection of planes easy is associated with more oozing hence achieving proper hemostasis is extremely important.
- Closing the vagina with interrupted sutures or leaving the central part open after taking both the angles carefully, may facilitate pelvic drainage and prevent post-operative pelvic collection.

E) B-Lynch procedure: (Fig. 7.1a and b)

It is a fundus compression suture that is placed at the time of laparotomy, after hysterotomy and delivery of the fetus. Bimanual uterine compression is tried first to see if bleeding can be controlled by compression. If it seems so, the suture is placed by using no. 2 chromic catgut on a heavy round body needle as shown in the diagram.

There are several case reports since the original publication of a series of 5 cases of severe PPH managed in this manner[21]. At CS, since there is already a hysterotomy incision, placing of this suture may be expeditious. This suture has an ease of application, and potential for conserving fertility but needs to be established by larger studies.

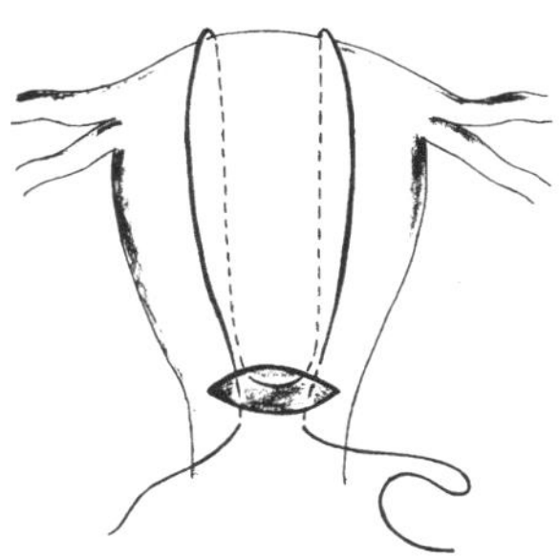

Fig. 7.1a. B-Lynch suture viewed from the anterior uterine surface

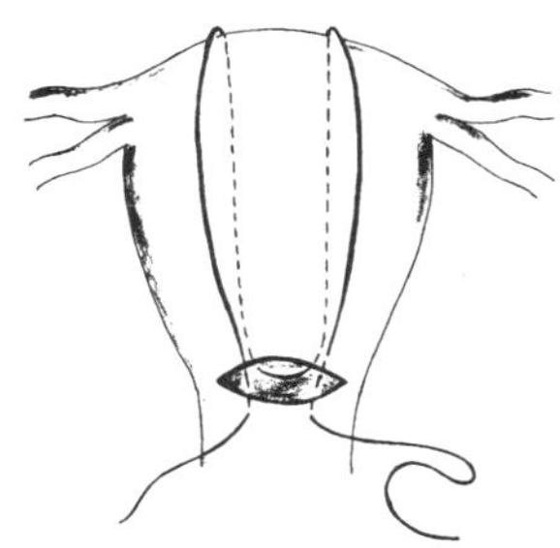

Fig. 7.1b. B-Lynch suture viewed from the posterior uterine surface

F) Pelvic Packing

In this troublesome event of bleeding despite hysterectomy, packs may be placed at the origin of the bleeding and brought the abdominal incision, to be removed 24-48 hours later. Logethetopolus umbrella pack has also been described to control such bleeding[6,21].

DIFFICULT ABDOMINAL CLOSURES

As discussed earlier, the abdominal incision may present with certain difficulties. Depending on the type of incision taken, or the additional problems encountered, certain problems may be faced :

a) Peritoneal closure: Closure of the visceral and parietal peritoneum no longer seems necessary[7,8,24].

b) Intraperitoneal drain placement: may be required rarely, such as in patients with HELLP syndrome, ascites due to severe pre eclampsia or other medical conditions. We prefer using a closed drainage system in such cases.

c) Rectus muscle bleeders: can be often troublesome and lead to a hematoma, hence should not be ignored. If cauterization does not stop the bleeding it is better to ligate or underrun the bleeder with chromic catgut.

d) Subcutaneous tissue: obliteration of space either by suture or by suction seems to reduce wound disruption[8]. Suction drains may be better for persistent oozing, but closure of camper fascia using 3-0 plain catgut or vicryl running suture has been shown to reduce the risk of hematoma formation[24].

e) Mass closure using Smeade-Jones technique: It has been recommended for patients at high risk of post-operative dehiscence[24]. If a vertical midline incision is used, it is one's preference to use no. 1 or 2-monofilament nylon in continuous non-locking suture for mass closure to have better outcome.

f) Skin closure: If a previous scar exists, in most situations it is advisable to take the repeat skin incision through it, or excising it. Removal of fibrosed tissue to have fresh bleeding edges will reduce the risk of post-operative wound disruption, even if subcuticular closure is opted for. We prefer to use interrupted sutures if the patient is obese, has medical risk factors, is immunocompromised or there is persistent oozing in subcutaneous tissue.

DIFFICULTIES WITH TUBAL LIGATIONS

Female sterilization is still one of the most popular methods of limiting family size. Particularly in women undergoing repeat cesarean section, certain issues may arise:

a) Decision on TL:

The patient should ideally be counseled and an informed consent for sterilization taken before onset of labor, in the antenatal period. However certain situations where the CS is being done for fetal indications (e.g. distress, IUGR, preterm breech) may make the decision difficult. In such situations a clear discussion about fetal prognosis should be undertaken, and in case of doubt it may be better to withhold doing the TL till later.

b) Accessing the tubes:

Usually is not difficult, but prior surgery or pelvic pathology may lead to dense adhesions where it may not be possible to access one or both tubes. In such cases, modification of standard Pomeroy technique, such as simple ligation of cornual end of tube may be possible. Any such departure from usual method or inability to perform the procedure on one or both the sides should be later explained to the patient and documented on the hospital record.

c) Hemostasis:

Occasional cases of broad ligament hematoma following slippage of a ligature of TL, or injury to venous plexuses have been described, but can be avoided by careful technique. It is wise to recheck the ligated cut ends after repositing the uterus if it was exteriorized prior to the TL.

COMPLICATIONS OF CESAREAN SECTION

Although CS is becoming increasingly safe, there are certain risks inherent to the anesthesia, surgical procedure and others, which cannot be disregarded.

Risk Factors for complications at CS have been identified[24]

a) Excessive speed - It is often wiser to take a couple of minutes extra rather than ignore or bypass certain surgical details, which can later lead to much more trouble.

b) Lack of Experience - Indisputably, practice makes one perfect at surgical technique, but in rural situations it is often lack of personnel that leads to serious problems. Even in developed health care settings like the NHS need for greater consultant involvement has been emphasized for improving obstetric outcomes.

c) Gestational age below 32 weeks - A higher association with malpresentations, PROM, placenta previa, poorly developed lower uterine segment and hazards of prematurity are contributory factors.

d) Low station of the vertex - such as a deeply engaged head following prolonged or obstructed labor, often leads to difficulty in fetal extraction.

e) Ruptured membranes preoperatively - often are associated with risk of endometritis, risk of fetal injury at the incision due to the uterus gripping the fetus and other associated factors.

MATERNAL MORTALITY

Hibband had reported that in 1789, there was not a single mother in the city of Paris who had survived a cesarean section in the previous 90 years. In modern times the mortality rate attributable to the operation is reported to range from zero to 59 per 100,000[5]. Studies show that CS delivery is associated with a 5-fold increase in maternal mortality compared with vaginal delivery, after the exclusion of severe antenatal complications and medical disorders. The ratio of risk corrected for the reasons for the CS are approximately 5:1 CS versus vaginal delivery, and 1.5:1 for emergency intrapartum versus elective CS[26]. Confidential enquiry into Maternal Deaths in the UK 1991-1993 found hypertensive disorders, pulmonary embolism, hemorrhage, sepsis and anesthesia to be the main causes of obstetric deaths. They also raised the issue whether increased mortality was related to unplanned CS delivery, and lack of senior obstetric input into many of the unplanned cesarean deliveries, which resulted in fatalities[24].

In India, with overall mortality rates still being unacceptably high, and an inequitable distribution of health care resources, it is even more difficult to quantitate maternal mortality attributable to CS itself, and that due to concomitant obstetric/medical factors or delay in appropriate antenatal planning and rigorous intrapartum care[27].

MATERNAL MORBIDITY

Although there is an undesirable mortality associated with CS, in most countries the actual death rates when seen prospectively are quite low[6,24,27]. Most intraoperative complications rarely lead to death, and are most often reflected as morbidity. In fact, many complications if recognized and managed appropriately may not even lead to morbidity. The subsequent discussion will highlight the various complications associated with cesarean, and are appropriate measures to be taken to prevent or treat these.

COMPLICATIONS OF ANESTHESIA

General Anesthesia:

The triennial maternal mortality reports from UK provide insight into the nature of anesthesia deaths, most being in cases with general anesthesia[5, 24]. Emergency CS increases the risk almost 4-fold, and appropriate anesthesia management would avoid the majority of these deaths[5].

a) *Mendelson's syndrome:* In 1946, Mendelson hypothesized Aspiration of acidic gastric contents to produce a pulmonary injury syndrome characterized by pulmonary edema and hypoxemia. Pregnancy increases the threat of aspiration.

   Various factors include[5]

   - Mechanical displacement of the gastro esophageal junction and pylorus by the gravid uterus delaying gastric emptying, and increasing gastric volume (more so after 34th week of gestation)
   - Elevated plasma progesterone and decrease plasma motilin leading to smooth muscle relaxation and slowed gastric motility.

   Prophylactic measures include

   - Histamine H_2 receptor antagonists such as cimetidine and ranitidine which increase the gastric pH-but need to be given at least 45 minutes prior so as to act.
   - Metoclopropamide, Ondanesteron to increase lower-esophageal sphincter tone and speed gastric emptying require 15 minutes
   - Sodium citrate, a non-particulate antacid is highly effective in increasing the gastric pH and should be used intrapartum or via endogastric tube
   - Prefer regional anesthesia whenever possible
   - Avoid head low position
   - Consider all parturients at high risk for aspiration and excercise caution.

b) *Difficult intubations*

   Airway difficulties such as esophageal intubation, failed intubation, or regurgitation and inhalation of stomach contents have been identified as factors in general anesthesia related deaths[5]

   Preventive measures :

   - Recognition of high risk or difficult intubations, including severe preeclampsia-eclampsia where cord edema may lead to problems.
   - Presence of senior or second experienced anesthesiologist whenever possible.
   - Use of rapid anesthetic induction and intubation.
   - Use of cricoid pressure (Sellick's maneuver) prior to loss of reflexes- it can prevent gastric regurgitation even with high gastric pressures.
   - Verification of accurate tracheal intubation by auscultation is not always full proof, and when available the carbon dioxide analyzer allows immediate verification of

proper endotracheal intubation, since the typical CO_2 waveform cannot be produced by esophageal intubation[5]

- Pulse oximetry warns of hypoxemia prior to the development of cyanosis.

c) *Fetal Problems:* Proper general anesthetic for CS should protect both mother and fetus. Longer general anesthetic induction to delivery times may adversely affect the neonate. Longer uterine incision to delivery times is also associated with neonatal depression. Measures to avoid fetal depression include:

- Maintenance of uterine perfusion.
- Uterine displacement (preferably to left) by wedge under back prevents vena caval obstruction.
- Increasing inspired maternal oxygen concentration improves neonatal oxygenation.
- Supplementation with low dose halogenated agents (halothane, isothane, enflurane) decreases maternal intraoperative recall while allowing increased inspired oxygen concentration, without depressing the newborn.

Regional Anesthesia

Choice of anesthesia ideally is to be made by consensus between obstetrician, parturient and the anesthetist but most prefer regional anesthesia as 100% oxygenation can be maintained, drugs crossing the placental barrier are avoided and infact epidural may already be in place for labor analgesia. However regional anesthesia also has its hazards :

a. *Hypotension :* Pregnancy by itself is associated with profound changes in peripheral resistance, blood volume and cardiac output. Supine hypotension is a known problem in advanced pregnancy. When regional blocks are used, special precautions need to be taken to avoid lowering the BP:

- Adequate prehydration (2 liters crystalloid)
- Left lateral tilt
- Avoidance of persistently low (< 80 mm of Hg) systolic BP to prevent fetal problems.
- Aggressive use of agents (such as IV ephedrine 5 to 10 mg) to restore BP as soon as it drops below the baseline, while additional fluids are administered.

b. *Local anesthetic toxicity* has been identified as a factor in regional anesthesia related deaths[5]. Seizures and cardiac arrest can follow accidental injection of local anesthetic into a distended epidural vein during epidural anesthesia. Fatal cardiac arrests are associated with bupivacaine more commonly.

c. *High spinal blocks* and fatal "total spinal blocks" are less frequent due to appreciation of reduced requirements for spinal and epidural local anesthetic drugs during pregnancy and precautions discussed above to avoid hypotension. However, spinal shock characterized by profound hypotension, respiratory distress, loss of consciousness and cardiac arrest can follow a mismanaged high block and is often preventable.

d. *Postoperative headache* or post-dural puncture headache may be seen following spinal or epidural anesthesia. It is thought to be due to continued cerebrospinal fluid leakage into the epidural space, and is always postural and dependent on needle size. Postoperative bed rest does not influence the incidence of post-dural puncture headache and most resolve spontaneously within 48 hours. Conservative measures include fluids, reassurance, analgesics and possibly an abdominal binder. Persistent headaches are treated with an epidural blood patch technique[5].

INTRAOPERATIVE COMPLICATIONS

1) Hemorrhage: Blood loss at CS averages 700-1000 ml[6,24] but transfusion is usually not required as majority of blood is derived from the placenta or uterus, which is rapidly decreasing in size. Although post partum hemorrhage (PPH) is traditionally defined as blood loss more than 500 ml, it is known that average blood loss during delivery progressively increases with the complexity of delivery mode[21]. Factors associated with hemorrhage (blood loss > 1.5 liters) at CS include[24]:
   - Placenta previa
   - Previous post partum hemorrhage
   - Obesity
   - Prolonged second stage of labor
   - Preeclampsia
   - General anesthesia
   - Amnionitis
   - Preterm cesarean section
   - Classical uterine incision
   - Anterior placenta previa, uterine scar (suspect possibility of accreta)
   - Combination of factors-increased risk
   - Intraoperative extension of uterine incision
   - Performance of CS by unsupervised trainees

   Strategies to minimize blood loss and to control hemorrhage have been discussed in detail in the previous section.

2) Extension of uterine incision : This is a frequent cause of hemorrhage, and can lead to serious complications.
   a) Low transverse incision
      - Lateral extension into uterine vessels can produce brisk hemorrhage, or lead to development of broad ligament hematoma if unrecognized.
      - Attempts to control hemorrhage may lead to ureteral damage (see below).
      - Downward extension into bladder may cause trigonal injury
      - Inadvertent vaginal incision leads to more bleeding, possible ureteral damage
   b) Other extensions: Extension into upper uterine segment, inadvertently or otherwise is associated with more bleeding, difficulty in suturing and increased operative time. Future pregnancies also should be terminated by CS birth only.

3) Urinary tract injury : Despite the close anatomical location, urinary tract injuries at CS are uncommon, with bladder damage being 0.3%, and ureteral injury < 0.1%[6,24].

a) Bladder injury
   - More common at repeat CS due to adhesions, fibrosis
   - The lower the risk of injury, the greater the risk of subsequent fistula
   - Most important is recognition during surgery, and if in doubt methylene blue instillation via perurethral catheter should be done.
   - Bladder is an organ that heals very well; a two-layered repair with 3-0 or 4-0 delayed absorbable suture will suffice.
   - Indwelling urinary catheter kept for longer time, till microscopic hematuria clears and prophylactic antibiotics will be enough to ensure complete recovery in most cases.

b) Ureteral injury
   - Rare, but may occur during attempts to control bleeding following lateral extension of transverse uterine extension, or an inadvertent vaginal incision in cases of prolonged labor.
   - Unlike the case with bladder injury, it is wise to involve urologist to evaluate suspected ureteral injury during surgery to minimize morbidity.
   - Indigo carmine testing, cystoscopy or cystostomy to visualise ureteral orifices may be required.

4) Bowel injury

Fortunately the gravid uterus displaces the bowel in such a manner that bowel injury is extremely rare. Prior surgery or pelvic inflammatory disease is an underlying factor in most cases where it occurs.

- Small bowel serosal damage may not require suturing. Deeper injuries can be repaired by suturing at right angles to the bowel axis in 2 layers, using 3-0 or 4-0 delayed absorbable suture for first layer. The second layer can be taken with the same suture or with 4-0 silk; of course, large lacerations or transection require resection-anastomosis.
- Colon injuries are even less common, and small tears can be over sewn as above. However more extensive damage may need a diverging colostomy.

5) Injuries of newborn

Atraumatic delivery is the goal of the obstetrician. When abdominal rate is chosen, it is often assumed that this will be the case. However, sometimes mechanical injury of the newborn may occur at the time of CS too. Possible causes of injury includes:

- Deep or uncontrolled uterine incision lacerating the fetal parts (scalp, ear in cephalic, buttock or thigh in podalic).
- Inappropriate or inadequate uterine incision trapping the fetal parts (discussed in section on uterine incisions)
- Haste or difficulty in fetal extraction (discussed under difficult baby deliveries)

Major injuries described in literature for CS births include[9]

- Head: laceration, skull fracture, dislocation of nasal cartilage

- Neck, Shoulder : fracture clavicle, unilateral brachial plexus injury, cervical vertebral dislocation
- Abdomen, Spine : liver hematoma, fractured spine
- Limbs : fractured tibia and radius, fractured femur.

Birth asphyxia is defined as a severe disturbance of oxygen supply to the fetus, which develops in the first or second stage of labor. To prevent hypoxic damage after an abrupt disruption of oxygen supply (e.g. Cord compression, abruptio placentae or rupture uterus) it is necessary to deliver the fetus within 15-20 mins of the acute event[33]. If the emergency CS takes longer than that, it may not be possible to prevent hypoxic damage.

6) Amniotic fluid embolism
Although an extremely rare entity, 80% maternal mortality associated with it makes it a dreaded complication. Risk factors such as tumultuous labor, medical disease, use of oxytocics may or may not be identifiable. Sudden onset of respiratory distress and circulatory collapse are often the first signs on table. This may subsequently be followed by onset of coagulopathy. Vigorous cardio-respiratory support, fluid and blood component therapy are the mainstay of treatment.

7) Unanticipated gynecological/surgical pathology
The abdomen has been described as a "Pandora's Box" and although one has opened it for delivering the fetus, other problems may be encountered:
    - Leiomyomas: may be found more often as the average age of pregnant women is rising and parity is declining. Resist the temptation to do a myomectomy as the increased size and vascularity in pregnancy invites trouble. Only small myomas in the line of incision, or pedunculated subserous tumors should be removed.
    - Ovarian tumors: with exteriorization of uterus, adnexal masses may be noticed but are rare. Majority of ovarian tumors in pregnancy are benign, with luteomas of pregnancy and theca lutein cysts being the most common and needing no treatment. Benign cystic teratomas or mucinous cysticteratomas or mucinous cystadenomas are next common and should be removed sparing ovarian tissue if possible[6,9]. Malignant ovarian tumors are rare, of which dysgerminomas is the most frequently reported in pregnancy. The treatment of these neoplasms should be as it would be in the non-pregnant state.

EARLY POSTOPERATIVE COMPLICATIONS

1) Reactionary Hemorrhage
As discussed earlier, bleeding is the most frequent complication noted in cesarean births. Risk factors and overall plan of management are as detailed in the previous section. However, reactionary hemorrhage is often seen, as a response to rise in blood pressure post operatively, especially if there was intraoperative hypotension. Sometimes after the effect of oxytocic agents has worn off, a patient prone to uterine atony may start bleeding in the postoperative ward. Slippage of ligatures or retraction of a large vessel is an uncommon cause, as the uterine musculature itself acts as a "living ligature" to control most bleeding, yet should be thought of if the patient is bleeding or has a rising abdominal girth with hypotension.

2) Retention of urine

Most operators prefer to use an indwelling Foley catheter till the patient is ambulatory, and hence urinary retention is less frequently seen. If not used, it is necessary to be vigilant as a full bladder may inhibit uterine contraction and predispose to PPH. Hot water bag, analgesics and early ambulation can take care of retention if it occurs.

3) Paralytic ileus

Excessive handling of the bowel is rare at CS, but infection or predisposing factors or electrolyte imbalance may lead to this complication.

4) Disseminated Intravascular Coagulation (DIC)

Known risk factors for coagulopathy are usually identifiable such as :

- Severe preeclampsia-eclampsia
- HELLP syndrome
- Retained dead fetus
- Prolonged obstructed labor
- Placenta praevia
- Abruptio placentae
- Amniotic fluid embolism
- Heritable coagulation disorders
- Massive blood transfusion

Depending on the etiological factors, specific treatment may be directed along with rigorous blood and component therapy.

5) Pulmonary Embolism

With changing trends in health, thromboembolism is an important cause of mortality and morbidity after cesarean. Unfortunately, upto 70% of those who suffer a fatal pulmonary embolism may exhibit no warning signs[24]. In the absence of risk factors, early mobilization and adequate hydration are enough for thromboprophylaxis. The RCOG Working Party (1995) has given guidelines for risk-assessment and type of thromboprophylaxis employed. Moderate risk factors include:

- Age > 35 years
- Weight > 80 Kg
- Para 4 or more
- Current infection
- Significant varicose veins
- Preeclampsia
- Immobility > 4 days
- Major illness
- Emergency CS in labor
- Post partum hemorrhage

They recommend use of heparin prophylaxis for 5 days if any of these factors is present either as

- Unfractionated heparin 5000 mg subcutaneously twice daily
- Enoxaparin 20 mg subcutaneously once daily

High-risk women (3 or more risk factors, hereditary hypercoagulable conditions) should receive heparin for 6 weeks[24].

6) Infection

In the past much debate has raged on infection prophylaxis, many trials conducted and reports published. However, many variables can alter the risk of infection. It is indisputable that postpartum endometritis is a frequent complication in women delivered by CS, with rates ranging from 5 to 85% depending on population studied[28]. Recognized risk factors for infectious morbidity[24,28]:

- Prolonged ruptured membranes
- Prolonged labor
- Emergency intrapartum surgery
- Multiple vaginal examinations
- Use of invasive monitoring like fetal scalp electrodes
- Bacterial vaginosis
- Maternal obesity (for wound infections in particular)
- Maternal disease (diabetes, pre eclampsia)

Types of infectious morbidity reported are:

- Endometritis
- Wound infection
- Urinary tract infection
- Febrile morbidity
- Pelvic parametritis, abscesses are rare.

Criteria to diagnose postpartum endometritis include:

- Oral body temperature above 101^{0}F/38^{0}F
- Tachycardia
- WBC count > 14,000 per mm^3
- Greater than 10% increase in immature polymorphonuclear leucocytosis
- Marked uterine tenderness

Infection Prophylaxis :

Cochrane overviews of over 69 randomized controlled trials of antibiotics given at the time of CS have shown a stastically significant reduction in postpartum morbidity and other serious morbidity, wound infection and other serious infection[24]. Hence, antibiotic prophylaxis is the norm for all CS, but no particular antibiotic has been shown to be superior to all the others. Optimal time of admission is at the time of bacterial contamination. A single IV dose after clamping the cord may suffice in low risk cases.

Other measures[8, 20,24]

- Meticulous hemostasis-prevents nidus of infection on blood clots
- Good surgical technique
- Preoperative skin preparation
- Clipping hair rather than shaving
- Avoid manual removal of placenta

- Close Camper's fascia
- Limiting number of people in theatre
- Reporting of cases
- Careful asepsis for cathetrization, early removal of catheters.

7) Abdominal wound problems
   Difficulties with closure are detailed in the previous section.
   Postoperative complication include:
   - Stitch hematomas
   - Stitch abscess
   - Cellulitis
   - Wound dehiscence
   - Burst abdomen

LATE POST OPERATIVE COMPLICATIONS

1) Rupture of uterus : Vaginal Birth after cesarean (VBAC) has been an important tool to control rising CS rates. However increases in the prevalence of uterine rupture are causing concern about morbidity and mortality in subsequent pregnancy after a CS[29, 30]. The bottom line is that compared with a patient with no previous uterine surgery, the pregnant patient with a scarred uterus is at significantly increased risk, regardless of the mode of delivery[30].

2) Need for repeat CS
   From a time when all patients with CS were advised repeat CS, to VBAC, now to trials of VBAC after two or more cesareans[29]; the pendulum is swinging back again. Some authors have expressed concern that aggressively trying to reduce the rate of cesarean delivery may lead to more complications for mothers and their babies[31]. Recent large studies demonstrate that elective CS appears safer than trial of scar or trial of breech delivery[27]. However it is proper examination and communication in each individual case, which will help to take the decision for future obstetric performance.

3) Intrauterine adhesions
   Endometritis, manual removal of placenta or accidental suturing of posterior wall can all lead to intrauterine adhesions. If very extensive, this may lead to Asherman's syndrome.

4) Periuterine infection
   Pelvic adhesions, tubal damage or even infertility may occur as a sequel of pelvic infection. Predisposing factors are excessive handling of adenexa, prolonged ruptured membranes and other factors leading to infections.

5) Fistulae
   Unrecognized or incompletely treated urinary tract or bowel injury may lead to fistulae formation, but this is very rare.

6) Psychological Sequelae
   In many parts of the developed world, a debate is being entertained whether a woman has a right to choose her mode of delivery[27]. Women requesting CS range from 4 to 38%

across the globe. For Indian women however vaginal delivery is still the preferred mode of delivery[32]. They consider it to be natural, non invasive, less costly, less morbid and an enriching experience. Hence, failure to accomplish vaginal delivery may have a negative impact on the woman's psyche. Conversely, a traumatic birthing experience may also lead to psychological stress[4].

7) Medicolegal Issues

Golden rules for avoiding malpractice litigation may be followed, but with a maloccurence you may still be sued[30]. Hence keeping good communication as the foundation, tricky situations like CS for congenital anomalies[3], or for premature breech[18] should be handled after weighing pros and cons with full disclosure to the would be parents.

CONCLUSION

As obstetricians, it is our endeavor to have a healthy mother and baby at the end of pregnancy. If CS is the better mode to achieve this, we may opt for it while keeping in mind the inherent risks and difficulties of it as a surgical procedure.

REFERENCES

1. Gregory KD, Curtin SC, Taffer SM, Notzon FC. Changes in indication for cesarean delivery: United States, 1985 and 1994. Am J Public Health, 88 (19) : 1384-7, 1998.
2. Glantz JC, Mc Nanley TJ. Active management of Labor : a meta- analysis of cesarean delivery rates for dystocia in nullipara. Obstet Gynecol Surv, 52 (8) :497-505,1997.
3. McCurdy CM Jr, Seeds JW. Route of delivery of infants with congenital sanomalies. Clin. Perinatal, 20(1) : 81-106, 1993.
4. Reynolds JI. Post-traumatic stress disorder after childbirth: the phenomenon of traumatic birth. CMAJ 156(6); 831-835,1997.
5. Hood DD. Anesthesia for Cesarean section: Minimizing risk and complications. In: Obstet Gynecol Clinics North America, Vol 15(4); 639-652,1988.
6. Rogers R.E./ Complications at Cesarean section. In; Obstet Gynecol clinics North America, Vol 15(4); 673-684,1988.
7. Holmgren G, Sj"oholm L, Stark M. The Misgav ladach methjod for cesarean section : method description. Acta Obstet Gynecol Scand, 78(7); 615-21,1999.
8. Hema KR, Johonson R. Techniques for performing Cesarean Section. Best Pract Res clin Obstet Gynecol, 15(1) ; 17-47,2001.
9. Stedman CM, Kline RC. Intraoperative complications and unexpected Pathology at the time of Cesarean Section. In: Obstet Gynecol Clinics North America, 15(4);745-766,1988.
10. Shipp TD, Zelop CM, Repke JT et al. Lieberman, Intrapartum uterine rupture and dehiscence in patients with previous lower uterine segment vertical and traverse incisions. Obstet Gynecol: 94; 735-740,1999.
11. Patterson LS, O'connell CM, Baskett TF. Maternal and Perinatal morbidity associated with classic and inverted T cesarean incisoions. Obstet Gynecol; 100(4); 633-637,2002.
12. Warenski JC. A technique to facilitate delivery of high floating head at cesarean section. Am J. Obstet Gyecol;139;625,1981.

13. DeClereq A: Technique to facilitate delivery of high floating head at cesarean section (letter). Am J. Obstet Gynecol 142;118,1982.
14. Wani R J. cesarean section. In Wani R J. essential Obstetrics, Bhalani Book Depot, Mumbai, 505-512, 1997.
15. Fasubaa OB, Ezechi OC, Orji EO, Ogunniyi SO, Akinedele ST, Loto OM, Okogbo FO. Delivery of the impacted head of the fetus at cesarean section after prolonged obstructed labor: a randomized comparison study of two methods.
16. Myerscough P.R. Breech presentation. In:Munro Kerr's Operative Obstetrics, 10th Edn. Balliere Tindall, London. 70-88, 1992.
17. Hytten FE. Breech presentation: Is it a bad omen? Br J Obstet Gynecol 89; 879;1982.
18. Anderson G, Strong C. the premature Breech: Cesarean Section or trial of labor? J Med Ethics; 14(1): 18-24, 1988.
19. Myerscough PR. Cesarean Section: Sterilization: Hystrectomy. In: Munro Kerr's Operative Obstetrics, 10th Edn, Balliere Tindall, London. 295-319,1992.
20. Atkinson MW, Owen J, Wren A, Hauth JC. The effect of manual removal of the placenta on post cesarean endometritis. Obstet Gynecol, 87(1); 99-102,1996.
21. Dildy 3 G.A. postpartum Hemorrhage: New management options. Clinical Obstet Gynecol, Vol 45(2); 330-343, 2002.
22. Dimri S, Mankha U, Sharma JB. Morbidly adherent placenta: A Serious Abnormal Placentation. Obst & Gnae, Vol7(2):69-71, 2002.
23. Clark SL, Koonings PP, Phelan JP. Placenta previa/accreta and prior cesarean section. Obstet Gynecol, 66,88-92,1985.
24. Murphy K.W. reducing the complications of cesarean section. In: Bonnar J.(ed). RA in Obstet Gynecol, Vol 20, Churchill Livingstone, Edinburgh, 141-152, 1998.
25. Mc Curdy CM, Magann EF, Mc Curdy CJ, Saltzman AK. The effect of placental management at cesarean delivery on operative blood loss. Am J Obstet Gynecol. 167;1363-1367, 1992.
26. Lilford RJ, Van Coeverden de Gnot HA, Moore PJ, Bingham P. The relative risks of cesarean section(intrapartum and elective) and vaginal delivery: a detailed analysis to exclude the effects of medical disorders and other acute pre-existing physiological disturbances. Br. J. Obstet Gynecol;97; 883-892,1990.
27. Paterson-Brown S. Elective Cesarean section- a woman's right to choose? In: Studd J(ed) Progress Obstet Gynecol Vol 14; 202-215, 2000.
28. Faro S. infectious disease relations to cesarean section. Obstet Gynecol Clinics N Am; 15(4); 685-694,1988.
29. Lieberman E. Risk factors for uterine rupture during a trial of labor after cesarean. Clinical Obstet Gynecol; 44(3); 609-621, 2001.
30. Flamm B. Vaginal birth after cesarean: Reducing medical and legal risks. Clinical Obstet Gynecol; 44(3); 622-629, 2001.
31. Sachs B, Kobelin C. the risks of lowering the cesarean delivery rate. New Engl. J Med;340(1), 54-57, 1999.
32. Vijayanath A, Deka D.Indian women's choice regarding elective cesarean section. J Obstet Gynecol Ind; 53(5); 458-460,2003.
33. Schneider H. [Birth asphyxia-an unsolved problem of perinatal medicine]. Z Geburtshilfe Neonatol; 205(6); 205-212,2001.

8 | CHAPTER

Vaginal Birth After Cesarean Delivery

Suchitra N. Pandit, Sejal Desai

FRAMEWORK

- Introduction
- Risk factors for uterine rupture during trial of labor after previous cesarean birth
  - Factors known at the outset of pregnancy
  - Current pregnancy characteristics
- Lower segment vs. classical scar
- Prerequisites for a trial of labor
- Management of a patient with a previous cesarean delivery
  - Antepartum management
  - Intrapartum management.
- Diagnosis of rupture of cesarean scar in labor
- ACOG Guidelines
- Reducing medical and legal risks
- Vaginal birth after cesarean section – a continuing controversy
- The future

INTRODUCTION

The advent of cesarean delivery was followed immediately by dilemmas in the management of the patient who had a history of a previous cesarean section. At that time the performance of a repeat cesarean section meant exposing the patient to a significant risk of losing her life. But on the other hand even a scarred uterus was believed to be a contraindication for labour out of fear of uterine rupture. This must have led Edwin B. Cragin to announce his famous statement in his address to the Eastern Medical Society of the city of New York on May 12, 1916.

"Once a cesarean, always a cesarean". The dictum was greeted with mixed responses worldwide. However, it is important to place Cragin's dictum in a historic context. It is noteworthy that this was an era, when all cesarean sections were performed using a classical incision on the uterus. Even then, the issue of vaginal birth after cesarean section was constantly investigated.

The introduction of the low transverse uterine incision by Kerr[1] in 1926 was the largest boost for the advocates of vaginal birth after cesarean in the early decades of 1900s. Case[2] explained that the 'Kerr' incision prevented peritonitis by limiting the seepage of infected material from the wound into the peritoneal cavity and thus lowered maternal mortality[2].

Initially for these increasing cesarean deliveries, the future pregnancies would nearly always be managed by repeat caesarean section. However Schmitz[3] reported 62 out of 448 women with a history of previous cesarean section, who underwent vaginal delivery at Lewis Memorial Maternity Hospital. Schmitz reasoned that if the risk of uterine rupture was 4% and the maternal mortality from rupture was 11% then the maternal mortality (0.44%) is less with trial of Labour than with a repeat cesarean section.

Whereas repeat cesarean section was the American method of choice, a trial of labour after a pervious cesarean section was common place in Europe in the mid 20th century. Merrill and Gibbs[4] reported from the University of Texas at San Antonio that subsequent vaginal delivery was safely accomplished in 83% of their patients with prior cesarean deliveries. This rekindled interest in VBAC (vaginal birth after cesarean delivery) at a time when only 2% of American women who had previously undergone cesarean section were attempting vaginal delivery.

Though the use of VBAC increased significantly, there have been several reports published that suggest that VBAC may be riskier than anticipated[5]. Such reports raised concern about the safety of VBAC and have contributed to heightened controversy.

RISK FACTORS FOR UTERINE RUPTURE DURING A TRIAL OF LABOUR AFTER CESAREAN DELIVERY

The ability of clinicians to provide a more individualized risk of uterine rupture based on each woman's characteristic could enhance the safety of a trial of labour after cesarean. There are certain specific factors associated with the risk of uterine rupture during a trial of labour after cesarean.

A. Factors known at the outset of pregnancy

1) Type of scar: The rate of uterine rupture with a low transverse incision has been estimated as 1% in contrast to a much higher value of 12% in the presence of a classical

scar[6]. Also in one of the largest study, Shipp et al[7] compared the rate of ruptures in women with low vertical incisions with those having low transverse incisions. The rate of rupture was found to be similar (0.8% among women with low vertical incisions compared with 1.0% among women with low transverse incision).

2) Number of previous cesareans: Studies examining the effect of the number of previous cesareans on risk of uterine rupture present conflicting results. But overall more than one previous scar does increase the risk of rupture. Miller et al[8] in a study of more than 12,000 women including 1586 women with two or more previous cesareans, reported a three fold higher risk of rupture than in women with more than one previous scar (1.8% v/s 0.6%). Thus there are substantial data suggesting that even two cesareans may be associated with a substantial increase in risk of rupture and hence number of scars should be considered when determining the potential risks of a trial of scar.

3) Previous vaginal deliveries: In a case control study examining uterine rupture by Leung et a[9] it was concluded that a previous vaginal delivery did protect against uterine rupture. While the odds ratio was 0.5, the difference was not statistically significant. The date are insufficient to draw definitive conclusions but the largest study to date found a significant protective effect of previous vaginal delivery in women with one previous cesarean and the suggestion of an effect in women with two previous scars.

4) Interdelivery interval : Shipp et al[10] hypothesized that a short interval between a cesarean section and subsequent trial of labour might increase the risk of uterine rupture because of inadequate time for healing. For women with an interdelivery interval of 18 months or less, the rate of uterine rupture was 2.3% compared with a rupture rate of 1.0% for women with longer interdelivery intervals.

5) Postpartum fever after cesarean section: It has been proposed that febrile morbidity at the time of a cesarean section might predispose to poor wound healing and fever after the previous cesarean is a contraindication to a trial of labour[6,11].

6) Maternal age: A single study conducted by Shipp et al[12] suggests that a maternal age older than 30 years may be associated with a higher risk for rupture.

7) Uterine anomalies: In a study by Ravasia et al[13] the rate of uterine rupture was 8% in women with known mullerian duct anomalies compared to 0.6% for women without these anomalies.

In our opinion, type of scar, number of previous cesarean sections and postoperative complications are the most important factors and these are further influenced by other factors.

B. Current Pregnancy Characteristics:

1) Macrosomia: It has been suggested that the risk of uterine rupture might increase with the infant birth weight because of the accompanying uterine distension[14]. A small

increase in risk is possible, but the presence of a macrosomic infant is not associated with a large increase in risk of uterine rupture.

2) Gestation beyond the estimated date of delivery: No significant increase in the risk of rupture has been reported for women delivering after their estimated date of delivery.

3) Thickness of the lower uterine segment: It has been proposed that ultrasound examination of the uterus might be a useful tool for identification of women at high risk for uterine rupture. In a study by Rozenberg et al[15] the risk of uterine rupture increased directly with the thinness of the lower uterine segment. The risk was 0% with a lower uterine segment more than 4.5mm, 0.6% with a lower uterine segment 3.6 to 4.5mm thick, 6.6% with a lower uterine segment 2.6 to 3.5mm thick and 9.8% with a lower uterine segment less than 2.5mm thick. Whether this could be used as a screening test for identification of candidates for trial of labour is still controversial. Clinical implications of whether a patient should be subjected to a repeat cesarean just because of a thin scar is controversial, but we should be vigilant while allowing these patients to undergo trial of labor.

LOWER SEGMENT SCAR VERSUS CLASSICAL SCAR

The lower segment scar is more sound than the classical scar. The apposition of the cut margin is more perfect as the margins are thinner compared to the classical incision. Healing is better as the lower segment of the uterus remains inert. The stretching of the scar during future pregnancy and labor is more along the line of scar unlike the classical scar where it is at right angles. The chances of placental implantation on the scar in future pregnancy are less common. Thus overall the scar is sound leading to lesser chances of rupture.

PREREQUISITES FOR TRIAL OF LABOUR

The eligibility for a trial of labor following a previous cesarean section should be decided upon after assessing the available options and selecting the appropriate choice for the individual. There is always a group in whom trial of labor is contraindicated, another group who though eligible for the trial are likely to have lesser success rate and a final group who have a high chance of achieving vaginal delivery.

Various factors affect the trial of labor following previous cesarean section. Recurrent causes like contracted pelvis, uterine anomalies, cervical dystocia have lesser success rates whereas previous cesarean done for malpresentations, fetal distress have a fair chance for vaginal delivery. Previous vaginal deliveries rule out an obvious contracted pelvis. The number of previous cesarean deliveries should also be taken into consideration before deciding for trial of labor. Details about the type of previous uterine incision should be known. Therefore documentation of this information is an important prerequisite to a trial of labor. On the other hand, several series have been reported in which the type of uterine incision was unknown and this did not significantly alter the incidence of subsequent vaginal birth[16,17].

Gestational age also influences the mode of delivery as a preterm baby may be delivered vaginally. Postoperative complications, which could have affected the integrity of scar, like history of febrile illness in the postoperative period, discharge from the wound or any wound gaping should be inquired.

MANAGEMENT OF A PATIENT WITH PREVIOUS CESAREAN DELIVERY

Antenatal period

Antenatal registration: The patient should be considered as "high risk' and hence should have an early antenatal registration. Patient should preferably register in a hospital which is fully equipped to manage the patient in antenatal & intranatal periods. The hospital should have a skilled Obstetrician, neonatologist, anesthetist and an accessible operation theatre at all hours.

Thorough History taking: A meticulous history taking is must for planning out further management of the patient. Certain factors should be taken into consideration like the indication of previous cesarean section, place of delivery, any antenatal problems in previous pregnancy and whether any trial of labor was given. Previous operative notes should always be asked as it can tell us if there was any technical difficulty in the primary operation leading to lateral extensions or tears in the surrounding tissue. It would also give us information about the suturing method of the previous uterine scar whether it was a single or double layer closure and the nature of the suture material. Uterus can be sutured in one single layer or a double layer technique. Various studies done show that either procedure has similar risk of rupture or dehiscence in the subsequent gestation[18,19,20].

History of any postoperative complications like wound infection and fever should be elicited. Enquiry should be done about the interval between the previous & present pregnancy. Present pregnancy complications like twins, hydramnios or macrosomia also puts stretching effect on the scar.

Examination : Beside usual evaluation, examination of the abdominal scar especially its position, presence of keloid or hypertrophied scar and any incisional hernia is crucial. Any puckering or thickened scar may be suggestive of prior wound infection or secondary suturing.

Antenatal follow-up : Advice the patient to follow up regularly. Give her haematinics and high protein diet to rectify anemia. Any puckering or thickened scar may be suggestive of prior wound infection. Investigate the patient and get an ultrasound for obstetrical parameters as well as for examination of the scar. As mentioned earlier, the risk of uterine rupture increased directly with the thinness of the scar [15]. If possible all previous cesarean section patients should be admitted two weeks prior to expected date.

Counseling of the patient : The patient should be well counseled regarding the risks involved in the vaginal as well as cesarean delivery. Though she should be given the liberty to make her choices for mode of delivery, the management should be individualized. The odds of a vaginal birth against repeat cesarean section should be weighed and thoroughly explained to the patient.

Intrapartum management

With increasing number of women subjected to trial of labor, intrapartum issues need to be highlighted especially the safety of induction of labor and its augmentation.

Induction of labor : Spontaneous labor is preferred in women who have experienced previous cesarean section. But some women do require induction or cervical ripening.

The use of prostaglandins is an accepted management in women with a cervix unsuitable for labor induction. Concern has been expressed regarding the safety of these agents in the scarred uterus for fear of increased risk of uterine rupture. Several studies have been published investigating Prostaglandin E_2 for cervical ripening in women with prior caesarean section. Mackenzie et al[21] published a series using prostaglandin gel to ripen the cervix in 143 women with a prior caesarean delivery. This was followed by oxytocin induction or augmentation of labour. A 76% vaginal delivery rate was reported and there were no uterine dehiscence or ruptures. In a similar study by Norman and Ekman[22], 0.5mg PGE_2 gel was used intracervically achieving a 63% vaginal delivery rate with no cases of uterine rupture. A large retrospective observational study by Stone et al[23] compared 94 women with a scarred uterus who received PGE_2 gel for induction, with 866 nulliparous women induced similarly. Similar rate of successful vaginal delivery was noted in both groups. Only two uterine dehiscences' were documented in patients undergoing trial of labour.

Oxytocin : Intravenous oxytocin infusions are widely used in obstetrics to induce or augment labour. In modern obstetrics a previous lower segment caesarean section per se is not a contraindication to the use of oxytocin for induction or augmentation of labour[6,24,25,26,27]. When standard management guidelines are adhered to, oxytocin can be used effectively without increased maternal or fetal risk.

Flamm et al[25] reported a series of 1776 women with previous caesarean section and undergoing trial of labour of whom 485 (27%) received oxytocin for either induction or augmentation of labour. There were no significant differences in maternal or perinatal mortality in terms of obstetric outcomes in the study and control group. There was no difference in the incidence of uterine rupture between the two group although the rate of full thickness uterine rupture was higher in the oxytocin group (4/1000 v/s 1/1000).

The timing and dose of oxytocin are also factors that could influence the risk of rupture. In a study by Goetzl et al[28] women with uterine rupture had a somewhat higher mean oxytocin dose and duration of oxytocin exposure, but the differences did not reach statistical significance. Also the data of Leung et al[9] and Grubb et al[29] suggest that induction or augmentation witn oxytocin in the latent phase of labour may increase the risk of scar separation during labour.

Misoprostol : Use of Misoprostol for induction of labour in women with previous caesarean section is contraindicated because of an extremely high rate of disruption of the previous uterine scar.

Labour management :

Patients undergoing trial of labour should be monitored vigilantly. Protocols for intrapartum management of patients undergoing a trial of labour are recommended at all institutions where women having a previous cesarean scar are allowed to labour.

Trial of scar should be conducted in well-equipped units where the facilities exist for an emergency cesarean section. On admission these patients should have an intravenous line and blood should be cross-matched. Patient should be appropriately counseled and consent for VBAC should be taken. Fetal monitoring should be done on continuous or intermittent basis on an electronic fetal monitor. Progress of labour should be charted on a partogram.

Monitoring of maternal pulse and blood pressure is extremely essential to diagnose impending scar dehiscence or rupture. Oxytocin may be used with vigilant monitoring.

Use of intrauterine pressure catheters during trial of labour following a previous cesarean section has been considered as an aid to the early detection of uterine scar rupture. The studies performed to investigate this concept have not demonstrated any benefit from this form of monitoring (85-88). Thus the routine insertion of an intrauterine pressure catheter for the purpose of uterine rupture detection is not justified[30,31,32,33].

It is always prudent to cut short the second stage with generous episiotomy, outlet forceps or vacuum extraction.

Assessment of uterine scar integrity : The practice of post partum scar palpation to discern uterine scar integrity following a vaginal delivery has been advocated by some. Apart from the technical difficulties in this procedure, no study has ever demonstrated any benefit form routine manual exploration of the scared uterus. Gemer et al[34] detected only one out of the thirteen cases by transcervical scar assessment. The procedure may in fact do more harm than good, with the potential for infection, converting a dehiscence into a larger rupture or even falsely identifying a separation in the thin soft anterior wall of lower uterine segment.

In an asymptomatic woman, the management of a dehiscence discovered fortuitously is conservative and most women do well without intervention. Manual exploration of the lower segment cannot be advocated as a routine procedure, but may be indicated in women when persistent post partum bleeding suggests a possible uterine rupture, which requires surgery.

DIAGNOSIS OF RUPTURE OF CESAREAN SECTION SCAR IN LABOUR

Rupture of a scar refers to separation of the old uterine incision throughout most of its length with rupture of fetal membranes. All or part of the fetus is usually extruded into the peritoneal cavity. Dehiscence of the uterine scar is defined as incomplete separation of the uterine scar but with fetal membranes and peritoneum intact.

There are certain specific signs and symptoms of scar rupture or impending scar rupture. There may be sudden onset of continuous pain over the uterine scar, which is also present in between the contractions. However painless rupture of a fibrous scar is also possible. Bleeding from the genital or urinary tract may be present. Bladder involvement is likely to edge proximity of bladder to the lower uterus segment. The most important feature is sudden onset of abnormalities in the fetal heart trace.

With established rupture there is cessation of uterine contractions and superficial palpation of the fetal parts distinct from the uterus.

Management of a ruptured uterus :
On diagnosis of scar dehiscence or rupture, resuscitative measures should be instituted immediately. Patient should be shifted to the theatre for a laparotomy. The aim should be delivery of the fetus and repair of the rent with ligation of any bleeding vessels.

However if the bleeding is uncontrollable, bilateral internal iliac ligation or caesarean hysterectomy may be resorted to depending on the condition of the patient. Sterilization is performed at the same time if prior consent has been obtained.

Follow up :
If sterilization is not done, women are advised contraception and can be followed up for laparoscopic sterilization 6 weeks later. If the woman is interested in further child bearing, thorough counseling should be done. She should be forewarned of the associated risks and an elective caesarean section should be performed by 37–38 weeks of gestation.

THE ACOG GUIDELINES FOR VAGINAL BIRTH AFTER CESAREAN SECTION

The American college of Obstetricians and Gynecologists in 1999 have observed that VBAC is associated with a small but significant risk of uterine rupture with poor outcomes for both mother and the baby. This led to a more circumspect approach to trial of labour by even the most religious supporters of VBAC. There was rising need to reevaluate VBAC recommendations.

The current VBAC recommendations by The American college of Obstetricians & Gynecologists (ACOG)[35] are given below, which although urging caution also strongly supports VBAC.

Recommendation of the ACOG (1999) for selection of candidates for VBAC.

Selection criteria

- 1 or 2 prior low transverse caesarean deliveries.
- Clinically adequate pelvis
- No other uterine scars or previous rupture
- Physician available throughout labour capable of monitoring labour and performing an emergency caesarean delivery.
- Availability of anaesthesia and personnel for emergency caesarean delivery.

During the end of the 20th century several studies involving thousands of women undergoing trials of labour largely confirmed that there is a success rate of approximately 60-80% of achieving a vaginal delivery and the rate of uterine rupture is approximately 1%[9,36].

REDUCING MEDICAL & LEGAL RISKS

There are various controversial medical and legal aspects of VBAC. It should be emphasized that compared to a patient with no previous uterine surgery, the pregnant patient with scarred uterus is at significantly increased risk, regardless of the mode of delivery.

Reducing Medical Risk

- Watch out for previous classical or T-shaped uterine incisions as these scars may rupture even before the onset of labour.
- Be more vigilant when dealing with uterine scar of unknown type.
- Beware of placenta praevia/accreta. The combination of previous cesarean section with a placenta praevia significantly increases the risk of a morbidly adherent placenta. When imaging studies indicate probable placenta accreta, the patient should be consented for possible cesarean hysterectomy and blood products should be kept ready.
- Avoid misoprostol in VBAC.
- Do not use outpatient cervical ripening in VBAC.
- Exercise caution with more than one previous caesarean section.
- Be cautions with oxytocin in VBAC.
- Be alert for clinical signs and fetal monitor signs of uterine rupture.

Reducing legal risk

- **Informed consent for VBAC:** Patients considering VBAC should be informed that the risk of uterine rupture during trial of labour is approximately 1% and if the uterus does rupture there is a significant risk to both mother and baby. Informed consent should also point out that the alternative to trial of labour, i.e. planned caesarean section is not risk free.
- **Cost analysis of VBAC:** The debate concerning the cost effectiveness of trial of labour with elective caesarean delivery is still going on. A universal policy can never exist advocating one mode of delivery for all women pregnant after a previous caesarean section. A VBAC programme will prove cost effective only in select women with a previous scar who have a high likelihood of success because the greatest expenses remain with patients who experience adverse outcomes that are frequently associated with trial of labour.

VAGINAL DELIVERY AFTER PREVIOUS CAESAREAN DELIVERY: A CONTINUING CONTROVERSY

Due to rising rates of caesarean delivery, considerable attention has been focused on vaginal birth after caesarean section. The dictum "Once a caesarean, always a cesarean" is now changed to 'Once a cesarean, always a hospital delivery'. The problem of high cesarean rate will have to be attacked on two fronts i.e. reducing the primary section rate and reducing the incidence of repeat cesarean birth.

A trial of labour approach decreases the total number of cesarean births resulting in a less expensive and shorter hospital stay. Additionally, the resources of the blood bank, nursing care and anaesthesia services are economized.

THE FUTURE

Till date there are no prospective, controlled, randomized studies comparing outcomes between vaginal birth after caesarean section and elective repeat caesarean delivery. Also, routine elective caesarean results in an excess of maternal mortality and morbidity and high cost to the medical infrastructure.

At this time, what is needed is more careful screening of patients and a heightening of the eligibility requirements for patients to pursue a trial of labour. The VBAC controversy is bound to demonstrate shifting, evolving even cyclic patterns.

The fact that vaginal delivery after a caesarean section is a safe and effective approach for may patients is a well established fact. This does not mean that it is appropriate for all women contemplating a pregnancy in the presence of a uterine scar. The management should be individualized with the obstetric decision making based on evidence-based medicine.

REFERENCES

1. Kerr JM. The technique of caesarean section with special reference to the lower uterine segment incision. Am J Obstet Gynecol 1926; 12: 729 – 731.
2. Case BD, Corcoram R, Jeffcoate N et al. Caesarean section and its place in modern obstetric practice. J. Obstet Gynaecolo Br. common w. 1971; 78: 203 – 214.
3. Schmitz HE, Gajewski CJ. Vaginal delivery following caesarean section Am J Obstet Gynaecol. 1951; 61: 1232 – 1242.
4. Merrill BS, Gibbs CE. Planned vaginal delivery following caesarean section, Obstet Gynecol 52; 50: 1978.
5. Leveno KJ. Controversies in Ob : Gyn should we rethink the criteria for VBAC? Contemporary Ob-Gyn, Jan 1999.
6. Rosen MG, Dic, Weshoff CL. Vaginal birth after caesarean, a mata analysis of morbidity and mortality. Obst & Gyn 1991; 77: 465 – 470.
7. Shipp TD, Zelop LM, Reoke JT et al. Intrapartum uterine rupture & dehiscence in patients with prior lower segment vertical and transverse incisions. Obstetrics and Gynaecology 1999; 94: 735 – 740.
8. Miller D, Diaz F, Paul R. Vaginal birth after Caesarean : a 10 year experience. Obstetrics and Gnaecology 1994; 84: 255 – 258.
9. Leung As, Farmer RM, Leung EK et al. Risk factors associated with uterine rupture during trial of labour after caesarean delivery : a case control study. Am J Obstet Gynaecol 1993; 168: 1358 – 1363kin son JC.
10. Shipp T, Zelop LM, Repke JT et al. Interdelivery interval and risk of symptomatic uterine rupture Obstet Gynaecol 2001; 97(2): 175 – 177.
11. Lavin JP, Stephns RJ, Miodovnik M et al. vaginal delivery in patients with a previous caesarean section. Obstet Gynaecol. 1982; 59: 135 – 148. et al.
12. Shipp T, Zelop C, Repke JT et al. Maternal age as a predictor of symptomatic uterine rupture during a trial of labour after previous caesarean delivery. Am J Obstet Gynaecol 2001; 184: 571.
13. Ravasia DJ, Brain PH, Pollard JK. Incidence of uterine rupture among women with mullerian duct anomalies who attempt vaginal birth after caesarean delivery. Am J Obstet Gynaecol, 1999; 181: 877 - 881.

14. Kaltreider D, Krone W. delivery after caesarean section. Clini Obstet Gynaecol. 1959; 2: 1029Beall M, Eglinton GS, Clark SL et al. vaginal delivery after caesarean section in women with unknown types of uterine scar. J. Reprod. Med. 1984; 29: 31 – 35.

15. Rosenberg P, Goffinet F, Phillppe HJ , Misand I. Thickness of lower uterine segment : its influence in the management of patients with previous caesarean sections. European Journal of Obstetrics & Gynaecology & Reproductive biology 1999; 87: 39 – 45.

16. Preutt K. M, Kirshon B, Cotton D. B, Unknown uterine scar and trial of labour. American journal of obstetrics and Gynecology 159, 807-810.

17. Beall M, Eglinton GS, Clark S et al (1984). Vaginal delivery after caesarean section in women with unknown type of uterine scar. Journal of reproductive medicine 29, 31-35s.

18. Jelsema RD, Wittingen JA, Vander Kolk KJ. Continuous, nonlocking, single-layer repair of the low transverse uterine incision. J Reprod Med. 1993 May;38(5):393-6.

19. Enkin MW, Wilkinson C. Single versus two layer suturing for closing the uterine incision at caesarean section. Cochrane Database Syst Rev. 2000;(2):CD000192.

20. Rayburn WF, Schwartz WJ 3rd. Refinements in performing a cesarean delivery. Obstet Gynecol Survev. 1996 Jul;51(7):445-51.

21. Mackenzie IZ, Bradley S, Embrey M P (1984) vaginal prostaglandins and labour induction for patients previously delivered by caesarean section. British Journal of Obstetrics and Gynaecology. 91, 7-10.

22. Norman M, Ekman G (1992) preinductive cervical ripening with prostaglandins E2 in women with one previous caesarean section scar. Acta Obstetricia et Gynaecologica Scandinavica 71, 351-355.

23. Stone JL, Lockwood CJ, Berkowitz G et al (1994) Use of cervical prostaglandin E2 gel in patients with previous caesarean section. American Journal of perinatology 11,309-312.

24. Flamm B, Goings J, Fuelberth N, Fischermann E, Jones C, Hersh E (1987) Oxytocin during labour after previous caesarean section, results of a multicentre study. Obstetrics and Gynaecology 70,709-712.

25. Flamm B (1985) vaginal birth after caesarean section, controversies old and new. Clinical Obstetrics and Gynaecology 28,735-745.

26. Horenstein JM, Phelan JP (1984) previous caesarean section, the risks and benefits of oxytocin usage in trial of labour. American journal of Obstetrics and Gynaecology 151,564-569.

27. Flamm BL, Dunett C, Fischermann E et al (1984) vaginal delivery following caesarean section: use of oxytocin augmentation and epidural analgesia with internal tocodynamic and internal fetal monitering. American journal of Obstetrics and Gynaecology 148, 759-763.

28. Goetzl L, Shipp T, Cohen A, et al. Oxytocin dosing and risk of uterien rupture in trial of labour after caesarean delivery. Obstet Gynaecol. 2001; 97(3): 381 – 384.

29. Grubb DK, Kjos SL, Paul RH. Latent labour with an unknown uterine scar. Obstet Gynaecol. 1996; 88: 351-355.

30. Jones R, Nagashima A, Hartnett-Goodman M, Goodlin R (1991) rupture of low tranverse caesarean scars during trial of labour. Obstetrics and Gynaecology 77, 815-817.

31. Rodriguez M, Masaki D, Phelan J, Diaz F. Uterine rupture : are intrauterine pressure cathers useful in the diagnosis?(1989). American journal of Obstetrics and Gynaecology 161, 666-669.

32. Beckley S, Gee H, Newton JR (1991) Scar rupture in labour after previous caesarean section : the role of uterine activity measurement . British journal of Obstetrics and Gynaecology 98, 265-269.

33. Devoe L, Croom C, Youssef A, Murray C (1992) the prediction of controlled uterine rupture by the use of intrauterine pressure catheters. Obstetrics and Gynaecology 80, 626-629.

34. Gemer O, Segal S, Sassoon E, (1992) detection of scar dehiscence at delivery in women with prior caesarean section. Acta Obstetricia et Gynaecologica Scandinavica 71, 540-542.

35. ACOG. Vaginal birth after previous caesarean delivery. ACOG July 1999; 1017 – 1023 practice Bulletin 5.

36. Holland JG, Dupre AR, Blake PG et al. Trial of labour after caesarean delivery , experience in the non-university level II regional hospital setting .Obstete Gynaecol. 1992; 79, 936-939.

9 | CHAPTER

Cesarean Delivery After A Prior Cesarean Birth

Sanjay B. Rao

FRAMEWORK

- Introduction
- The antenatal approach
- Surgical perspectives
  - Abdominal incision
  - Other intraoperative considerations
  - Closing the abdominal incision
- Repeat cesarean delivery after a failed trial of labor
- Risks of a repeat elective cesarean delivery
- Fetal considerations in an elective repeat cesarean birth
- Sterilization at repeat cesarean delivery
- Conclusion

INTRODUCTION

Over the past few decades, trends towards performing repeat cesarean sections in contemporary obstetric practice have become more liberal. These changes could be attributed largely to the advent of prophylactic antibiotics, improvised anesthesia and easier availability of blood and component therapy. Worldwide, preferences have gradually metamorphosed towards nuclear families. The baby's right to survival has been increasingly recognized. Consequently many of the indications for Cesarean section are often solely concerned with fetal interests[1]. The reluctance to permit a trial of labour after a previous cesarean section could be influenced by various reasons. In developed countries especially, maternal awareness is likely to play a large role. Cesarean section is now being regarded as a safe and convenient procedure. The modern obstetrician is less tolerant to facing the unpleasant complications of scar dehiscence and possible litigations.

Repeat cesarean sections account for the major share of the present day indications for caesarean sections. In India, it ranges from 8.48% to 41.9%[2,3]. A review of literature reveals that repeat cesarean sections account for 35% of all cesarean sections in U.S.A, 23% in Norway and 8% in Hungary[3].

THE ANTENATAL APPROACH

Planning well in advance could help the obstetrician to optimize the maternal and fetal outcome in repeat cesarean sections. It would be prudent to identify patients who would be likely to undergo a repeat cesarean section during the antenatal visit. Previous operative records should be screened for vital information regarding the indication of the previous Caesarean section, details of the operative techniques especially the uterine incision, extension if any and the type of closure. Any major post-operative complications should make the obstetrician more alert about the current pregnancy. The progress of the neonate and its milestones should also be recorded. Even in busy antenatal clinics, health care providers – doctors and midwives should try to discuss management issues with clients and provide information to clear doubts. This develops a rapport and reduces litigation problems in the long run.

For elective repeat Caesarean sections it is important to be reasonably sure of the composite period of gestation. Besides accurate dating, this could also be reconfirmed by an ultrasound scanning. For a vigilant obstetrician it is vital to recognize the exact location of the placenta. If the placenta overlies the previous scar it should be worthwhile doing Doppler studies to exclude abnormal penetrations like an accreta, increta or percreta. An accurate hemoglobin estimation and confirming the availability of blood according to the group would avoid last minute delay in the event of acute blood loss. Prior consultation with the anesthetist would help to identify medical risk factors and decide the type of anaesthesia which be best suited for the client. Another important issue would be to discuss with the couple, the options of undergoing sterilization during repeat caesarean section. Counseling about risks and benefits should be done in advance especially when the client is more relaxed and receptive to information. This may be difficult when she presents in established labor.

SURGICAL PERSPECTIVES

The abdominal incision

The choice of the abdominal incision in repeat cesarean section and its closure should be individualized to the characteristics of the woman and also the circumstances demanding operative intervention. There should be an earnest attempt to strike a delicate balance between cosmetic and surgical advantages. Most obstetricians would prefer to make an incision over the previous scar and excise the old skin scar for better aesthetic results. In the event of there being two parallel vertical scars, the new incision should be avoided in between the two due to reduced blood supply and the risk of poor healing. In a series of 25 women undergoing repeat cesarean section, Bowen and Chamock found that the use of the 'double-bladed scalpel' yielded better healing and cosmetically better scars[4]. In Pfannensteil incisions, the fascial sheath can be extended by scissors or alternatively both the subcutaneous tissue and fascia can be divided by traction in opposite lateral directions by the surgeon and assistant, the so-called 'rip-technique'. However, this method may be difficult to practice with pre-existing scars[5]. Moreover with previous Pfannenstiel incisions there is a likelihood of extensive fibrosis in the rectus sheath or between the rectus muscle bellies and parietal peritoneum. The inferior epigastric vessels may cause troublesome bleeding necessitating haemostatic sutures. Next, the parietal peritoneum ought to be incised as high as possible exercising caution and care. This would avoid encountering the urinary bladder which may tend to be displaced upwards or the loops of the small intestine which may be adherent to the original scar. Palpation of the peritoneum held between two artery forceps will prevent inadvertent damage. It is also important to ensure that the bladder is in its pelvic location preferably by a pre-operative insertion of a No. 14F or No. 16F self-retaining Foley's catheter connected to a closed drainage system.

The possibility of intra-peritoneal adhesions during a repeat cesarean section is difficult to predict and varies in every case. However a previous history of genital tract infection or puerperal sepsis or post-operative hematoma formation is likely to increase the risk of intra peritoneal adhesions. With increasing number of repeat cesarean sections, there is a likelihood of dense lower segment adhesions with the bladder, bowels and omentum. These adhesions should be separated gently by sharp and blunt dissection to approach the lower uterine segment. Identifying the course and insertion of the round ligaments serves as a reliable anatomical landmark to define the limits of the lower uterine segment.

Other intraoperative considerations

Once the parietal peritoneum is negotiated the uterovesical pouch is much shallower than in a primary cesarean section. Along with sharp dissection care should be taken in sponging down the bladder off the lower uterine segment, because it may be rather more adherent than usual and thus suffer more damage.

The previous scar can be identified in most cases. It is preferable to make the repeat incision just above the previous scar. This would facilitate better approximation of the myometrial edges even in the event of extensions of the uterine incision following delivery of the baby.

The two most commonly practiced methods to expand the uterine incision are the blunt technique using the operator's fingers and the sharp technique using scissors to expand the incision. The expected advantages of the blunt method are increased speed and reduced bleeding from the myometrial edges[6]. However, this method could result in more damage laterally to major vessels[7]. With the sharp technique there is a precise controlled expansion of the uterine incision thereby protecting the uterine artery and parametrial veins[7].

Unless strongly indicated, the transverse lower segment incision could be made even with a previous lower segment vertical incision; the obvious advantages would be placing the incision along the direction of uterine muscle fibres, a less vascular field of surgery and better myometrial approximation. Though a transverse incision is more physiological, the choice of incision with a previous classical scar is left to the discretion of the obstetrician concerned. A repeat classical upper segment incision could be made in cases of preterm deliveries with a poorly formed lower segment, severe adhesions in the lower segment reducing accessibility, a large cervical fibroid or post-mortem cesarean sections.

In most situations, repeat cesarean sections should be performed by an experienced obstetrician as far as possible. Expertise helps to limit the induction-delivery interval and the mean operating time. Longer uterine incision-delivery intervals (more than 8 mins under general anaesthesia and 3 mins under both general or spinal anaesthesia) could increase the risk of low APGAR scores and neonatal acidosis.Though traditionally the placenta is removed manually at the time of caesarean section, the ideal method should not differ from the controlled cord traction used at vaginal delivery. A review of the Cochrane database shows that manual shearing of the placenta does not allow retraction of the myometrial fibres and leads to increased blood loss[9]. The practice of mop curettage of the uterine cavity could also theoretically increase the risk of bacterial contamination and post-operative endometritis[10].

Exteriorization of the uterus in repeat caesarean section could be difficult at times due to dense adhesions. Some obstetricians prefer exteriorization especially during the learning curve. The main advantage would be a wider exposure of the uterine incision. It also offers better visualization of adnexal structures and may help to detect a co-existent ovarian pathology. Exteriorization if attempted should be informed to the anaesthesia provider to watch for hemodynamic changes following traction to the infundibulopelvic ligaments. Some women experience nausea and pain. Studies by Handler and Bromage show that traction on the uterine sinuses and raising the incision to a level higher than that of the heart increases the hydrostatic gradient and promotes venous air embolism[11,12]. However more research would be desirable to arrive at a uniform consensus on the practice of exteriorization. Most conventional obstetricians prefer the traditional two layered uterine suturing technique recommended by Kerr in 1926[13]. However, in modern obstetric practice a large number of randomized trials suggest that single layer closure is associated with less tissue damage, includes less foreign material and takes less operative time[14]. The outcome of assessment factors such as hemostasis or occurrence of endometritis in none of these trials showed that the two-layered closure was superior to the single layer closure. In a repeat cesarean section it would be best to follow a flexible approach. In elective repeat caesarean with a thicker lower segment the approximation would be better in two layers. In an emergency repeat cesarean section with a well formed lower segment, a single layer closure would provide a good apposition in most situations. Often interrupted haemostatic sutures may be required in repeat cesarean section to control bleeding in a vascular lower segment with previous adhesions.

Closing the abdominal incision

Conventionally, closure of the Pfannenstiel or vertical incision is performed in anatomical layers. Evidence based randomized controlled trials on the other hand do not recommend routine closure of peritoneum, as this could predispose to adhesions[15,16]. The operative time is also reduced without alteration in short term morbidity[17]. During closure meticulous haemostasis is the key to prevent rectus sheath hematomas. Some obstetricians prefer to use a closed drain system when there is perioperative infection or a large moist potential space is left. High strength and low tissue reactivity of polyglycolic acid or polyglactin sutures are ideal for rectus sheath. Alternatively polypropylene (prolene) or polydioxanane (PDS) also cause very little reaction and retain their strength reliably especially in vertical incisions. These sutures decompose in tissue by hydrolysis rather than phagocytosis. Asepsis, minimal and meticulous handling of tissues results in better healing. Approximation of layers without 'strangulation' produces the best scars. This retains the blood supply with the least tension. Wound healing is best if sutures are 10 mm from the edge and 10 mm apart. This is due to the fact that collagenolysis occurs over an area of 10 mm from the wound edge. Wound closures constructed within this zone leads to weaker scars.

REPEAT CAESAREAN SECTION AFTER A FAILED TRIAL OF LABOUR

Most obstetricians today prefer to offer a trial of labour to women with a previous lower segment Caesarean for a non-recurrent indication. However there is evidence to show that the morbidity associated with a failed trial of labour is more serious than that of an elective repeat LSCS. A study reported by Scott TD et al showed that 75% of women with previous LSCS undergoing trial of labour delivered vaginally[19]. Of these, 0.8% had a major complication and 1.5% had minor complications. In contrast, the major complication rate was 0.1% and minor complications seen in 2.4%. Those who failed a trial of labour had the highest risk of major complications. Often there is a possibility of inadequate starvation and hence a risk of Mendelson's syndrome. Failed trial could lead to maternal exhaustion, distress and a higher risk of sepsis. Delivery of the head could be difficult if deeply engaged and result in tears or extension of the repeat lower segment incision. Suturing and approximation of the edges could be a difficult task and also entail a higher risk of post-partum hemorrhage.

RISKS OF ELECTIVE REPEAT CAESAREAN SECTION

Although there are several confounding variables, available data suggests that the maternal mortality rate associated with elective repeat Caesarean section is approximately 2-4 times that of vaginal delivery. However the maternal mortality rate associated with elective repeat Caesarean section in developed countries was much lower as depicted in the table[20].

MATERNAL MORTALITY V/S DELIVERY MODE

Mode	Maternal mortality
Cesarean section (overall)	40.9/100000 births
Vaginal delivery (overall)	9.8/100000 births
Elective repeat cesarean section	17.9/100000 births
Uncomplicated vaginal delivery	4.9/100000 births

Evidence from literature suggests that major surgical complications and maternal mortality is more likely with repeat cesarean sections. The operating time is longer in women with multiple cesarean sections. Kirkenen reported a 13% incidence of caesarean hysterectomy in a cohort of 64 women with multiple caesarean sections[21]. Chazotte and Cohen reported a serious complication rate of 2.4% in their review of 711 women. This included 9 uterine ruptures and 5 cases of placenta accreta[22]. There are several reports which also discuss the negative impact of caesarean section on subsequent fertility[23,24] and psychological status[25].

For an individual patient, the incidence of placenta praevia increases with increasing number of caesarean sections[26]. The presence of placenta praevia in a woman with previous caesarean section is also a recognized risk factor for placenta accreta. There is an increased tendency for placental implantation in the vicinity of the uterine scar with secondary trophoblast invasion of the myometrium. Clark et al reported a 24 % increase of placenta accreta in women with one previous caesarean section and placenta praevia. This incidence rose to 67% with 4 previous caesarean sections[27]. With the need to perform caesarean hysterectomy there is an increased maternal morbidity.

FETAL CONSIDERATIONS IN ELECTIVE REPEAT CESAREAN SECTION

The effect of cesarean section on the fetus centers around iatrogenic preterm birth and respiratory distress. With careful dating criteria, the incidence of iatrogenic preterm birth can be reduced. Also there are differences in respiratory function when infants are born by caesarean section as compared to those delivered vaginally. Reduced lung gas volumes, elevated mid-volume total pulmonary resistance and lower lecithin/sphingomyelin ratios in the pharyngeal aspirate have been reported[28,29].

STERILIZATION AT REPEAT CESAREAN SECTION

Issues concerning tubal ligation at the time of repeat Caesarean section should be discussed with the couple during the antenatal period. In India, the gender of the baby still plays a major role in influencing the decision to opt for a permanent contraception at the time of repeat Caesarean section. Fear of neonatal death or social factors predispose to refusal of sterilization. A study by Verkuyl DA in Zimbabwe found that sterilization could be offered even during unplanned Caesarean section in a country with limited health resources. The study concluded that women may not regret the decision at a later date[30].

CONCLUSION

Every case of a repeat caesarean section poses a new challenge even to the experienced obstetrician. Prior preparedness and anticipation of problems helps to minimize the risks involved in the surgery. It would be best to manage these cases in well-equipped hospitals for a safe maternal and neonatal outcome.

REFERENCES

1. Ian Donald : Practical Obstetric Problems 5th edn: PG publishing Pvt Ltd: Caesarean Section ch XXIV:825-861.
2. Singh J, Lakshmi Devi Y: Obstet Gynecol 34:849,1984.
3. Arora R, Oumachigui A; A Obstet Gynecol 41: 192,1991.
4. Bowen ML and Chamock FML. Instruments and methods. Obstetrics and Gynaecology 1994; 83:476-477.
5. Goodlin RC. An incision technique for emergency caesarean section. Surgery,Gynaecology and Obstetrics 165,544-546.
6. Clark SL Caesarean delivery in: Hawkins GDV, Clark SL, Cunningham FG, Gilstrap LC, editors. Operative Obstetrics. Norwalk, Connecticut: Appleton and Lange,1995:301-322.
7. Jananoul R. Incision of the pregnant uterus and delivery of low birth weight infants. Am J Obstet Gynecol 1985;152:971-974.
8. Datta S, Ostheimer GW, Weiss JB et al. Neonatal effect of prolonged anaesthetic induction for caesarean section. Obstetrics and Gynaecology 1981;58:331-335.
9. Wilkinson C, Enkin MW. Manual removal of the placenta at caesarean section (Cochrane Review) in. The Cochrane library, Issue 2. Oxford: Update software 2000.
10. Rayburn WF, Schwartz WJ. Refinements in performing a caesarean delivery. Gynaecology and Obstetric surgery 1996; 51: 445-451.
11. Handler JS and Bromage PR. Venous air embolism during caesarean delivery. Regional anaesthesia 1990;15:170.
12. Lowenwirt IP, Chi DS and Handwerker SM. Nonfatal venous air embolism during caesarean section; a case report and review of literature. Obstetrical and Gynaecological survey 1994;49:72-76.
13. Kerr JMM. The technique of caesarean section with special reference to lower uterine segment incision; .American Journal of Obstetrics and Gynaecology1926;12:729-734.
14. Hauth JC, Owen J and Davis RO. Transverse uterine incision closure: one versus two layers . American Journal of Obstetrics and Gynaecology 1992;167:1108-1111.
15. Pietrantoni M, Parsons MT, O'Brien WF et al(1991) Peritoneal closure or non-closure at caesarean section. Obstetrics and Gynaecology 77;293-296.
16. Luzuy F, Inon O, Beguin F(1994) A randomised study of closure of the peritoneum at caesarean delivery. American Journal of Obstetrics and Gynaecology 170;341-345.

17. Oher G, Younis JS, Lang N, Levit A(1996) double layer closure of uterine incision with visceral and parietal peritoneal closure: are they obligatory steps of routine caesarean sections? Journal of Maternal-Fetal medicine;5:366-369.

18. Kirk RM. Surgical techniques and technology. In Aljafri AM and Kingsworth A(eds) Fundamentals of surgical practice,p87-108. London: Ashford Colour Press,1998.

19. Scott TD, Flora R, Deveny TC: Elective repeat caesarean delivery vs trial of labour: A comparison of morbidities in a community hospital setting 5(4):188,1998.

20. Pettiti DB, Cefalo RC, Shapiro S et al. (1982) In-hospital maternal mortality in the United States time trends and relation to method of delivery. Obstetrics and Gynaecology 59,6-11.

21. Kirkenen P(1987) Multiple caesarean sections: Outcomes and complications. British Journal of Obstetrics and Gynaecology 95,778-782.

22. Chazotte C, Cohen WR(1990) Catastrophic complications of previous caesarean section in: American Journal of Obstetrics and Gynaecology 163,738-742.

23. Hurry DJ, Larsen B, Charles D(1984) Effects of postcaesarean section febrile morbidity on subsequent fertility: Obstetrics and Gynaecology 64,256-260.

24. Herminski E, Graubard BI, Hoffman HJ et al(1985) Caesarean section and subsequent fertility results from the 1982 national survey of faily growth. Fertility and Sterility 43,520-528.

25. Garfel M, Lelong N, Karminski M(1987) Psychological consequences of caesarean childbirth in primiparas. Journal of Psychosomatic Obstetrics and Gynaecology 6,197-209.

26. Weckstein LN, Amssermann JSH, Garite TJ(1987) Placenta accreta:a problem of increasing clinical significance. Obstetrics and Gynaecology 69,480-482.

27. Clark SL, Koonings PP, Phelan JP(1985) Placenta praevia-accreta and previous caesarean section. Obstetrics and Gynaecology 66,89-92.

28. Boon AW, milner AD, Hopkins IE(1981) Lung volumes and lung mechanics in babies born vaginally and by elective and emergency lower segment caesarean section. Journal of Paediatrics 98,965-968.

29. Callen P, Goldsworthy S, Gravest et al(1979) mode of delivery and the lecithin-sphingomyelin ratio. British Journal of Obstetrics and Gynaecology 86,965-968.

30. Verkuyl DA : Sterilisation during unplanned Caesarean section for women likely to have a completed family – should they be offered? Experience in a country with limited health resources. Aust NZ Obstet-Gynaecol 2002 Nov; 42(5) : 526-9.

10 | CHAPTER

Anesthesia In Contemporary Cesarean Practice

Grace Korula

FRAMEWORK

INTRODUCTION

Medicine has advanced tremendously in the last couple of hundred years. Two major disciplines where these advances have been noteworthy are obstetrics and anesthesia. Obstetric care was revolutionized during the last couple of hundred years with childbirth being institutionalized. Along with advances made in the obstetric care, anesthesia was also developing into a very systematic discipline. Without the advances made in anesthetic techniques childbirth, and especially cesarean birth would never have been as safe as it is today.

Labor has been portrayed as a painful, life-threatening and fearsome event since the earliest recorded history. When the anesthetic effects of ether and chloroform were discovered in the mid 1800's, many argued that this human intervention in the miracle of birth was sin against the will of God. According to Scripture, childbirth pain originated when God punished Eve and her descendants for Eve's disobedience in the Garden of Eden. If God had wished labor to be painless, he would have created it so.

The first use of modern anesthetic for childbirth occurred a scant 3 months after Morton's historic demonstration of the anesthetic properties of ether at the Massachusetts General Hospital in Boston, Massachusetts. James Young Simpson used diethyl ether to anesthetize a woman with a deformed pelvis for childbirth. Queen Victoria undaunted by the arguments chose one day to use an anesthetic during labor. The first woman anesthetized for childbirth in the United States was Fanny Longfellow, wife of the American poet Henry Wadsworth Longfellow. She wrote "I am very sorry you all thought me so rash and naughty in trying the ether. Henry's faith gave me courage and I had heard such a thing had succeeded in abroad where the surgeons extend this great blessing more boldly and universally than our timid doctors.... This is certainly the greatest blessing of this age".

Techniques of obstetric anesthesia improved with the passing years, paralleled by improvements in techniques of blood transfusion, advent of more effective antibiotics and improvements in surgical technique.

In this chapter the various techniques available for anesthesia in cesarean delivery are discussed: the basic technique itself, its advantages & disadvantages, and the necessary safeguards one should remember to be able to practice safe obstetric anesthesia. The anesthetic techniques in patients with coexisting disease are also given a brief mention. An obstetrician should be 'aware' of the basic anesthetic techniques used in cesarean delivery and this chapter is therefore designed and structured to appeal to the obstetrician.

Before these issues are discussed, consideration must be given to some important aspects of maternal and fetal physiology as they have a major impact on the provision of safe anesthesia irrespective of the method used.

MATERNAL PHYSIOLOGICAL CHANGES

Pregnancy causes profound changes in maternal physiology. These physiological alterations are designed by nature for ease of fetal nourishment during pregnancy. These physiological changes however, are extremely important to remember, both for the obstetrician and the anesthetist. Changes occur in a variety of maternal systems but only the pertinent changes are discussed below.

Cardiovascular system adaptation

The maternal cardiovascular system undergoes considerable changes during pregnancy.

Blood volume increases by 40% at term; plasma volume increases more than red cell volume, resulting in lower hemoglobin concentrations. Cardiac output (CO) rises during the second trimester to meet the increased oxygen consumption to a 20% increase at term[1]. CO exceeds 50% during labor and remains elevated until the third postpartum day. Heart rate increases and peripheral vascular resistance and diastolic blood pressure (BP) decrease[2]. Central venous pressure is unchanged[3]. The growing uterus receives 20% of the cardiac output. The uterine enlargement causes compression of the inferior vena cava and the aorta, resulting in maternal hypotension and fetal distress. This aorto-caval compression is of considerable significance.

It was Ahltorp who for the first time described the supine hypotension syndrome[4]. All pregnant women are prone to developing supine hypotension syndrome because the posterior aspect of the enlarging uterus is in close proximity to the great vessels of the abdomen. If venous return to the right atrium is significantly impaired, cardiac output falls and this may be followed by hypotension. Angiography reveals that compression of inferior vena cava is common in pregnant patients at term[5]. Even so, not all women develop supine hypotension; only 60% of women become symptomatic when supine. Even at term, less than 10% of women actually develop overt supine hypotension syndrome[6]. This is because, in many women the collateral circulation through the epidural and azigous veins is sufficient to maintain an adequate cardiac output. Secondly, pressure on the vena cava not only causes decreased venous return to the right heart, but also causes elevated pressures in the uterine veins, which may compromise placental perfusion. Again the incidence of decreased placental perfusion is not the rule in all women because a significant part of the uteroplacental blood flow drains into the ovarian veins, which drain above the site of obstruction in the vena cava[7].

This has an important bearing during labor. The aorto-caval compression syndrome, which is position related, is entirely preventable. Therefore, during labor, the gravida can lie on her side, lie in the semi recumbent position or when this is not possible, a wedge or folded sheet can be placed under the hip to result in a lateral tilt which will relieve the aorto-caval compression.

During regional anesthesia, there is an associated sympathetic blockade because of which the parturient is unable to compensate effectively for the drop in blood pressure. Also, during general anesthesia, the ability of the mother to compensate for the hypotension can be interfered with and in addition, the inhaled anesthetics may produce hypotension themselves.

Another important implication of the hemodynamic changes is that the engorgement of the epidural vasculature makes puncture of an epidural vein more likely. The decrease in epidural space by the engorged vessels leads to decreased drug requirement. Pregnant patients need only two-thirds of the amount of anesthetic agent used in non-pregnant patients.

Respiratory system adaptations

In a pregnant patient, the enlarging uterus elevates the diaphragm thereby increasing the thoracic diameter. By term, the thoracic cage is fully expanded and inspiration is almost exclusively produced by diaphragmatic descent[3]. As the expanding uterus displaces the diaphragm cephalad, it decreases the functional residual capacity (FRC). Vital capacity (VC) and inspiratory capacity remain unchanged, because of an increase in antero-posterior thoracic diameter[8]. Tidal volume increases by 40% and respiratory rate by 15% resulting in a raise in alveolar ventilation by 70%. The elevated progesterone level has been assumed to stimulate the rise in alveolar ventilation. The increase in alveolar ventilation produces respiratory alkalosis with compensatory renal excretion of bicarbonate and correction of pH. Therefore, oxygenation is improved, as a consequence[9]. Despite maternal alkalosis, the P50 of the oxyhemoglobin dissociation curve increases throughout pregnancy, most probably because of an increased 2,3-diphosphoglycerate concentrations[10]. This increase in P50 facilitates the delivery of oxygen from maternal hemoglobin to fetal hemoglobin as well as to maternal tissues.

The clinical implication due to the decreased FRC is that the parturients are more susceptible to hypoxia and hypercarbia during apnea while pushing and after induction of general anesthesia. The supine and lithotomy position assumed during birth aggravates the onset of hypoxia. Severe hyperventilation during pain leads to hypocarbia, causing uterine artery vasoconstriction. The decreased FRC implies that preoxygenation and induction of anesthesia with inhalation agents occur more rapidly, as does emergence. Administration of supplemental 100% oxygen is mandatory during fetal distress and prior to induction of general anesthesia.

Another important fact that should be remembered is that there is capillary engorgement of the respiratory tract, which leads to edema, and increased friability of the mucous membranes with increased tendency to severe hemorrhage during insertion of nasogastric or endotracheal tubes. So, care should be taken during nasogastric tube insertions especially in preeclamptic patients, where an associated vocal cord edema may be present.

Gastrointestinal system adaptations

There are a number of changes that occur in gastrointestinal system during pregnancy that have an important bearing on anesthetic considerations.

During pregnancy, the stomach is shifted cephalad and the intrabdominal portion of the esophagus is often displaced into the thoracic cavity[11], thus reducing the efficiency of the lower esophageal sphincter. The enlarged uterus increases the intragastric pressure and the gastro-esophageal angle flattens.

Elevated progesterone levels decrease gastric motility and food absorption is delayed. The placental secretion of gastrin results in higher gastric acidity and gastric volume. Therefore, during pregnancy, there is prolonged bowel transit time, delayed gastric emptying, increased intrabdominal pressure and relaxation of the gastro-esophageal sphincters[12].

These gastrointestinal changes result in an increased danger of vomiting and aspiration of gastric contents in the parturient. Regardless of the number of hours after last food intake, all parturients are considered to have a full stomach. It is therefore, recommended that no solid food be given to parturients and that liquids be restricted to a small amount of ice chips or sips of water. Although histamine$_2$-blocking agents (cimetidine, ranitidine) have been used in elective cesarean section patients with success, the time required to change gastric acidity is unpredictable and too long to be effective in labor patients. Metoclopramide increases gastric motility and lower esophageal sphincter tone, and has central antiemetic effects. Oral clear liquid antacids 0.3 M sodium citrate, 30 mL, is sufficient to buffer gastric acidity acutely. It may ameliorate pulmonary irritation from gastric acid, if aspiration occurs.

Whenever possible, regional anesthesia is chosen over general anesthesia. Clear oral liquid antacid, 30 mL, is administered 10 minutes prior to induction. The patient is preoxygenated with 100% oxygen for 3 minutes; anesthesia is induced with a fast-acting IV agent, followed by a muscle relaxant, with cricoid pressure and intubation, inflating the cuff immediately. If difficult intubation is anticipated, awake intubation with topical spray and mild sedation is indicated.

FETAL CONSIDERATIONS

Drugs given to the parturient during pregnancy or labor may affect the fetus or the newborn by a direct pharmacological transfer or indirectly because of their effect on maternal physiology, placental perfusion, and the maternal acid base balance.

There is no absolute barrier to the passage of drugs across the placenta. Passage of a drug from the mother to the fetus is governed by its physio-chemical properties and the dynamics of the two circulations. The rate and extent to which free drug crosses the placenta depends on several factors: lipid solubility of the drug, placental permeability and the concentration gradient for the unbound diffusible drug.

Regional anesthesia may affect the fetus either by direct drug transfer across the placenta or indirectly through a change in the maternal physiology. The dose of a local anesthetic drug crossing the placenta is mainly dependant on the maternal plasma concentration and this in turn is determined by the absorption from the epidural space, which is rapid. Lignocaine has been detected in the maternal circulation within three minutes of epidural injection, with peak concentrations occurring at approximately 20 minutes[3]. Once in the maternal bloodstream, unbound drug crosses the placenta readily since these drugs are lipophilic. The local anesthetic drugs used for regional anesthesia are weakly basic drugs and therefore highly bound to the a_1-acid glycoprotein. Of these, bupivacaine is more protein bound and therefore less drug is free to cross the placenta[13].

Subtle neurobehavioral changes have been observed with use of these drugs for regional anesthesia. Kuhnert et al. compared neonatal neurobehavior following use of these drugs for vaginal or cesarean delivery[14]. The changes detected were very subtle and the authors commented that type of delivery affected the scores more than the type of local anesthetic used, with worse scores following vaginal delivery compared with cesarean section. Recently, using sensitive tests of neonatal neurobehavior, these drugs have been studied at an elective cesarean section and it has been observed that none produced any significant adverse effects on the newborn[15].

The use of drugs for regional anesthesia may also affect the fetus due to the indirect effects on the maternal physiology. Uterine and placental blood flow is determined by maternal blood pressure and the degree of vasoconstriction in uteroplacental blood vessels. Any fall in the systolic blood pressure results in a reduction in the uteroplacental blood flow. Local anesthetic drugs administered spinally or epidurally block the preganglionic sympathetic fibers causing vasodilation, which may result in hypotension. Marked decrease in the maternal blood pressure related to anesthesia can be avoided if appropriate preventive measures are used.

The importance of maternal position has already been discussed and use of a wedge to avoid supine hypotension should be the rule. Left uterine displacement is extremely vital to avoid aorto-caval compression. Regional block induced hypotension can also be avoided by infusing an adequate amount of intravenous fluid before the institution of the anesthetic agent. A fluid preload is commonly given before regional blocks to prevent or attenuate maternal hypotension.

The type and the amount of the 'preloading agent' has been studied in various trials. Hartmann's solution/Ringers lactate or normal saline are usually given to increase the blood volume and cardiac output; Dextrose is not used because it as been associated with increased incidence of fetal acidosis[3]. Also, dextrose containing solutions should be avoided as they lead to maternal hyperglycemia, which in turn leads to fetal hyperglycemia. The fetal hyperglycemia causes fetal hyperinsulinemia; this might cause neonatal hypoglycemia at birth, as the maternal source of glucose is lost[12].

The amount of intravenous fluid for preload has increased over the years as various investigators have proved the efficacy of larger volumes in maintaining maternal blood pressure within normal range. In a study of 60 women scheduled for a elective cesarean section, two liters of a balanced salt solution were infused immediately before institution of an epidural block[16]. Central venous pressure rose from a mean level before hydration of 4.05 ± 0.5 cm H_2O to 5.72 ± 0.5 cm H_2O after the block had been established. At the same time, less than 10% of patients had a decline in their systolic blood pressure and there was no indication for vasopressor therapy in any of these women. The amount of fluid required is dependant on the extent of the sympathetic block induced increase in vascular capacity. With blocks for a normal delivery, the initial infusion should be at least 15% of the blood volume. However, for a cesarean section, the initial fluid bolus should be of the order of 30% of the pregnant blood volume (i.e. at least 1500 ml)[12].

There can be a marked difference in the 'preload' requirement between women undergoing elective cesarean section and in those women requiring surgery after being in labor for some time. Women undergoing an elective cesarean section after an overnight fast are likely to have a lower blood volume because of lack of fluid intake and therefore block induced hypotension is more likely to occur[17]. In women undergoing elective cesarean section after a period of fasting, the spinal blockade develops more rapidly than epidural blockade and some authors have suggested that the incidence and severity of maternal hypotension, and therefore uterine hypoperfusion is greater[18]. Women who have been in labor for a variable period of time have received intravenous hydration during labor and are therefore at a lesser risk.

Another important cause of decreased uteroplacental perfusion is maternal hyperventilation. Most obstetric anesthetists administer supplementary oxygen to the mother before cesarean section under regional anesthesia. It was once a common practice to use a combination of oxygen and nitrous oxide during cesarean section. However in a study when different concentrations of oxygen were administered to women undergoing cesarean section, it was seen that lowest fetal oxygen concentrations occurred when mother's arterial oxygen concentration was below 100 mm Hg[19]. Maximum benefit as far as the fetal oxygen status was associated with maternal oxygen tensions of 300 mm of Hg. This can be achieved by providing at least 50% oxygen through the endotracheal tube[19]. If a regional anesthesia is employed, this can be achieved with 100% oxygen given through a facemask. Houle reported better fetal oxygenation and acid base balance when mothers breathed 100% oxygen for at least 10 minutes before delivery, compared to mothers who breathed only air[20]. Ramanathan et al randomized mothers who had received epidural anesthesia for cesarean section to breathe air or supplementary oxygen in concentrations of 47%, 74% and 100%[21]. It was observed that PaO2 in maternal blood and umbilical venous & arterial blood increased with increasing inspired oxygen concentrations. Mothers, who breathed air, and their babies, also demonstrated a metabolic acidosis not seen in the groups receiving supplementary oxygen.

General anesthetic agents affect the fetus more than the drugs given as a part of regional anesthesia. The use of general anesthesia for cesarean section is associated with lower Apgar scores, a greater need for active resuscitation of the neonate, and more admissions to the neonatal unit than following epidural anesthesia. However, no long-term adverse effects have been reported as long as trained staff provides neonatal care.

Thiopentone is the agent used most commonly for induction of anesthesia in pregnancy and for cesarean delivery under general anesthesia. Thiopentone is a weak acid, a highly lipid soluble drug and therefore the free unionized drug crosses the placenta rapidly. Thiopentone has been detected in umbilical venous blood within 30 seconds of maternal intravenous administration[3]. Peak fetal Thiopentone concentrations occur between 90 and 120 seconds after maternal intravenous injection. Following its passage across the placenta, Thiopentone has similar effects on the fetus as on the mother, the extent depending on the dose delivered to the fetus and therefore on the induction-delivery interval (IDI). The usual dose of

Thiopentone used for inducing general anesthesia is 4 mg/kg; at this dose there is no untoward effect on neonatal Apgar score[12]. However, the timing of the delivery is an important determinant of the newborn's status at birth.

Propofol is not yet licensed for use in obstetric anesthesia. It is lipophilic and protein bound, therefore crosses the placenta readily. It is not used for cesarean deliveries. Although ketamine is much less lipid soluble than Thiopentone it crosses the placenta readily. Induction with ketamine 2 mg/kg has been associated with low Apgar scores and inadequate ventilation. It is rarely used for induction of general anesthesia.

Halothane was been employed for maintenance of general anesthesia but is no longer used in obstetric practice and more recently has been superseded by other inhalational agents. Placental transfer of halothane is rapid, causing a dose dependent direct neonatal depression.

Neuromuscular blocking drugs are fully ionized and cross the placenta very slowly. The small amount of the drug that does cross the placenta is usually excreted renally and the drug has no clinical effect on the baby.

When general anesthesia is used, there are several important considerations viz. maternal hypotension, maternal oxygenation and ventilation and the induction delivery and incision delivery intervals.

All induction agents used for general anesthesia cause maternal vasodilatation and myocardial depression. In doing so, they may lower the blood pressure. This is more marked following an overdose in presence of hypovolemia or fixed cardiac output states. Adequate fluid resuscitation is therefore necessary before surgery. Aorto-caval compression should be avoided by left uterine displacement. However, provided the aorto-caval compression is avoided, maternal blood pressure and fetal acid base status may be better maintained with general anesthesia compared to regional anesthesia techniques[22].

Another important cause of reduced uteroplacental perfusion is excessive maternal ventilation. Excessive maternal hyperventilation during general anesthesia reduces the $PaCO_2$, causing vasoconstriction of uteroplacental blood vessels and a reduction in placental perfusion[23]. This should be borne in mind and overzealous ventilation during cesarean section should be avoided.

There are two time frames that are critical during cesarean delivery, especially under general anesthesia. They are the induction to delivery interval and the incision to delivery interval[24]. Neonatal welfare, as indicated by umbilical gas and acid base status, is influenced by both the time period from induction of anesthesia to delivery, the IDI, and the time from the incision of the uterus to the delivery of the baby, the uterine incision to delivery interval, the UDI.

When regional anesthesia is used, prolonged IDI does not adversely affect the neonate provided placental perfusion is maintained. Under general anesthesia however, an IDI of greater than eight minutes has been associated with lower Apgar scores[24].

However, a UDI of more than 180 seconds in both general as well as regional anesthesia is associated with low one-minute Apgar scores and fetal academia. This is because once the uterus is incised, the spatial relationship between the intervillous space and the myometruim is disrupted and the transfer of oxygen to the fetus is curtailed[12].

TECHNIQUES OF ANESTHESIA FOR CESAREAN SECTION

Development of obstetric anesthesia as a discipline has contributed greatly in making cesarean delivery safe. Techniques of obstetric anesthesia have evolved considerably over the years and various anesthetic techniques have been refined and improved. There are two basic techniques employed for cesarean delivery: General anesthesia and Regional anesthesia. Each of these techniques has their own advantages and disadvantages. Both these techniques are discussed below.

It must be stressed at this point that an obstetrician must have knowledge of basic anesthetic drugs, their effects on the mother and the fetus and also some knowledge of the techniques themselves. It enables the obstetrician to make better-informed decisions regarding patient management. This chapter does not deal with all the anesthetic issues in depth but only the most relevant ones are discussed here. The basic anesthetic techniques used for cesarean delivery are described below.

Regional anesthesia

Regional anesthetic techniques are increasingly being used for cesarean deliveries in many obstetric centers. The popularity of regional anesthesia stems from the improvements and refinements made in pharmacological armamentarium, equipment, monitoring and clinical management. Regional block provides effective anesthesia with significant maternal and fetal advantages over general anesthesia and enables the mother to experience the joy of childbirth. Regional anesthesia permits active participation in childbirth and most parturients find the experience more satisfying than general anesthesia.

Techniques used as a part of regional anesthesia include:

- Epidural anesthesia
- Spinal anesthesia
- Combined spinal epidural anesthesia

Epidural anesthesia is the favored technique used for elective cesarean section. It is also preferred in a variety of medical disorders associated with pregnancy (this aspect is discussed later in the chapter). Epidural anesthesia may be administered in lateral or sitting position.

A small skin wheal is created with a local anesthetic between the second and third lumber vertebrae. The epidural needle (either 16 or 18 gauge needle) is introduced through the skin wheal between the second and third lumber interspace and advanced. It is very important to identify the epidural space; the most commonly used and the most reliable technique is the loss of resistance technique. Once the loss of resistance is felt with the syringe and the epidural space is identified, the local anesthetic drug is injected (The drug i.e. the test dose is usually given after the catheter is introduced - the catheter introduction can pierce the dura). The total dose is fractionated and administered to minimize the risk of complications occurring after an accidental placement of the needle (subarachnoid or intravascular placement). Test dosing is one of the useful methods to prevent or detect aberrant catheter placement[25]. The addition of a small drop of epinephrine to a 5-ml test dose of local anesthetic has been advocated; tachycardia after the test dose would indicate intravenous placement. This is however still controversial in obstetrics[12]. A total of 15-25 ml of local anesthetic is administered, preferably with the patient in left lateral position to minimize risk of aorto-caval compression.

After administration of the complete drug, the epidural catheter is advanced into the epidural space and then taped in place. The patient is then put in the supine position with left uterine displacement.

After drug administration and ascertaining that catheter placement is correct, the upper and lower levels of the blocks should be checked and documented before the start of the surgery. Although, maternal pain during surgery occurs in less than 10% of cases, all patients should be forewarned of this possibility and complaints of intraoperative pain should be heeded and managed[26]. Pain may result from inadequate anesthesia, visceral input, subcostal or referred shoulder tip pain, or precordial pain[3].

Spinal anesthesia also has been a favored technique for cesarean delivery. It has several advantages as a technique for regional anesthesia. The advantages of spinal anesthesia include a faster onset, reliability of needle placement, relative ease of the technique, reduced postoperative sequelae and the virtual elimination of the risk of local anesthetic toxicity[27, 28]. The potential disadvantages include an increased likelihood of hypotension and post dural puncture headache. The incidence of post dural puncture headaches has been dramatically reduced by use of small gauge non-cutting spinal needles.

Spinal/Subarachnoid block can be administered in sitting or lateral position. A small wheal is created in the skin with a local anesthetic over the chosen lumber interspace(usually L3-L4 or L2-L3). A fine gauge spinal needle is introduced and advanced for a calculated distance and the CSF flow identified. Both bupivacaine and lignocaine are used but the latter is disadvantaged by a short duration of action (45-60 mins). Bupivacaine is available as hyperbaric and isobaric solutions. The hyperbaric solution is preferred because of its reliable spread to midthoracic level and appropriate duration of action. Isobaric solution compares favorably, although it may occasionally produce a high block, especially when injected in the sitting position.

After the needle is withdrawn, the patient is turned supine and left uterine displacement ascertained. A facemask is applied and 100% oxygen is administered. Blood pressure is periodically checked to detect the occurrence of hypotension at the earliest when the left uterine displacement is augmented and so is the intravenous fluid administration.

Combined spinal-epidural anesthesia has become popular in many obstetric centers for elective cesarean section. It was first described by Brownridge in 1981 and since then has gained popularity for a number of advantages[29]. It combines the advantages of spinal anesthesia for surgery with the flexibility afforded by epidural catheterization[30]. The technique is more reliable than epidural block alone, with minimal risk of perioperative conversion to general anesthesia due to inadequate anesthesia.

After conventional anesthesia, the epidural catheter is employed if required to extend anesthesia cephalad, but principally dosed for postoperative pain relief. Epidural space is identified by the loss of resistance technique using the standard Tuohy needle. A 25-27 gauge spinal needle is introduced through this to pierce the duramater. Spinal local anesthetic drug is injected through this after confirmation by flow of CSF. The spinal needle is removed and the epidural catheter is introduced through the Tuohy needle which is in the epidural space. The level of block can be controlled by incremental epidural dosing. This has the advantage of better hemodynamic stability, fewer side effects, and faster recovery at the expense of a longer preparation time for surgery.

There are several advantages of regional anesthesia, which make it a popular technique of anesthesia. Some of the advantages are listed below :

- Lower incidence of maternal mortality
- Reduced postoperative morbidity
- Less neonatal resuscitation
- Awake, alert mother
- Immediate maternal bonding
- Early establishment of breast feeding

Complications of regional anesthesia

They include total spinal block, subdural block, intravenous injection, hypotension and shivering.

Total spinal block or high block may occur due to excessive and unpredictable spread of spinal anesthesia, accidental subarachnoid injection of epidural solution, or following a spinal anesthesia after a failed epidural block[31]. Total spinal block may occur unexpectedly despite failure to aspirate cerebrospinal fluid, a negative test dose, and a previously normal epidural response. The classic symptoms of a total spinal block include rapidly ascending sensory change, paralysis, apneoa, hypotension and unconsciousness[32]. Avoidance of aorto-caval compression and early protection of airway to avoid aspiration must not be forgotten. Maternal monitoring should be intensive and circulatory support should be given. A good prognosis follows early resuscitation, ventilation, and circulatory support accompanied by anesthesia or sedation until block regresses to a safe level.

Subdural block is well recognized and the reported incidence ranges from 1% to one in 1400 in the obstetric population[33]. The subdural space lies between the dura and the arachnoid mater and contains a minute quantity of serous fluid. The subdural space is present throughout the spinal meninges and also extends intracranially. Subdural entry is usually indistinguishable from an uneventful epidural injection, although sometimes a prominent backflow of solution or immediate headache is noted. Subdural block shows a varied spectrum of clinical manifestations, from early or delayed high sensory block with minimal systemic disturbance to immediate life threatening apnea and hypotension. Ventilation and intubation is required if consciousness, respiration or swallowing is impaired.

Intravenous injection is another complication, which might occur due to accidental injection. This is more likely in pregnancy due to engorgement of the epidural venous plexus and relatively low venous pressure. The sequelae of accidental intravenous injection of local anesthetic can be serious (seizures, respiratory and cardiac arrest), and has caused several maternal mortalities[34]. More recently, there has been a decline is the incidence of reported deaths due to a greater awareness and better prevention of accidental intravenous injection[35]. The pathophysiology of central nervous system and cardiac toxicity has been exhaustively reviewed[36]. Early features include tinitus, visual disturbance, oral and perioral tingling and numbness, metallic taste and slurring of speech but these symptoms may be unreliable as they may be masked by sedative drugs or be absent prior to sudden onset of convulsions or cardiac arrest. The entire obstetric team should be trained to recognize and manage these symptoms of serious toxicity.

Hypotension is the most common immediate complication of regional anesthesia. In the supine position in late pregnancy, partial or complete inferior vena caval compression near its bifurcation is likely in about 90% of patients and prevention of aorto-caval compression is pivotal to the safe management of regional blocks[5]. The full left lateral or left lateral tilt should be assumed till the surgery commences, after which uterine displacement is achieved by either table tilt or wedging under the right hip and buttock.

As mentioned earlier, hypotension associated with regional anesthesia is more likely with elective surgery than with laboring patients[17]. After the spinal anesthesia, blood pressure falls rapidly, usually within 3 to 10 minutes and the 10° head down position does not reduce the incidence. Intravenous fluid preloading should be done as discussed above. Preloading with crystalloid appears to be only of minor benefit because of rapid extracellular redistribution, crystalloid increases blood volume by only about 20% of the volume administered[37]. Aggressive rapid volume loading also significantly increases central venous pressure, reduces colloid osmotic pressure and hematocrit. The maximum benefit, however, is achieved with a crystalloid volume of about 10 ml/kg. Dextrose containing fluid should be avoided because maternal hyperglycemia and hyperinsulinemia predispose to subsequent neonatal hypoglycemia[12]. There are some studies, which suggest preloading with colloid, which has a longer intravascular half-life, and more effectively expands blood volume but its disadvantages include cost and occasional anaphylactoid reactions. Vasopressors are widely used to combat hypotension during regional anesthesia and their prophylactic administration is more effective than preloading[38]. But the use of vasopressor alone is usually not recommended as they may cause fetal acidosis. The commonly used vasopressor is Ephedrine. This can be given in incremental doses of 5 mg intravenously if hypotension occurs. For prophylaxis 15-30 mg can be given intramuscularly before giving regional anesthesia.

Shivering also occurs in some patients who have been administered regional anesthesia.

The etiology of shivering is multifactorial. Some of these factors are anxiety, inadequate skin covering, skin and body cavity exposure and blood loss during surgery. During regional blocks, the loss of sympathetically mediated skin and peripheral vasoconstriction may result in heat loss but a more important factor is the redistribution of heat from the central core to the periphery, which results in a rapid fall of core temperature[39]. Surface prewarming or forced air warming, both of which reduce redistribution of heat from central compartment, is effective in preventing shivering. In patients with and epidural catheter in situ, administration of epidural fentanyl (25 mg or more) reduces the proportion of parturients who shiver[40].

Post dural puncture headache (PDPH) occurs after spinal anesthesia and can be an annoying complication. Following a spinal anesthesia, there is CSF leakage through the dural hole producing a low CSF pressure[41]. The low pressure following CSF leakage through the dural hole leads to traction on the pain sensitive structures in the brain with associated cerebral vasodilatation when the patient is upright[42]. The headache lasts until the hole in the dura spontaneously heals and CSF pressure is restored; the headache lasts for a few days but rarely more than a week. The patient is advised bed rest as assuming a horizontal position alleviate the pain[41]. Normal hydration should be maintained as dehydration makes the symptoms worse. Over hydration, as is commonly prescribed, to help the body make more CSF, does not decrease the headache. Narcotic analgesics and in some cases, non-steroidal anti-inflammatory drugs should be administered to decrease the severity of pain. Some authors suggest the use of caffeine to help constrict vasodialated blood vessels[42]. Boluses or infusion of epidural normal saline can help to transiently increase the epidural pressure, slowing the speed at which CSF leaks through the dural hole[43]. This may speed the natural healing process. Although epidural saline can be a useful technique, higher success rates are often achieved with epidural blood patches[44].

An association has been noticed between the needle size and the incidence of post dural puncture headache. The incidence of PDPH can be as high as 80% if puncture occurs with a 16G needle[45]. Some authors have suggested that the incidence of PDPH can be reduced to almost 0% with the use of specially designed, non-cutting point, fine gauge needles. However, most recent series report incidences of 1%-3% even with these smaller gauge needles[46]. The fact that not every patient has a headache after dural puncture, even with 16G needles, would indicate that the degree of inter-patient variability and difference in technique of insertion also have a profound effect on incidence. The factors which have been identified in affecting the incidence of PDPH are the size of needle (decreased incidence with smaller needles), design of needle (decreased incidence with a non-cutting tip as compared with a cutting tip), relationship of bevel to the dural fibers (decreased incidence if needle bevel is parallel to dural fibers), angle of puncture of the dura (less with acute angles), and the choice of local anesthetic agent (lignocaine > bupivacaine > tetracaine) [46]. The nomenclature of needle size derives from the "Standard Wire Gauge" used to measure electrical wires. The commonly used sizes of spinal needles are 22G-27G. However, spinal needles are available in a variety of sizes from 19G-30G.

Contraindications to regional anesthesia are few and are mentioned in the box below :

- Bleeding disorders
- Uncorrected hypovolemia, and shock
- Major hemorrhage
- Anticoagulation and severe preeclampsia induced thrombocytopenia
- Disorders of the spine
- Local anesthetic allergy
- Local infection
- Maternal disease (e.g. specific cardiac diseases)
- Refusal to consent

Regional anesthesia is an advantageous technique for cesarean section and is safe provided necessary precautions are taken.
A basic protocol is suggested below :

- Administer a non-particulate oral antacid within one hour of induction of anesthesia
- Transport patient to the operating room in lateral position
- In the operating room, ensure left uterine displacement.
- Administer preloading intravenous fluid with a dextrose free balanced salt solution
- Check resuscitation equipment and drugs before instituting block
- Institute desired block
- Administer 100% oxygen via face mask
- Monitor blood pressure periodically and treat hypotension with vasopressors.

General anesthesia

With improvement in the techniques of regional anesthesia, general anesthesia is no longer the preferred technique for cesarean delivery. But, there are many clinical situations where general anesthesia is preferred. In contrast to regional anesthesia, general anesthesia has the advantages of a more rapid induction, less associated hypotension and cardiovascular instability and better control of airway and ventilation.

Concern regarding general anesthesia is primarily because of the morbidity and mortality associated with it. Death is usually due to hypoxia secondary to problems with tracheal intubation or from aspiration pneumonitis. More recently, however, there has been a considerable decrease in the mortality associated with general anesthesia due to improved techniques[41]. Still, however, the indication for general anesthesia must be valid and a note of it should be made in the patient notes.

Preoperative assessment of the patient prior to general anesthesia is extremely mandatory. It is important to assess the patient in a structured manner. Ideally for all high-risk patients who are likely to need general anesthesia in labor, the obstetrician should request an antenatal anesthetic evaluation. This allows a proper assessment of the patient with study of previous notes and investigations. During such an evaluation, a proper history should include obstetric details, details of previous anesthetic charts, medical illnesses, and a history of known drug allergies. A thorough examination should be done including a mandatory assessment of airway. An attempt should be made to predict difficult intubation in patients at this stage. The three best predictors of difficult intubation are inability to visualize the posterior pharyngeal wall when the mouth is wide open and the tongue protruded, a thyromental distance of less than 7 cms with full head extension and not being able to protrude the jaw so that the lower incisors fail to overlap the upper incisors[42,43,44]. Assessment of mouth opening, neck movement and body mass index may also help to predict difficulties with intubation[45]. It should be remembered that failed intubation may still occur in a woman with a previous successful tracheal intubation during pregnancy[46].

Aspiration pneumonitis is a major cause of maternal mortality and morbidity during administration of general anesthesia. Therefore of paramount importance during general anesthesia is the antacid prophylaxis. Heartburn and regurgitation occur in 80% of pregnant women at term and nearly all pregnant women at term can be regarded to have an incompetent oesophageal sphincter[47]. The incidence of aspiration pneumonitis has reduced over the years due to antacid prophylaxis, preoxygenation, cricoid pressure and tracheal intubation.

Antacid prophylaxis for elective surgeries can be given in the form of ranitidine (H_2 blocker) or omeprezole (proton pump inhibitor) given orally on the previous night and if necessary repeated on the morning of the surgery. For emergency surgeries, oral 30 ml of 0.3 M sodium citrate is given immediately before the induction of anesthesia. But the action of sodium citrate lasts only for 30 minutes with normal gastric emptying; therefore the risk of aspiration remains high in some women[48]. Addition of Metoclopramide caused no improvement in the risk but the latter was reduced if in addition to sodium citrate, patients also received ranitidine 50 mg intravenously immediately after the decision of surgery was made[49].

Preoxygenation is necessary in all obstetric patients needing general anesthesia. The object of preoxygenation is to replace the alveolar nitrogen with oxygen to give a period of apnea without hypoxemia. A common problem with preoxygenation is failure to make an adequate seal between the mask and face, which allows room air to be inspired. It also prevents the reservoir bag from distending and therefore expiratory valve fails to open, causing rebreathing of nitrogen. The bag must distend to ensure an adequate seal between the patient's face and the mask.

Cricoid pressure is used to prevent regurgitation during induction of anesthesia in patients at risk of pulmonary aspiration. Sellick first described the maneuver of cricoid pressure in 1961[50]. Cricoid pressure is applied with the single-handed technique using a force of 10 N (1 kg); use of too strong a force is more likely to flex the head and make the laryngoscopy more difficult[51]. Normally, the upper oesophageal sphincter prevents regurgitation into the pharynx; during intravenous induction of anesthesia the sphincter relaxes just before the loss of consciousness[52]. Cricoid pressure should therefore be applied to the awake patient before loss of consciousness. Use of a very strong force at cricoid pressure may be very uncomfortable and this may cause retching; therefore light cricoid pressure should be applied to awake patients (10 N or 1 kg)[53]. The pressure may be increased to 30 N (3kg) after loss of consciousness[54]. Forces of over 40 N can cause airway obstruction, difficulty in passing the tube and impaired view at laryngoscopy without neck support[53]. Anesthetic trainees can be taught to apply correct pressure by practicing on weighing scales.

Induction of anesthesia is done following preoxygenation and application of cricoid pressure. Three minutes after the start of adequate preoxygenation anesthesia is induced with 4-7 mg/kg of Thiopentone given intravenously over about 20 seconds. Thiopentone is the agent of choice for induction of cesarean delivery as it maintains a balance between maternal unconsciousness with minimal neonatal depression and hemodynamic instability[55]. Following administration of Thiopentone, loss of consciousness is noted and suxamethonium 1.5 mg/kg is given and flushed with the intravenous infusion. Suxamethonium gives rapid intubating conditions within 60 seconds and usually wears off within 6 minutes[55]. With loss of consciousness, the cricoid pressure is increased to a firm pressure but laryngoscopy is not attempted for about 60 seconds or until suxamethonium fasciculations have stopped and full neuromuscular blockade has been achieved.

Intubation may be attempted after achieving full neuromuscular blockade. Ventilation of the lungs should not be attempted during this time. Insertion of the laryngoscope is now done with the handle pointing towards the patient's right shoulder. The handle is subsequently turned towards the midline and at the same time the tongue is pushed towards the left. After intubation and cuff inflation, the tube position must be checked, the chest excursions observed and the breath sounds examined.

Maintenance of anesthesia is done with inhalational agents and short acting non-depolarising muscle relaxants. Volatile anesthetic agents cross the placenta and are taken up by fetal tissue. Provided the mean alveolar concentration is below a critical level and the induction delivery time is less than 8 minutes, minimal neonatal depression is caused[56]. Above a critical alveolar concentration, the volatile agents cause a dose dependant relaxation of the uterus. Nitrous oxide is also taken up by the fetus but no untoward effects have been noted with 50% concentration provided the induction delivery interval is not prolonged[55].

Recovery from general anesthesia after the completion of the surgery should be done with equal amount of care and concern. The neuromuscular block is reversed, the volatile agents and nitrous oxide are discontinued and ventilation with 100% oxygen continued until spontaneous breathing returns. The carbon dioxide concentration may be allowed to rise at the end of surgery so that spontaneous ventilation is aided. The pharynx is cleared by gentle suction. After the patient regains consciousness, the endotracheal tube is deflated and the tube is removed. Supplemental oxygen is administered till the patient is fully awake.

Complications of general anesthesia are mainly relating to difficulties with intubation and aspiration pneumonitis.

As already mentioned an attempt should be made to assess the difficulty at intubation during preoperative assessment. [The three best predictors of difficult intubation are inability to visualize the posterior pharyngeal wall when mouth is wide open and tongue protruded, a thyromental distance of less than 7 cms with full head extension and not being able to protrude the jaw so that the lower incisors fail to overlap the upper incisors[42,43,44]].

In the obstetric patient, intubation can be frequently difficult especially with lateral body tilt, cricoid pressure and vocal cord edema. To minimize the difficulty, the head and neck must be properly positioned and the neuromuscular block must be allowed to develop before intubation is attempted. During the second attempt at intubation, some authorities suggest that the cricoid pressure should be released[57]. No more than two attempts at intubation should be done; it is important to abandon attempts at intubation and make the diagnosis of failed intubation at an early stage before hypoxemia sets in. Once the diagnosis of failed intubation is made, senior anesthetic assistance should be immediately called and the cricoid pressure maintained. An oral airway should be inserted and manual ventilation should be attempted using 100% oxygen via a face mask. If ventilation proves difficult, the amount of cricoid pressure may be reduced to half and ventilation tried again as excessive pressure may obstruct the airway. If ventilation is still not satisfactory, the oral airway should be replaced with a laryngeal mask airway. If after the insertion of the laryngeal mask, ventilation is still not possible, the next step is to insert a cricothyrotomy canula. The final option in this drill is to perform a tracheostomy.

Spontaneous ventilation returns after the effects of the suxamethonium wear off. The further plan of action depends on the urgency for delivery. It should be remembered that failed intubation and failed ventilation are life-threatening situations and all anesthetists managing obstetric patients should be fully conversant with their management.

Another important and potentially life threatening complication is aspiration pneumonitis. The reasons why term pregnant patients are more prone to this complication are already mentioned in the text above. Every attempt should be made to avoid and prevent this complication. The clinical consequence of pulmonary aspiration depends on the amount of aspirate, the pH of the aspirate and its extent of distribution in the pulmonary tissue[58]. Aspiration of a large volume of gastric contents may lead to acute lung injury within a period of two hours. Other clinical features include dyspnea, tachypnea, tachycardia, productive cough with a pink frothy sputum and hypotension. In patients suspected to have aspiration, immediate pharyngeal suction must be performed. This should be done with the mother on the side to prevent further aspiration. If the mother is awake, coughing is effective at expelling small fragments of aspirated material. If however, the mother is unconscious, intubation and tracheal suction must be done. Cardiovascular support may be needed and so is mechanical ventilation in cases of hypoxemia not responding to above management. The patient must be nursed and managed in an intensive care unit.

A basic protocol for cesarean section is suggested below:

- Check consent and preoperative assessment records, if any
- Administration of a oral sodium citrate 30 ml 0.3 M with ranitidine 50 mg IV
- Left uterine displacement
- Start IV infusion with a large bore intravenous access

- Preoxygenate for 3 minutes with high flow oxygen
- Apply cricoid pressure
- Induce with Thiopentone and suxamethonium
- Intubate, inflate and ventilate
- Maintain anesthesia with volatile anesthetics
- Avoid maternal hyperventilation.

ANESTHESIA FOR SPECIAL SITUATIONS

There are a lot of patients requiring cesarean section; some of those are normal while others have associated high risk factors. The associated high risk factors may be obstetric or non-obstetric. A number of patients with medical illnesses require cesarean section, for various reasons. Choosing the correct anesthetic technique for such patients is of paramount importance as it has an important bearing on the morbidity following the surgical childbirth. Some of the common and important situations are discussed below:

Preeclampsia and Eclampsia

Preeclampsia and Eclampsia are leading causes of maternal morbidity and mortality. The pathophysiology changes in preeclampsia involve nearly every organ system. There is a generalized vasoconstriction, and despite retention of sodium and water and generalized edema, the intravascular volume is usually decreased. Glomerular filtration rate, renal blood flow, renal function, and urinary output may be reduced. Fibrin deposits are present within the glomeruli and most of the small blood vessels of the body. Uteroplacental perfusion is decreased and fetal distress is common. Eclamptic patients are usually treated with magnesium sulphate. Magnesium sulphate decreases the amount of acetyl cholinesterase at the neuromuscular junction, and depresses the excitability of the muscle membrane. The therapeutic maternal levels of magnesium sulphate are 4-7 mEq/L.

The use of epiduaral or spinal anesthesia in a patient with preeclampsia or eclampsia is controversial. In a large series of eclamptic patients, it was shown that regional anesthesia should be avoided as it may further compromise uteroplacental circulation secondary to sympathetic block and maternal hypotension[59]. However, studies stating the avoidance of spinal anesthesia in preeclampsia have been poorly controlled studies[60]. Other investigators have recommended continuous epidural anesthesia in severe preeclampsia and eclampsia to help control blood pressure and to increase renal and uterine perfusion[61].

In patients with evidence of acquired coagulopathy or in patients where regional anesthesia cannot be offered, general anesthesia is indicated e.g. severe coagulopathy, maternal hypovolemia or depressed level of consciousness. The standard technique for general anesthesia is modified to avoid prolonged paralysis due to the interaction of magnesium with muscle relaxants. If muscle relaxants are given, their doses should be carefully titrated, and their effects monitored with a nerve muscle stimulator[61]. Additionally, drugs such as methoxyflurane and ketamine should be avoided. Endotracheal intubation and surgical stimulation under light anesthesia can produce dramatic increase in the blood pressure and therefore extreme care should be taken[62]. Efforts should be made to obtund the hypertensive response to tracheal intubation as this may increase the risk of cerebral hemorrhage. It should be noted that the b-blocker esmolol produces fetal bradycardia and should not be used predelivery but is of value in preventing a rise in blood pressure on extubation.

Cardiac disease

Anesthesia for pregnant patients with heart disease requires an understanding of the pathophysiologic changes associated with pregnancy as well as the changes induced by the cardiovascular condition. There are considerable adaptations that occur in pregnancy and patients with cardiac disease may not tolerate them. The cardiac output increases by about 30-50% as a result of increases in both stroke volume and heart rate. These changes peak during the third trimester (28-32 weeks) and cardiac output increases again during labor.

Drugs used during obstetric anaesthesia can affect cardiovascular performance either directly or indirectly through the autonomic nervous system. If an appropriate analgesic or anesthetic technique is selected for a parturient, the hemodynamic consequences of the chosen method can sometimes be used to the advantage of the parturient with cardiovascular disease.

Patients with cardiac disease should be managed with a multidisciplinary approach. Heart diseases can be broadly classified into congenital and acquired types. The most common cause of acquired heart disease in India and other developing countries is Rheumatic heart disease. Congenital heart diseases may be further classified into cyanotic and acyanotic heart diseases. Most patients with acyanotic congenital heart disease have a successful outcome to pregnancy.

The most commonly affected valve in rheumatic heart disease is the mitral valve. If uncorrected the stenosis at the level of the valve increases over a period of time. As the stenosis increases, the flow through the stenotic valve decreases and causes an increase in the left atrial pressure. This over a period of time leads to secondary pulmonary hypertension culminating in right ventricular failure. Another complication that patients with mitral stenosis develop is atrial fibrillation. Patients are initially managed with medical therapy but if medical treatment fails, balloon valvuloplasty may be required. Some patients with severe disease may require mitral valve replacement. Anticoagulants are used in these patients to decrease the risk of thrombus formation. If the patient is not receiving oral anticoagulants, epidural anesthesia may be given. Many authors recommend epidural block as the technique of choice in providing anaesthesia for caesarean section in these patients[69, 70]. However, during cesarean section, the level of the block should be increased cautiously to avoid sudden decrease in systemic vascular resistance, which some patients may not be able to tolerate.

Patients with regurgitant lesions fare well in pregnancy, as the vasodilatation and slight increase in the heart size tend to reduce regurgitation. For these patients, epidural anesthesia is recommended. In these patients an increase in systemic vascular resistance should be prevented. Epidural block is the technique of choice for anaesthesia for caesarean delivery[71].

Acyanotic lesions are more common types seen in pregnancy than acyanotic ones. One of the most common congenital heart diseases seen in pregnancy is atrial septal defect. Epidural anesthesia should be preferred in these patients. For patients with ventricular septal defects undergoing cesarean section, either regional or general anesthesia may be used but as far as the regional block is considered, epidural should be preferred compared to the spinal anesthesia. Patients with aortic stenosis have a fixed cardiac output and are unable to compensate for decreases in the systemic vascular resistance except by increasing their heart rate. The choice of anesthesia for these patients has been a matter of controversy but general anesthesia may be used.

For patients with tetralogy of Fallot undergoing caesarean section both light and deep levels of general anaesthesia have been advocated[71]. Tachycardia or infundibular spasm can be prevented by the administration of cardio-selective β-blockers.

Patients with Eisenmenger's Syndrome present with pulmonary hypertension with right-to-left or left-to-right shunt at aorto-pulmonary, ventricular or atrial level. A decrease in the ratio of systemic to pulmonary vascular resistance results in increasing cyanosis. In these patients pregnancy and delivery are associated with a high mortality rate[72]. For caesarean section the anesthetic technique of choice is general anaesthesia using drugs that do not depress cardiovascular function.

In patients with Coarctation of the aorta, the main cardiovascular consequence is a chronically increased left ventricular afterload that causes hypertrophy of the left ventricle. General anaesthesia is preferred for cesarean section[71].

Choice of anesthetic for cesarean delivery in parturient with heart diseases should be assessed individually with special attention to the functional impairment and use of invasive monitors. General anesthesia with endotracheal tube provides airway protection and mechanical ventilation eliminates the work of breathing and reduces oxygen consumption. The complications of general anesthesia may include decreased venous return, ventricular dysfunction, and compression of pulmonary vessels, hypoxemia, hypo/hypercarbia and acidosis. Regional anesthesia allows spontaneous ventilation with little disruption of ventilation-perfusion relationship. Epidural catheter technique offers continuous, titrated anesthesia or analgesia with gradually advancing block and hemodynamic stability.

Thus, the decision to use a particular anesthetic technique for cesarean delivery should be individualized based on anesthetic, obstetric and/or fetal risk factors and the preference of the patient and anesthesiologist. Resources for the treatment of potential complications should be available.

Diabetes Mellitus

Anesthetic requirements in diabetic women are common as many patients require instrumental or operative delivery. In these patients, regional anesthesia is preferred[73]. It should be remembered that fluid preload should not preferably contain dextrose. Strict control of blood glucose is mandatory to prevent hypoglycemia in the neonate. The complications of diabetes e.g. autonomic neuropathy, stiff joint syndrome make general anesthesia more risky than the regional anesthesia.

Thrombophilia and pregnancy

Thrombophilias are conditions, which predispose the patient to develop thomboembolic disease. Thrombophilias may be congenital or acquired. The congenital thormbophilias are due to anti thrombin III deficiency, deficiency of protein C or protein S, and activated protein C resistance. The most common cause of acquired thrombophilia is antiphospholipid antibody syndrome. The choice of anesthesia in these classes of patients is to be individualized after careful assessment of risks and benefits.

Generally, regional anesthesia is avoided for fear of producing hematomas. General anesthesia on the other hand may actually increase the risk of thrombosis[63]. Patients with platelet counts of greater than 100 X 109/ml can be safely administered regional blocks, especially if the clotting studies are normal. It is generally considered safe to perform a regional block on patients receiving aspirin and prophylactic doses of subcutaneous heparin[64]. When full doses of heparin are being used, a regional block should not be performed for at least six hours after the last dose and an aPTT level should be checked.

Other diseases

For patients with epilepsy, regional block can be used. If general anesthesia is used, drugs with epileptogenic potential should be avoided e.g. ketamine.

For patients with renal disease, regional blocks may be used. However, care should be taken to maintain renal perfusion while at the same time not causing fluid overload. If a general anesthesia is used for cesarean section, suxamethonium should be used with caution if the serum potassium level is high. Atracurium is the non-depolarizing muscle relaxant of choice for maintenance as its elimination is independent of renal function.

Patients suffering from bronchial asthma should be preferably given regional anesthesia as it decreases the respiratory work and reduces maternal stress and hyperventilation, which may cause bronchospasm. When general anesthesia is required, a rapid sequence induction should be used to prevent aspiration although in some patients bronchospasm may result.

Local anesthesia for Cesarean section

Local anesthetic infiltration for caesarean delivery is a rarely used technique. It has application in situations where both general and regional anaesthesia is contraindicated and in situations when health resources are limited e.g. anesthetic expertise is lacking/limited, anesthetic equipment or gas supplies are unavailable[73,74]. It may also find usefulness in certain clinical scenarios e.g. familial dysautonomia, myotonic dystrophy[74]. The advantages of local infiltration anesthesia are that: it allows for immediate commencement of surgery in emergency situations, avoids sudden hemodynamic changes that occur with regional blocks and it protects patient's airway reflexes[73].

In this technique, infiltration is begun in the subcutaneous plane to anesthetize the skin. The fat layer is relatively devoid of innervation and a large amount of local anesthetic may be wasted by infiltrating this layer, which is relevant to the often large total dose used; this should therefore be avoided. As far as the fascia is concerned, direct infiltration can be used, however, bilateral rectus sheath blocks may be used. Retropubic space can be a difficult area to anaesthetize and may require additional infiltration retropubically and into the pyramidalis muscles. Parietal peritoneum can also be a difficult area to anaesthetize and several techniques have been described: The injection of several ml of solution through the fascia (before its division) helps to separate the layers and to anaesthetize the parietal peritoneum. Once the peritoneum is opened, 10-15ml of local anesthetic is instilled into the peritoneal cavity. Visceral peritoneum / uterus do not need infiltration, but doing so separates the visceral layer of the peritoneum from the lower uterine segment[75].

While performing this technique, the maximum dose of the drug instilled should be kept in mind; the volume required may be as high as 100 ml. Not all of this may be required initially, and further infiltration may be necessary after delivery to close the superficial layers. Lignocaine 0.5% or chloroprocaine 1% with 1:200,000 adrenaline is adequate for infiltration anaesthesia and both agents are rapid in onset. The addition of adrenaline allows for the use of a greater overall dose. Longer acting agents such as bupivacaine have a slower onset time and a lower free drug concentration in the fetal blood[76]. The addition of hyaluronidase has been described[77] but may increase absorption.

In their series of 141 caesarean sections, Ranney and Stannage reported 61 patients having a second, 14 a third and 2 a fourth operation[78]. Only three patients wanted to have general anaesthesia for their repeat procedure.

REFERENCES

1. Capless EL, Clapp J. Cardiovascular changes in early phase of pregnancy. Am J Obstet Gynecol 1989; 161:1449-1453.
2. Robson SC, Hunter S, Boys R, Dunlop W. Serial factors influencing changes in cardiac output during human pregnancy. Am J physiol 1989; 256:H1060-H1065.
3. James Eldrige: Maternal changes in pregnancy. In: Anesthesia for Obstetrics & Gynecology Robin Russel eds. BMJ books 2000;1-30.
4. Ahltorp G. On problems in supine hypotension in pregnant women. Acta Obstet Gynecol Scand 1935;15:295-341.
5. Kerr MG, Scott DB, Samuel E. Studies on the inferior vena cava in late pregnancy. Br Med J 1964;1: 532-533.
6. Kinsella SM, Lohmann G. Supine hypotensive syndrome. Obstet Gynecol 1994;83:774-787.

7. Bieniarz J, Yoshida T, Romero-Salinas G, et al. Aortocaval compression by the uterus in late human pregnancy.IV. Circulatory homeostasis by preferential perfusion of the placenta. Am J Obstet Gynecol 1969;103:19-31.

8. Alaily AB, Carrol K. Pulmonary ventilation in pregnancy. Br J Obstet Gynecol 1978;85: 518-524.

9. Spatling L, Fallenstein F, Huch A, Huch R, Rooth G. The variability of cardiopulmonary adaptation to pregnancy at rest and during exercise. Br J Obstet Gynecol 1992;99: 1-40.

10. Kambam JR, Handte RE, Brown WU, Smith BE. Effect of normal and preeclamptic pregnancies on the oxyhemoglobin dissociation curve. Anesthesiology 1986;65:426-427.

11. Bassey OO. Pregnancy heartburn in Nigerians and Caucasians with theories about etiology based manometric recordings from the esophagus and stomach. Br J Obstet Gynecol 1977;84:439-443.

12. Gerard Bassel: Anesthesia for cearean section. In Clinics of Obstetrics and Gynecology eds. 1985;722-735.

13. Abboud TK, Afrasiabi A, Sarkis F, et al. Contininoius infusion epidural analgesia in parturients receiving bupivacaine,chlorprocaine, or lidocaine-maternal, fetal and neonatal effects. Anesth Analg 1984; 63: 421-428.

14. Kuhnert BR, Harrison MJ, Linn PL, Kuhnert PM. Effects of maternal epidural anesthesia on neonatal behavior. Anesth Analg 1984;63:301-308.

15. Roenblatt DB, Belsey EM, Lieberman BA, et al. The influence of maternal analgesia on neonatal behavior: II Epidural Bupivacaine. Br J Obstet Gynecol 1981;88: 407-413.

16. Lewis M, Thomas P, Wilkes FG. Hypotension during epidural analgesia for cesarean section:arterial and central venous pressure changes after acute intravenous loading with two litres of Hartman's solution. Anesthesia 1983;38:250.

17. Antoine C, Young BK. Fetal Lactic acidosis with epidural anesthesia. Am J Obstet Gynecol.1982;142: 55-59.

18. Caritis SN, Abouleish E, Edelstone DI, Mueller-Heubach E. Fetal acid base state following spinal or epidural anesthesia for cesarean section. Obstet Gynecol 1980: 56:610-615.

19. Marx GF, Mateo CV. Effects of different oxygen concentrations during general anesthesia for elective cesarean section. Can Anesth Soc J 1971;18:587.

20. Fox GS, Houle GL. Acid base studies in elective cesarean section during epidural and general anesthesia. Can Anesth Soc J 1971;18:60-71.

21. Ramnathan S, Gandhi S, Arismendy J, Chalon J, Turndorf H. Oxygen transfer from mother to fetus during cesarean section under epidural anesthesia. Anesth Analg 1982;61:576-581.

22. James FM, Crawford JS, Hoplkinson R, Davies P, Naiem H. A comparison of general anesthesia and lumber epidural analgesia for elective cesarean section. Anesth Analg 1977;56:228-235.

23. Shnider SM, Moya F. The hyperventilation controversy. In: Shnider SM, Moya F. eds The anesthesiologist, mother and newborn. Baltimore: Williams and Wilkins, 1974:98.

24. Datta S. Ostheimer GW, Weiss JB, Brown WU, Alper MH. Neonatal effect of prolonged anesthetic induction for cesarean section. Obstet Gynecol 1981;58:331.

25. Mulroy MF, Norris MC, Liu SS. Safety steps for epidural injection of local anesthetics: review of literature and recommendations. Anesth Analg 1997;85:1346-1356.

26. Paech MJ, Godkin R, Wbster S. Complications of obstetric epidural analgesia and anesthesia: a prospective analysis of 10995 cases. Int J Obstet Anesth 1998;7:5-11.

27. Davies SJ, Paech MJ, Welch H, Evans SF, Pavy TJG. Maternal experiece during epidural or combined spinal epidural anesthesia for cesarean section: a prospective, randomized trial. Anesth Analg 1997;85: 607-613.

28. Lussos SA, Datta S. Anesthesia for cesarean delivery. Part I: General considerations and spinal anesthesia. Int J Obstet Anesth 1992;1:79-91.

29. Brownridge P. Epidural and subarachnoid analgesia for elective cesarean section. Anesthesia. 1981;36:70.

30. Rawal N, Van Zundert A, Holmstrom B, Crowhurst JA. Combined spinal epidural technique. Reg Anesth 1997;22:406-423.

31. Morgan B. Unexpectedly extensive conduction blocks in obstetric epidural analgesia. Anesthesia 1990;45:148-152.

32. Reynolds F, Speedy HM. The subdural space: the third space to go astray. Anesthesia;45:120-123.

33. Hawkins JL, Koonin LM, Palmer SK, Gibbs CP. Anesthesia related deaths during obstetric delivery in United States, 1979-1990. Anesthesiology 1997;86:277-284.

34. Hogan Q. Local anesthetic toxicity : an update. Reg Anesth 1996;21(6S):43-50.

35. Rocke DA, Rout CC. Volume preloading, spinal hypotension and cesarean section. Br J Anesth 1995;75:257-259.

36. Gajraj NM, Victory RA, Pace NA, van Elstraete AC, Wallace DH. Comparison of an ephedrine infusion with crystalloid administration for preventing hypotension during spinal anesthesia. Anesth Analg 1993;76:1023-1026.

37. Glosten B, Hynson J, Sessler DJ, McGuire J. Preanesthetic skin surface warming reduces redistribution hypothermia caused by epidural block. Anesth Analg 1993;77: 488-493.

38. Shehabi Y, Gatt S, Buckman T, Isert P. Effect of adrenaline, fentany; amd warming of injectate on shivering following extradural analgesia in labor. Anesth Intens Care 1990;18:31-37.

39. Jones R J: The role of recumbency in the prevention and treatment of postspinal headache. Anesth Analg1974; 53:788-796.

40. Sechzer PH: Post-spinal anesthesia headache treated with caffeine. Part II: Intracranial vascular distension, a key factor. Curr Therap Res1979; 26:440-448.

41. Usubiaga JE: Effect of saline injections on epidural and subarachnoid space pressures and relation to postspinal anesthesia headache. Anesth Analg1967; 46: 293-296.

42. Bart AJ: Comparison of epidural saline placement and epidural blood placement in the treatment of post-lumbar-puncture headache. Anesthesiology 1978;48:221-223.

43. Halpern S, Preston R. Postdural puncture headache and spinal needle design. Meta-analyses. Anesthesiology 1994;81:1376-1383.

44. Naulty JS et al Anesthesiology 1990;72: 450-454.

45. Brown GW, Russel IF. A survey of anesthesia for cesarean section. Int J Obstet Anesth 1995;4:214 218.

46. Mallampati SR, Gatt SP, Guigino SP, et al. A clinical sign to predict difficult tracheal intubation: a prospective study. Can Anesth Soc J 1985;32:429-434.

47. Patil VU, Stehling LC, Zaunder HL. Fibreoptic endoscopy in anesthesia. Chicago: Year book Medical Publishers, 1983.

48. Calder I, Calder J, Crockard HA. Difficult direct laryngoscopy in patients with cervical spine disease. Anesthesia 1995;50:756-763.

49. Harmer M. Difficult and failed intubation in obstetrics. Int J Obstet Anesth 1997;6:25-31.

50. Hawthorne L, Wilson R, Lyons G, Dresner M. Failed intubation revisited: 17-yr experience in a teaching maternity unit. Br J Anesth 1996;76:680-684.

51. Vanner RG, Goodman NW. Gastro-oesophageal reflux in pregnancy at term and after delivery. Anesthesia 1989;44:808-811.

52. O'Sullivian G. Gastric emptying during pregnancy and the puerperium. Int J Obstet Anesth 1993;2: 216-224.

53. Stuart JC, Kan AF, Rowbottom SJ, Yau G, Oh TE. Acid aspiration prophylaxis for emergency cesarean section. Anesthesia 1996;51:415-421.

54. Sellick BA. Cricoid pressure to control regurgitation of stomach contents during induction of anesthesia. Lancet 1961;2:404-406.

55. Cook TM. Cricoid pressure: are two hands better than one? Anesthesia 1996;51: 365-358.

56. Vanner RG, Pryle BJ, O'Dwyer JP, Reynolds F. Upper oesophageal spincter pressure and the intravenous induction of anesthesia. Anesthesia 1992;47: 371-375.

57. Vanner RG. Tolerance of cricoid pressure by conscious volunteers. Int J Obstet Anesth 1992;1: 195 198.

58. Vanner RG, Asai T. Safe use of cricoid pressure (editorial). Anesthesia 1999;54:1-3.

59. Lussos SA, Datta S. Anesthesia for cesarean delivery. Part III: General Anesthesia. Int J Obstet Anesth 1993;2:109-123.

60. Warren T, Datta S, Ostheimer GW, Naulty JS, Weiss JB, Morrison JA. Comparison of the maternal and neonatal effects of halothane, enflurane, and isoflurane for cesarean delivery. Anesth Analg 1983;62:516-520.

61. Brimacombe JR, Berry AM. Cricoid pressure in chaos. Anesthesia 1997;52:924-926.

62. Lykens MG, Bowton DL. Aspiration and acute lung injury. Int J Obstet Anesth 1993;2:236 240.

63. Pritchard JA, Pritchard SA: Standardized treatment of 154 consecutive cases of preeclampsia. Am J Obstet Gynecol 1975;123: 543.

64. Howell P. Spinal anesthesia in severe preeclampsia: time for preappraisal, or time for caution? Int J Obstet Anesth 1998;7:217-219.

65. Sol MS, Gershon L. Obstetric Anesthesia In: Anesthesia Ronald Miller 2nd eds. Churchill Livingstone. 1986;1681-1720.

66. Hodgkinson R, Husain FJ, Hayashi RH: Systemic and pulmonary blood pressure during cesarean section in parturients with gestational hypertension. Can Anesth Soc J 1980;27:389.

67. Moir DD, Willocks J. Epidural analgesia in British obstetrics. Br J Anaesth 196840:129.

68. Marx GF, Hodgkinson R. Special considerations in complications of pregnancy. In Marx GF; Bassel GM eds, 297-334, Elsevier 1980.

69. Mangano DT. Anesthesia for the pregnant cardiac patient. In: Anesthesia for obstetrics. S Shnider & G. Levinson eds. 345-381, William and Wilkins, Baltimore 1986.

70. Gleicher N, Midwall J, Hockberger D, et al. Eisenmenger's syndrome in pregnancy. Obs Gynecol Surv 1979;3:721.

71. Crawford JS, Mills WG, Pentecost BL. A pregnant patient with Eisenmenger's syndrome. Br J Anaesth 1971;43:1091.

72. Bullingham A, Strunin L. Prevention of postoperative thromboembolism. Br J Anesth 1995;75:622 630.

73. Barker A, Barker M. Caesarean section under local analgesia. Tropical Doctor 1976; 6:23-25.

74. Leiberman JR, Cohen A, Wizniter A, Maayan C, Greemberg L. Cesarean section by local anesthesia in patients with familial dysautonomia. American Journal of Obstetrics and Gynecology 1991;165:110-1.

75. Mackey R. Local anaesthesia in obstetrics. Medical Journal of Australia. 1947; 2: 593.

76. Tucker GE, Mather LE. Properties, absorption, and disposition of local anesthetic agents. In: Cousins MJ, Bridenbaugh PO (eds). Neural Blockade in Clinical Anesthesia and Management of Pain, 2nd ed, JB Lippincott Co, Philadelphia,1988.

77. Busby T. Local anesthesia for cesarean section. American Journal of Obstetrics & Gynecology 1963; 87:399-404.

78. Ranney B, Stannage WF. Advantages of local anesthesia for cesarean section. Obstetrics & Gynecology 1975; 45: 163-167.

11 | CHAPTER

Neonatal Considerations in Caesarean Birth

Sankaranarayanan K., J A Mondkar

FRAMEWORK

INTRODUCTION

There has been a gradual rise in the incidence of caesarean sections during the last three decades. Today, caesarean is not performed as a last resort, but as a safe alternative to a vaginal delivery, which entails risks. However the caesarean delivery of a baby also has certain complications. The first section of this article describes the preparations for and technique of neonatal resuscitation during caesarean section deliveries. This article reviews the neonatal problems associated with a caesarean birth in two main sections: problems due to the caesarean procedure itself and problems secondary to the maternal or fetal condition, which necessitated the procedure.

NEONATAL RESUSCITATION

Approximately 5% to 10% of the newborns require some degree of active resuscitation at birth (e.g., stimulation to breathe) and approximately 1% to 10% born in the hospital are reported to require assisted ventilation. Every newborn has the right to resuscitation performed at a high level of competence.

Prior preparation

Once the decision to perform a caesarean section is intimated to the neonatologist, the following things should be kept ready :

1. To prevent heat loss
   - A radiant warmer is ideal.
   - Two sets of sterile prewarmed sheets.
   - Avoid hyperthermia

2. For Maintenance of airway
   - Towel rolls.
   - A suction device.
     Low-pressure suction, which is set at 100mm of Hg.
     Suction catheters/Feeding tubes 5F, 6F, 8F, 10F, 12F, 14F.

3. For Ventilation
   - Oxygen source: set at 5 liters/min., humidified and warmed.
   - Infant resuscitation bag: Type - Self-inflating.
   - Cushioned facemasks size 0, 1, and 2.

   The self-inflating bag is designed to inflate automatically as the grip on the bag is released. It does not require a compressed gas source to fill.

Resuscitation masks have rims that are either cushioned or non-cushioned.

Rim should cover the tip of the chin, the mouth, and the nose but not the eyes.

High concentrations of oxygen can be achieved with a self-inflating bag by using both oxygen tubing and an oxygen reservoir, which gives 90% to 100% O_2.

4. For Intubation
   - Laryngoscope (neonatal size), with straight blades size 0, 1. Extra bulbs and two batteries.
   - Endotracheal tubes with internal diameter of size 2.5, 3, 3.5 and 4.0 mm.

Use sterile disposable tubes
Approximate size of the ET tube is determined from the infant's weight

Weight	ETT size	Gestational age
< 1000 gms	2.5mm	< 28 weeks
1000-2000 gms	3.0mm	28-34 weeks
2000-3000 gms	3.5mm	34-38 weeks
> 3000gms	3.5mm	> 38 weeks

5. Drugs
   - Adrenaline: diluted to 1:10,000 (0.5ml in 4.5-ml normal saline.)
   - Sodium bicarbonate: 5 ml NaHCO3 diluted in 5ml of distilled water kept ready in a 10ml syringe.
   - Other drugs that should be available in the labor room are, Normal saline and Naloxone.

6. Miscellaneous
   - Umbilical venous catheters size 5F, 6F.
   - Scalp veins, size 24 G.
   - Stop-clock,
   - Gloves, scissors and adhesive tape.

At every high-risk delivery there should be at least one person who has the skills required to perform a complete resuscitation. He or she must be skilled in ventilation with bag and mask, endotracheal intubation, chest compressions, and the use of medications. Another person capable of initiating and assisting with resuscitation must be in the delivery room and must be primarily responsible for the infant. This person must be present even when a normal, healthy infant is expected.

Management of babies who cry immediately after birth

The following steps should be followed for all babies who cry immediately after birth.

1. Dry the baby thoroughly, including the scalp.
2. Remove wet linen.
3. There is no need to suction normal babies unless they have excessive secretions.
4. Wrap the baby in warm, dry linen and keep the baby warm. (Preferably with the mother).

5. The baby should be put to the mother's breast-feeding within half an hour of birth.
6. Inj. vitamin K 1mg IM. Should be given to all newborns.
7. Babies should not be given a bath until they are stable and successful breastfeeding has been established.

Management of babies who do not cry immediately after birth

Birth asphyxia is to be anticipated in the presence of the high risk antenatal or intrapartum risk factors as outlined in the following table:

Antepartum Factors	
Maternal diabetes	Multiple gestation
Pregnancy-induced hypertension	Pregnancy-induced hypertension
Size-dates discrepancy	Anemia or isoimmunization
Bleeding in second or third trimester	Maternal infection
Hydramnios	Premature rupture of membranes
Diminished fetal activity	

Intrapartum Factors	
Emergency caesarean section	Non reassuring fetal hearts rate patterns
Breech or other abnormal presentation	Premature labor
Precipitous labor	Meconium-stained amniotic fluid
Prolonged second stage of labor	Prolapsed cord
Abruptio placenta	Placenta previa

When a depressed newborn is expected, two persons who can work together as a team to perform all aspects of resuscitation should be in the delivery room. The only responsibility of these two people should be caring for the infant. This means that the person caring for the mother is not to be regarded as one of the two.

With multiple births, one such team is needed for each infant.

The Resuscitation Protocol

Evaluation is based on the following three signs :

1. Respiration
2. Heart Rate
3. Color

Efficient and effective resuscitation is brought about through a series of evaluations, decisions, and further actions.

Apgar score is not useful for decision-making at the beginning of resuscitation, but helpful for assessing the infant's condition and the effectiveness of the resuscitative effort. Thus, an

Apgar score should be assigned at 1 and 5 minutes of age. When the 5-minute Apgar score is less than 7, additional score should be obtained every 5 minutes for up to 20 minutes or until two successive scores are 8 or more.

The ABCs of Resuscitation remain the same even for the caesarean birth:

A. Establish airway:
   - Position the infant
   - Suction the mouth, nose, and in some instances the trachea
   - If necessary, insert an ET tube to ensure an open airway

B. Initiate breathing:
   - Use tactile stimulation to initiate respiration
   - Use PPV when necessary, using either bag & mask or Bag & ET tube

C. Maintain circulation:
   - Stimulation and maintain the circulation of blood with
     - Chest compressions
     - Medications

Initial Steps

The following steps must be taken after the birth of the baby.

a) Prevent heat loss

Place the infant under the radiant warmer.

Drying will also stimulate the baby, which may initiate or help maintain respiration.

Remove wet linen and the place the baby on a prewarmed towel.

If the baby requires suctioning for meconium then one may delay this stimulation while drying till the trachea is suctioned out.

- Avoid hyperthermia
- Open the airway

Opening the airway is accomplished by positioning the baby appropriately.

- The baby should be placed on his/her back with the neck slightly extended. Avoid overextension and under extension.
- Suction the infant.

b) If Meconium staining of amniotic fluid is present

Suction the mouth, pharynx, and nose as soon as the head is delivered (intrapartum suctioning) regardless of whether the meconium is thin or thick.

Do direct tracheal suctioning if respiration is absent, heart rate < 100 bpm, depressed babies or poor muscle tone.

Apply suction directly to a tracheal tube (ET tube) as it is withdrawn from the airway.

Repeat intubation and suctioning until little additional meconium is recovered or bradycardia occurs.

If bradycardia occurs, initiate positive-pressure ventilation despite the presence of some meconium in the airway.

c) If there is no meconium staining of amniotic fluid

Gently suction the mouth and then the nose.

Evaluate the respiratory effort. Adequate oxygenation of the infant (resulting in sufficient oxygen for the heart and tissues and for good color) primarily depends on adequate respiration. Give tactile stimulation.

Most newly born infants who require positive-pressure ventilation can be adequately ventilated with a bag and mask. Indications for positive pressure ventilation include apnea or gasping respirations, heart rate < 100 bpm, and persistent central cyanosis despite 100% oxygen[1].

Although the pressure required for establishment of air breathing is variable and unpredictable, higher inflation pressures (30 to 40 cm H_2O or higher) and longer inflation times may be required for the first several breaths than for subsequent breaths. Visible chest expansion is a more reliable sign of appropriate inflation pressures than any specific manometer reading. The assisted ventilation rate should be 40 to 60 breaths per minute (30 breaths per minute when chest compressions are also being delivered). Signs of adequate ventilation include bilateral expansion of the lungs, as assessed by chest wall movement and breath sounds, and improvement in heart rate and color. If ventilation is inadequate, check the seal between mask and face, clear any airway obstruction (adjust head position, clear secretions, open the infant's mouth), and finally increase inflation pressure. Prolonged bag-mask ventilation may produce gastric inflation; this should be relieved by insertion of an 8F-orogastric tube that is aspirated with a syringe and left open to air. If such maneuvers do not result in adequate ventilation, endotracheal intubation should follow.

After 30 seconds of adequate ventilation with 100% oxygen, spontaneous breathing and heart rate should be checked. If spontaneous respirations are present and the heart rate is 100 bpm, positive-pressure ventilation may be gradually reduced and discontinued. Gentle tactile stimulation may help to maintain and improve spontaneous respirations while free-flow oxygen is administered. If spontaneous respirations are inadequate or if heart rate remains below 100 bpm, assisted ventilation must continue with bag and mask or tracheal tube. If the heart rate is < 60 bpm, continue assisted ventilation, begin chest compressions, and consider endotracheal intubation.

The key to successful neonatal resuscitation is establishment of adequate ventilation. Reversal of hypoxia, acidosis, and bradycardia depends on adequate inflation of fluid-filled lungs with air or oxygen. Although 100% oxygen has been used traditionally for rapid reversal of hypoxia, there is biochemical evidence and preliminary clinical evidence to argue for resuscitation with lower oxygen concentrations. Current clinical data, however, is insufficient to justify adopting this as routine practice. If assisted ventilation is required, deliver 100% oxygen by positive-pressure ventilation. If supplemental oxygen is unavailable, initiate resuscitation of the newly born infant with positive-pressure ventilation and room air.

d) Chest Compressions

Heart rate in a neonate is assessed by auscultation of the precordium or by feeling the umbilical cord pulsations. The heart rate is counted for 6 seconds and then the value is multiplied by 10 to give the heart rate in beats per minute. Asphyxia causes peripheral vasoconstriction, tissue hypoxia, acidosis, poor myocardial contractility, bradycardia, and eventually cardiac arrest. Establishment of adequate ventilation and oxygenation will restore vital signs in the vast majority of newly born infants. In deciding when to initiate chest compressions, consider the heart rate, the change of heart rate, and the time elapsed after initiation of resuscitative measures. Because chest compressions may diminish the effectiveness of ventilation, do not initiate them until lung inflation and ventilation have been established.

The general indication for initiation of chest compressions is a heart rate < 60 bpm despite adequate ventilation with 100% oxygen for 30 seconds. Although it has been common practice to give compressions if the heart rate is 60 to 80 bpm and the heart rate is not rising, ventilation should be the priority in resuscitation of the newly born. Provision of chest compressions is likely to compete with provision of effective ventilation[1].

Compression Technique : Compressions should be delivered on the lower third of the sternum. Acceptable techniques are

1) 2 thumbs on the sternum, superimposed or adjacent to each other according to the size of the infant, with fingers encircling the chest and supporting the back (the 2 thumb-encircling hands technique), and
2) 2 fingers placed on the sternum at right angles to the chest with the other hand supporting the back. Data suggests that the 2 thumb-encircling hands technique may offer some advantages in generating peak systolic and coronary perfusion pressure and that providers prefer this technique to the 2-finger technique. For this reason, we prefer the 2 thumb-encircling hands technique for healthcare providers performing chest compressions in newly born infants and older infants whose size permits its use.

Consensus of the ILCOR (International liaison committee on resuscitation) Working Group[1] supports a relative rather than absolute depth of compression (i.e., compress to approximately one third of the anterior-posterior diameter of the chest) to generate a palpable pulse. The pediatric basic life support guidelines recommend a relative compression depth of one third to one half of the anterior-posterior dimension of the chest. In the absence of specific data about ideal compression depth, these guidelines recommend compression to approximately one third the depth of the chest, but the compression depth must be adequate to produce a palpable pulse. Deliver compressions smoothly. A compression to relaxation ratio with a slightly shorter compression than relaxation phase offers theoretical advantages for blood flow in the very young infant. Keep the thumbs or fingers on the sternum during the relaxation phase.

Coordinate compressions and ventilations to avoid simultaneous delivery. There should be a 3:1 ratio of compressions to ventilations, with 90 compressions and 30 breaths to achieve approximately 120 events per minute. Thus, each event will be allotted approximately 1/2 second, with exhalation occurring during the first compression following each ventilation. Reassess the heart rate approximately every 30 seconds. Continue chest compressions until the spontaneous heart rate is 60 bpm.

e) Indications for Endotracheal Intubation

- When prolonged PPV is required
- When bag-and-mask ventilation is ineffective
- When tracheal suctioning is required
- When diaphragmatic hernia is suspected.

Adding 6 to the infant's weight in kilograms will give the depth to which the endotracheal tube has to inserted. Signs that suggest accurate tube placement include adequate chest expansion, bilateral equal breath sounds, breath sounds heard better over the chest than the abdomen and no evidence of gastric distension. To minimize hypoxia during the procedure of intubation, the duration of the intubation should be limited to 20 seconds and the baby should receive appropriate ventilation in between the intubation attempts.

<u>Medications and volume expanders</u>

a) Epinephrine

Administration of epinephrine is indicated when the heart rate remains < 60 bpm after a minimum of 30 seconds of adequate ventilation and chest compressions. Epinephrine is particularly indicated in the presence of asystole. Epinephrine has both a and b adrenergic-stimulating properties; however, in cardiac arrest, adrenergic-mediated vasoconstriction may be the more important action. Vasoconstriction elevates the perfusion pressure during chest compression, enhancing delivery of oxygen to the heart and brain. Epinephrine also enhances the contractile state of the heart, stimulates spontaneous contractions, and increases heart rate.

The recommended intravenous or endotracheal dose is 0.1 to 0.3 mL/kg of a 1:10,000 solution (0.01 to 0.03 mg/kg), repeated every 3 to 5 minutes as indicated.

b) Volume Expanders

Volume expanders may be necessary to resuscitate a newly born infant who is hypovolemic. Suspect hypovolemia in any infant who fails to respond to resuscitation. Consider volume expansion when there has been suspected blood loss or the infant appears to be in shock (pale, poor perfusion, weak pulse) and has not responded adequately to other resuscitative measures. The fluid of choice for volume expansion is an isotonic crystalloid solution such as normal saline or Ringer's lactate. Administration of O-negative red blood cells may be indicated for replacement of large-volume blood loss. Albumin-containing solutions are less frequently used for initial volume expansion because of limited availability, risk of infectious disease, and an observed association with increased mortality.

The initial dose of volume expander is 10 mL/kg given by slow intravenous push over 5 to 10 minutes. The dose may be repeated after further clinical assessment and observation of response. Higher bolus volumes have been recommended for resuscitation of older infants. However, volume overload or complications such as intracranial hemorrhage may result from inappropriate intravascular volume expansion in asphyxiated newly born infants as well as in preterm infants.

c) Bicarbonate

There is insufficient data to recommend routine use of bicarbonate in resuscitation of the newly born. In fact, the hyperosmolarity and CO_2 - generating properties of sodium bicarbonate may be detrimental to myocardial or cerebral function. Use of sodium bicarbonate is discouraged during brief CPR. If it is used during prolonged arrests unresponsive to other therapy, it should be given only after establishment of adequate ventilation and circulation. Arterial blood gas levels or serum chemistries, among other evaluations, should direct later use of bicarbonate for treatment of persistent metabolic acidosis or hyperkalemia. A dose of 1 to 2 mEq/kg of a 0.5 mEq/mL solution may be given by slow intravenous push (over at least 2 minutes) after adequate ventilation and perfusion have been established.

d) Naloxone

Naloxone hydrochloride is a narcotic antagonist without respiratory-depressant activity. It is specifically indicated for reversal of respiratory depression in a newly born infant whose mother received narcotics within 4 hours of delivery. Always establish and maintain adequate ventilation before administration of naloxone. Do not administer naloxone to newly born infants whose mothers are suspected of having recently abused narcotic drugs because it may precipitate abrupt withdrawal signs in such infants.

The recommended dose of naloxone is 0.1 mg/kg of a 0.4 mg/ml or 1.0 mg/mL solution given intravenously, endotracheally, or if perfusion is adequate intramuscularly or subcutaneously. Because the duration of action of narcotics may exceed that of naloxone, continued monitoring of respiratory function is essential, and repeated naloxone doses may be necessary to prevent recurrent apnea.

e) Routes of Administration

The tracheal route is generally the most rapidly accessible route for drug administration during resuscitation. It may be used for administration of epinephrine and naloxone, but it should not be used during resuscitation for administration of caustic agents such as sodium bicarbonate. The tracheal route of administration may result in a more variable response to epinephrine than the intravenous route; however, neonatal data is insufficient to recommend a higher dose of epinephrine for tracheal administration.

Attempt to establish intravenous access in neonates who fail to respond to tracheally administered epinephrine. The umbilical vein is the most rapidly accessible venous route; it may be used for epinephrine or naloxone administration as well as for administration of volume expanders and bicarbonate. Insert a 3.5F or 5F radiopaque catheter so that the tip is just below skin level and a free flow of blood returns on aspiration. Deep insertion poses the risk of infusion of hypertonic and vasoactive medications into the liver. Take care to avoid introduction of air emboli into the umbilical vein.

Peripheral sites for venous access (scalp or peripheral vein) may be adequate but are usually more difficult to cannulate. Naloxone may be given intramuscularly or subcutaneously but only after effective assisted ventilation has been established and only if the infant's peripheral circulation is adequate. We do not recommend administration of resuscitation drugs through the umbilical artery because the artery is often not rapidly accessible and complications may result if vasoactive or hypertonic drugs (e.g., epinephrine or bicarbonate) are given by this route.

Intraosseous lines are not commonly used in newly born infants because the umbilical vein is more accessible, the small bones are fragile, and the intraosseous space is small in a premature infant. Intraosseous access has been shown to be useful in the neonate and older infant when vascular access is difficult to achieve. Intraosseous access can be used as an alternative route for medication/volume expansion if umbilical or other direct venous access is not readily attainable

Discontinuation of resuscitation

Inability to establish circulation after 15 minutes of active resuscitation.

Documentation of Resuscitation

Thorough documentation of assessments and resuscitative actions is essential for good clinical care, for communication, and for medicolegal concerns. The Apgar scores quantify and summarize the response of the newly born infant to the extrauterine environment and to resuscitation. Apgar scores are assigned at 1 and 5 minutes after birth and then sequentially every 5 minutes until vital signs have stabilized. The Apgar scores should not dictate appropriate resuscitative actions, nor should interventions for depressed infants be delayed until the 1-minute assessment. Complete documentation must also include a narrative description of interventions performed and their timing.

Continuing Care of the Family

The team caring for the newly born infant should inform the parents of the infant's condition at the earliest opportunity. The parents need to be informed of the procedures undertaken and their indications.

Algorithm for resuscitation of the newborn infant[1]

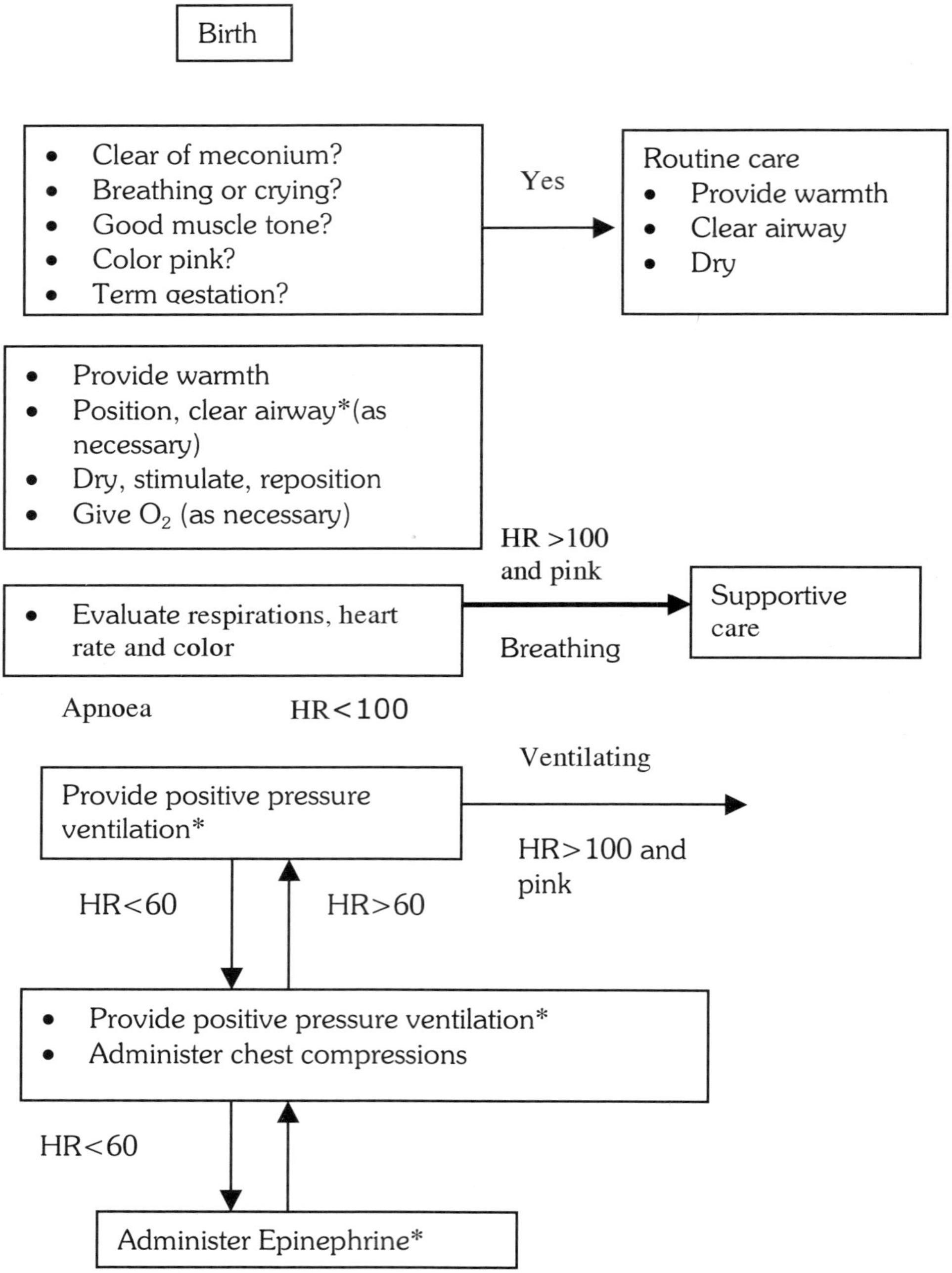

*Endotracheal intubation may be considered at several steps

COMPLICATIONS COMMON TO ALL CAESAREAN DELIVERIES

1) Transient tachypnea of the newborn.
2) Problems in initiation of lactation, which need constant support and supervision of feeding.
3) Anesthesia related problems.

Transient tachypnea of newborn

Cesarean section done prior to onset of labor is associated with an increased incidence of transient tachypnea of the newborn (TTNB)[2]. The proposed explanation for the clinical features of TTNB is delayed resorption of fetal lung fluid. It is commonly associated with caesarean section, because infants' thorax is not subjected to the same pressures as in vaginal delivery. It may be associated with prolonged maternal administration of hypotonic fluids. The syndrome of TTNB commonly presents as respiratory distress in term infants or preterm infants who are close to term. Clinical features comprise various combinations of mild cyanosis, grunting, flaring, retracting and tachypnea in the first few hours after birth. Arterial blood gases reveal varying degrees of hypoxemia, although respiratory failure is uncommon. The chest radiograph is the key to the diagnosis. The characteristic finding of prominent perihilar streaking may represent engorgement of the peri-arterial lymphatics. Differentiation from neonatal pneumonia or meconium aspiration can be extremely difficult. The transient nature of this disease is quite variable, for it may last anywhere from 12-24 hours in mild hours to beyond 72 hours in persistent cases. Although the majority of babies with TTNB require only supportive therapy, a small percentage may require ventilatory support.

Management of lactation in mothers delivering by caesarean section

A baby born by caesarean section should be placed on the mother's breast with the help of a health care provider or relative, as soon as the mother is responsive, after the effects of anesthesia wear out or within four hours after delivery, whichever is earlier. Immediate breast-feeding may get delayed under the following circumstances:

1) Heavily sedated mother.
2) An infant with a 5-minute Apgar score of less than 6.
3) A premature infant below 34 weeks gestation
4) An ill baby or one with a major defect requiring immediate surgery.

Even in these situations, expressed colostrum may often be fed to the baby via tube feeding or with a spoon and cup.

Anesthesia in high-risk maternal conditions and their effects on the neonate

Maternal diabetes : A preload administration of an intravenous bolus of 5% dextrose solution by the anesthesiologist could lead to serious rebound hypoglycemia in the neonate. The alternative would be for the diabetic patient to receive a solution that does not contain glucose.

Dysmaturity : Dysmaturity refers to an aging of the placenta and thus represents a notable risk to the fetus. Due to a diminished placental perfusion, the anesthesiologist should be careful to maintain maximal blood flow to the fetus, who may have no placental reserve. Therefore any method of analgesia that lowers maternal blood pressure may endanger the fetus. A secondary concern in dysmaturity is fetal entrapment of drugs administered to the mother when that fetus is acidotic in utero. The neonatologist should be alerted to this possibility, because an initially vigorous infant may give a false sense of security to the medical team. Caesarean section probably is done best with the patient under general anesthesia if there is definite evidence of fetal compromise identified by the obstetrician.

Prematurity : The premature infant has always been considered at increased risk for central nervous system depression from anesthesia and analgesia. Therefore the use of narcotic analgesics for discomfort in the first stage of labor should be severely restricted. Relief of pain in the first stage can be accomplished by use of selective regional analgesia while maternal and fetal homeostasis is maintained. The use of paracervical blocks in premature labors should be avoided because of the hazard of inadvertent intravascular injection of local anesthetic. This may result in fetal arrhythmias and even cardiac arrest in utero. Postnatally, these babies may have recurrent seizures.

Pregnancy induced hypertension : The placenta again is the affected end target organ, because generalized arterial disease is the primary problem. Women with mild toxemia do not have fetal embarrassment before delivery or during the intrapartum period unless complicated by some event such as severe hypotension or excessive uterine stimulation. These patients may obtain relief during the first stage of labor through the use of a mild narcotic analgesic. Segmental lumbar epidural blocks have minimal effects on blood pressure after fluid replacement. In severe preeclampscia, fetal compromise is present and maternal hypotension can have disastrous consequences for the fetus. Practically speaking, when the obstetrician notifies the anesthesiologist that there is fetal compromise and a significantly elevated maternal blood pressure, providing general anesthesia is the best option when a caesarean section is anticipated.

Elective caesarean delivery and anesthesia: Ideally, the use of general anesthesia should permit the mother to be unconscious and pain free without jeopardizing the fetus and neonate. Nitrous oxide relaxation technique is popular in the United States because it reduces the need for more potent inhalational anesthetics that cause myometrial and neonatal depression. Other approaches include the use of thiopental to produce unconsciousness and amnesia, followed by muscle relaxants, nitrous oxide and oxygen during the interval between induction and delivery. This method should produce ideal fetal and neonatal cases of known fetal, maternal or materno-fetal compromise[3].

NEONATAL CONSIDERATIONS IN CESAREAN DELIVERY FOR FETAL INDICATIONS

Fetal Distress

One of the common indications for an emergency caesarean section is fetal distress. The term fetal distress is too broad and vague to be applied with any precision to clinical situations. What the obstetrician and the neonatologist are worried about is the damage to the brain. For this to occur, the fetus must be exposed to profound hypoxia leading to just barely sub-lethal metabolic acidemia. Perinatal asphyxia and birth injuries together contribute to almost 19% of neonatal deaths. The following table depicts the mechanisms, which may lead to fetal acidemia:

MECHANISMS OF FETAL ACIDEMIA

Mechanisms	Examples of Disease States
More common pathways	
Poor maternal placental perfusion	Maternal hypotension Maternal vascular disease Increased uterine tone
Poor diffusion of gases across the placenta	Abruption Infarction Inflammation Villous edema
Less common pathways	
Poor fetal placental perfusion	Cord compression Cord prolapse Fetal anemia Fetal sepsis Fetal cardiac dysfunction
Maternal hypoxemia	Pneumonia
Rare pathways	
Maternal acidemia	Renal tubular acidosis Diabetic ketoacidosis Hypoventilation at caesarean section

Failure to initiate and sustain breathing immediately after delivery has been associated with hypoxic-ischemic damage to the central nervous system (CNS) and various other organs. The clinical manifestations of this injury have been termed as Hypoxic Ischemic Encephalopathy (HIE). HIE is of concern in an asphyxiated neonate because it can lead to serious long-term neurological sequelae among survivors.

Perinatal asphyxia may result in adverse effects on all systems with renal, CNS, cardiac and lung dysfunction occurring in 50%, 28%, 25% and 25% cases, respectively. The early outcome of an asphyxiated neonate depends on the extent of organ system dysfunction. Clinical management is directed at preventing hypoxia, hypercarbia and acidosis. Early arterial blood gas analysis and blood sugar level should be performed and acidosis and hypoglycemia treated. The infant's cardio-respiratory status should be monitored and signs of multi-organ system dysfunction sought and treated where appropriate.

The evaluation of the depressed newborn for a possible role of intrapartum asphyxia is based on the objective findings of the FHR tracing, umbilical cord blood gas, and newborn neurologic function. The American College of Obstetricians and Gynecologists (ACOG)[4] promulgated a statement in 1992 that set forth criteria necessary for subsequent neurologic impairment to be related causally to an intrapartum insult. These criteria for are as follows:

1) Profound umbilical artery metabolic or mixed acidemia (pH < 7.00)
2) Persistence of an Apgar score of 0 to 3 for longer than 5 minutes
3) Neonatal neurologic sequelae (e.g., seizures, coma, hypotonia)
4) Multiorgan system dysfunction (e.g., cardiovascular, gastrointestinal, hematologic, pulmonary, or renal).

Meconium stained amniotic fluid

Meconium stained liquor occurs in 10-20% of deliveries and increases to over 30% of deliveries after 42 weeks gestation. Meconium aspiration syndrome (MAS) occurs in 2-5% of infants born through meconium stained liquor.

Thick meconium stained liquor is liquor that has visible particles of meconium in it. Meconium stained liquor is uncommon in preterm infants and suggests infection. Pediatric staff should be present at caesarean deliveries where there is thick meconium staining of the liquor or where there is evidence of fetal distress.

If liquor is meconium-stained, suction oropharynx then nasopharynx following delivery of the head, on the perineum, with size 10 or 12FG suction catheter. There is no evidence that suctioning of vigorous term meconium-stained babies improves outcomes. If the newly born infant has absent or depressed respirations, heart rate < 100 beats per minute (bpm), or poor muscle tone, direct tracheal suctioning should be performed to remove meconium from the airway, using low flow wall suction set at 100-120mmHg (measured when tubing is occluded).

Post resuscitation care : All babies born with thick meconium who following resuscitation require IPPR or have respiratory distress should be admitted to the Nursery for observation and nursed in oxygen. Respiratory disease in these infants is a combination of aspiration, asphyxia and pulmonary hypertension so prompt provision of adequate oxygenation is essential. Babies at risk of pulmonary hypertension need to remain in optimal inspired oxygen to keep $PaO_2 > 80$ mmHg or $SaO_2 > 95\%$.

Intrauterine growth restriction

Infants with IUGR are a heterogeneous group with birth weight or length, or both, below the 10th percentile for gestational age. They may also be referred to as small-for-gestational age infants, in contrast to those who are appropriate for gestational age. The importance of this distinction, in addition to a number of issues influencing neonatal morbidity, is in the prediction of later growth: most appropriate-for-gestational age, low-birth weight infants experience catch-up growth during the first 2 years of life, in contrast to the slower, attenuated growth of small-for-gestational age infants who may have persistent height deficits throughout childhood and adolescence. The earlier in gestation that fetal growth is impaired, the less likely that complete recapture of lost growth will occur.

The mode of delivery is not necessarily dictated by the abnormalities recorded by biophysical or electro-physiological surveillance of the fetus. It would be judicious to avoid labor in those situations complicated by non-reactive NST result, absent or reversed diastolic flow or a positive contraction stress test (CST). Similarly, premature infants who are SGA, in particular those with a breech presentation and those, whose mothers have a completely unfavorable cervix, should be delivered by the abdominal route.

Perinatal problems of the IUGR neonate

Problem	Pathogenesis
1. Asphyxia	Acute fetal hypoxia imposed on chronic fetal hypoxia, placental insufficiency.
2. Meconium aspiration Syndrome	Hypoxic stress
3. Fasting hypoglycemia	↓ Hepatic glycogen, ↓ Gluconeogenesis, ↓ counter regulatory hormones, cold stress
4. Polycythemia, hyperviscosity	Placental transfusion, fetal hypoxia, ↑ Erythropoetin
5. Temperature instability	Cold stress, poor fat stores, hypoxia, hypoglycemia
6. Dysmorphology	TORCH syndrome complexes
7. Pulmonary hemorrhage	Hypothermia, polycythemia
8. Immuno-deficiency	Malnutrition "effect", TORCH
9. Decreased bone density	Possible substrate deficiency or altered vitamin D metabolism.

The implications of IUGR may extend beyond fetal life. Infants who have suffered intrauterine growth retardation, have an increased risk of hypertension, maturity-onset diabetes, and cardiovascular disease later in life[6,7,8]. Whether IUGR is causally related to these disorders or is a symptom of an underlying inborn metabolic disorder is not known.

Delivery of a preterm baby

Although, prematurity in itself is not an indication for a caesarean delivery, there are many situations involving the mother or the baby, which may necessitate abdominal delivery[9].

Routine caesarean delivery of all preterm or VLBW (Birth weight < 1500 grams) infants is not justified by current literature. Several large studies have failed to note improvement in perinatal morbidity or mortality with caesarean birth for indications other than classic obstetric ones. Trends favoring caesarean delivery disappear after adjustment for confounding factors. Grant et al. reviewed six trials that addressed immediate neonatal and maternal morbidities after vaginal versus caesarean delivery for infants born between 24 and 36 weeks. This review found increased risk of maternal morbidity with caesarean section without clear benefit for the infant. Neonatal intracranial hemorrhage appears to occur as often before and after caesarean as it does during labor and vaginal delivery.

For infants in breech presentation, there are intuitive reasons for caesarean birth, particularly to avoid trapping of the aftercoming head and other manipulations that could lead to trauma or hypoxia. Older retrospective studies that suggested a benefit for caesarean delivery led to the current custom of caesarean delivery for preterm breech fetuses, but support for this practice remains weak. Wolf et al. compared rates of survival without disability at 2 years for two cohorts of preterm (26 to 31 weeks) infants born between 1984 and 1989. At one hospital, the custom was vaginal, while the other preferred abdominal birth (n = 46). Multivariate analysis found that footling presentation was associated with a greater likelihood of poor outcome and antenatal steroid treatment more than 24 hours before birth with improved outcome but no effect of mode of delivery[9].

Preterm infants are at risk for specific diseases related to the immaturity of various organ systems. Common complications in these very premature infants include respiratory distress syndrome (RDS); intraventricular hemorrhage (IVH); bronchopulmonary dysplasia (BPD); patent ductus arteriosus (PDA); necrotizing enterocolitis (NEC); and sepsis, apnea, and retinopathy of prematurity (ROP). Extremely preterm infants are at greatest risk. There is wide geographic variation in the frequency of these sequelae, which may reflect differences in definitions as well as clinical practices.

Multiple gestations

Multiple births account for disproportionately high rates of perinatal morbidity and mortality caused primarily by the increased likelihood of low birth weight, which is the result of prematurity, intrauterine growth retardation or both[10]. Congenital malformations, abnormal presentations and prolapsed umbilical cord also contribute to the excessive risk. In addition maternal complications like polyhydramnios, preeclampsia, placenta previa and anemia, which are all more common in multiple gestation, also affect the fetuses. The perinatal death rate is four times that for singleton pregnancies and it increases correspondingly for gestations of a higher number.

Twin-to-twin transfusion syndrome is a complication unique to monochorionic twin gestations. It is thought to result from the transfusion of blood from one twin, the donor, to the other twin, the recipient, through placental vascular anastomoses. In the chronic form of TTTS, the donor gradually becomes anemic, hypovolemic, and growth retarded, whereas the recipient becomes plethoric, hypervolemic, and macrosomic. In advanced cases the recipient becomes hypertensive, and cardiomegaly develops to compensate for these changes. Because the incidence of TTTS is low, clinical comparisons of various treatments are difficult, and no treatment protocol is universally accepted. Nevertheless, serial amniocenteses have proved to be effective. Placental vascular laser surgery may improve perinatal outcome for monozygotic twins even further. However, only research on large series of TTTS will allow the development of definitive diagnostic criteria and therapies. Furthermore, because TTTS is often associated with severe neonatal complications, such as hydrops foetalis, delivery should preferably take place in a tertiary care center. Finally, in the case of intrauterine fetal death in a monochorionic twin pregnancy, careful pediatric follow-up of the surviving monozygotic twin is necessary, because cerebral and renal sequelae are common in these infants[11].

Hypertensive disorders in pregnancy

Hypertensive disorders occur in 6% to 8% of pregnancies and contribute significantly to stillbirths and neonatal morbidity and mortality. Expectant mothers with hypertension are predisposed toward the development of potentially lethal complications, notably abruptio placentae, disseminated intravascular coagulation, cerebral hemorrhage, hepatic failure, and acute renal failure. The causes of most cases of hypertension during pregnancy, particularly preeclampsia, remain unknown[12].

The major complications of PIH in the fetus are due to preterm labor, intrauterine growth restriction and hypoxia secondary to decreased perfusion of the utero-placental unit. Drugs used to treat eclampsia in the mother like magnesium sulfate prior to caesarean section can lead to neonatal depression and necessitate respiratory assistance.

Post term pregnancy

The fetus of a post term pregnancy is more susceptible to stress during labor than the fetus of a normal pregnancy. Women with post term pregnancy should be cautioned to come to hospital as soon as labor begins. Continuous electronic fetal heart rate monitoring should be used through out labor. The amount of amniotic fluid should be assessed by ultrasound. The presence of meconium stained amniotic fluid is important for several reasons:

1) Thick meconium stained amniotic fluid is evidence of fairly recent fetal stress.
2) If aspirated by the fetus, thick meconium can lead to a syndrome with high perinatal morbidity and mortality.
3) In the presence of thick meconium, abnormal fetal heart rate tracings are even more ominous.

The aspiration of meconium can be minimized by suctioning the fetus as soon as the head is delivered during caesarean section and before the delivery of the thorax. In the presence of hypoxemia and dysmaturity, the post term neonate is at considerable risk for the adverse effects of asphyxia. Finally hypoglycemia may be a manifestation of depleted nutrient stores caused by postmaturity.

Autoimmune disease and its fetal effects

Autoimmune thrombocytopenic purpura (ATP) is an autoimmune disorder that is encountered during pregnancy. Although the most feared complication of ATP is intracranial hemorrhage, the evidence for it is scanty. Nevertheless, considerable effort has been directed towards identification of the fetus with thrombocytopenia so that a planned caesarean section could be performed. Clinicians have developed three strategies for delivery for patients with ATP. Several authors advocate the use of fetal scalp sampling to determine the fetal platelet count with vaginal delivery being attempted if the platelet count is > 50,000/ml[3]. If it is less than > 50,000/ml[3], a caesarean section is performed. The major drawback is the incidence of falsely low platelet counts resulting in unnecessary caesarean birth. Some groups perform cordocentesis before the onset of labor with vaginal delivery if the fetal platelet count is > 50,000/ml[3]. The most serious complications of cordocentesis are hemorrhage from the cord and cord spasm leading to fetal bradycrdia. A third approach is expectant management with caesarean section being done for only the usual obstetric indications[13].

The newborn with thrombocytopenia is treated with platelet transfusions although, the survival of transfused platelets in ATP is short. High dose IVIg has been used to increase the fetal count. High dose IVIg therapy to the fetus is also a promising area for further research.

Other autoimmune disorders like the antiphospholipid antibody syndromes lead to recurrent fetal losses and intrauterine growth retardation. Systemic lupus erythematosus may lead to congenital heart block. Myasthenia gravis in the mother may lead to transient myasthenia in the baby, which may require intensive care including respiratory support[13].

Erythroblastosis foetalis

Erythroblastosis foetalis secondary to Rh isoimmunization is fortunately rare. The fetus affected by Rh isoimmunization may develop hydrops and die in utero. Preterm delivery, asphyxia, cardiac failure, surfactant deficiency leading to respiratory distress syndrome and, and hyperbilirubinemia are some of the major neonatal problems should the fetus survive till delivery. Disease severity, assessed by amniocentesis and umbilical cord blood sampling and gestational age remain the most significant determinants of the timing of delivery. Generally no benefit is gained by continuing pregnancy beyond 36-38 weeks; infact, continuation may be detrimental to the fetus. If facilities are available, intrauterine packed RBC transfusion is the treatment of choice with the last transfusion performed at around 35 weeks. An amniocentesis to determine the fetal lung maturity is also performed at 35 weeks. Both lecithin-sphingomyelin ratio and phosphatidyl glycerol levels are performed. If a mature profile is obtained, delivery is preferable. The site of delivery is also important. Mildly affected fetuses may be delivered in a hospital with facilities for exchange transfusion. Moderate and severely affected fetuses require expert neonatal care because hydrops and prematurity may complicate their presentation; therefore, a tertiary care center is the location of choice for the birth of these babies. Babies with hydrops tolerate labor poorly and may require to be delivered by the abdominal route. Once delivered, multisystem support may be required for babies with hydrops foetalis. Exchange transfusion and intensive phototherapy are also provided to treat the dangerously high bilirubin in these babies.

Non-immune hydrops

Since the development of Rh immune globulin in the 1960s for the prevention of Rh disease, approximately 90% of cases of hydrops foetalis are diagnosed as being due to non-immune cause. The prognosis in non-immune hydrops foetalis (NIHF) is poor with PNM rates that range from 50% to 90%. Maternal complications include preeclampsia, malpresentation and increased rate of caesarean delivery for fetal distress. The etiology of NIHF is never ending with cardiac malformations, arrhythmias accounting for the majority of cases. Chromosomal malformations, infections (TORCH), pulmonary anomalies, abdominal anomalies, skeletal anomalies, central nervous system anomalies account for some of the other causes[14]. In one series, the etiology was not found and the fetuses were labeled as having idiopathic NIHF.

After 34 weeks, the best treatment for the hydropic infant is delivery. The optimal timing of delivery should be discussed between the obstetrician and neonatologist. Other consultants like pediatric surgeons, cardiologists and cardio-thoracic surgeons may need to be involved. Parents need to be actively involved in the decision-making regarding the mode of delivery. Babies with hydrops tolerate labor poorly and may require to be delivered by the abdominal route.

Overall the prognosis in NIHF is poor, particularly if there are known structural defects or if the cause is not known. In these circumstances the PNM rate approaches 100%.

Suggested additional Equipment and supplies for delivery room resuscitation of newborns with hydrops foetalis

1) Four thoracocentesis/paracentesis kits
2) Normal saline infusion (avoid 5% albumin)
3) If severe anemia is suspected, O negative blood cross matched with mother
4) Three doses of epinephrine already prepared for estimated fetal weight
5) Furosemide 10 mg; recommended dose for severe hydrops foetalis is 2 mg/kg.
6) Heparinized blood gas syringe

Human immunodeficiency virus infection

To evaluate the relation between elective caesarean section and vertical transmission of human immunodeficiency virus type 1 (HIV-1), a meta-analysis was performed using data on individual patients from 15 prospective cohort studies[15]. Of 15,471 mother–child pairs enrolled in participating studies, 4585 met the exclusion criteria. The data included in the primary analysis were further restricted to mothers for whom the type of caesarean section (elective or non-elective) was known or who underwent vaginal delivery, to children whose HIV-1 status was known (infected or uninfected), and to the older (or oldest) child when there were younger siblings in the data set; 8533 mother–child pairs were eligible for inclusion in the primary analysis. Elective caesarean section was performed significantly more frequently in Europe than in North America from 1982 through 1996 ($P < 0.05$). The crude odds ratio for the relation between elective caesarean section and the infection status of the child was calculated for each study cohort. There was no evidence that the relation between the mode of delivery and risk of vertical transmission varied significantly among the studies (chi-square= 9.8 with 14 df by the Breslow–Day test of homogeneity; $P = 0.78$). A logistic-regression model was fitted to the data for 7840 mother–child pairs for whom data were complete, including the mode of delivery and the following three covariates: receipt of antiretroviral therapy, advanced maternal disease, and low birth weight of infants. After adjustment for these three covariates, elective caesarean delivery remained strongly associated with a lower risk of vertical transmission of HIV-1. The likelihood of vertical transmission was lower among women who underwent elective caesarean section than among women who underwent other specific types of delivery. This protective effect persisted when the data were stratified according to the receipt or non-receipt of antiretroviral therapy. When all caesarean sections were compared with all vaginal deliveries, instrumental vaginal deliveries, and non-instrumental vaginal deliveries, the likelihood of vertical transmission was decreased by the use of caesarean section, though not to the same degree as demonstrated for only elective caesarean section as compared with other modes of delivery.

Since a prolonged interval between rupture of the membranes and delivery has been shown to be associated with an increased risk of mother-to-infant, the interval between the rupture of membranes and delivery in relation to the risk of vertical transmission were performed. The crude rate of vertical transmission observed with elective caesarean section (8.4 percent) was lower than that associated with vaginal delivery after a short interval between rupture of membranes and delivery, either less than one hour (transmission rate, 11.7 percent) or less than four hours (transmission rate, 13.5 percent).

Since the standard of care in North America and the European countries represented in this analysis now includes zidovudine prophylaxis to prevent mother- to-infant transmission of HIV-1, the likelihood of vertical transmission and the rates of transmission were examined in greater detail according to whether antiretroviral therapy was used. When elective caesarean section and antiretroviral therapy during the prenatal, intrapartum, and neonatal periods were used, the likelihood of transmission was reduced by approximately 87 percent, as compared with the likelihood associated with the use of other modes of delivery and the absence of antiretroviral therapy. The rates of transmission were lower with elective caesarean section than with other modes of delivery whether or not antiretroviral therapy was given. The transmission rate with elective caesarean section but without antiretroviral therapy was 10.4 percent as compared with a rate of 19.0 percent with other modes of delivery but without antiretroviral therapy; the respective rates with antiretroviral therapy during the prenatal, intrapartum, and neonatal periods were 2.0 percent and 7.3 percent.

Herpes virus infections

Infection with herpes simplex virus (HSV) in newborn infants is associated with rates of illness and death of more than 50%. Even with early diagnosis and treatment with acyclovir the rates are distressingly high if the infection is disseminated or has involved the central nervous system before therapy is begun. Most often, the infant acquires HSV at the time of delivery, through direct contact with infectious secretions or lesions.

Recommendations of both AAP and ACOG are for caesarean section if primary, first episode or recurrent HSV lesions are present at the onset of labor. This recommendation for recurrent infection is controversial given the low attack rate of HSV to the neonate in the case of maternal recurrent disease. Nearly 1600 excess caesarean deliveries will be performed for every prevention of poor neonatal outcome.

Management of child born to a woman with active genital HSV infection[16].

Maternal primary or first episode:

1. Caesarean section with in 24 (preferably 4) hours of ruptured membranes.
   Culture eyes, nose, mouth, urine, and stools at 48 hours.
   Treat with acyclovir if any culture is positive or there are signs of neonatal HSV*.
2. Unavoidable vaginal delivery: Culture eyes, nose, mouth, urine, stools and CSF.
   Treat with acyclovir.

Recurrent infection, active at delivery:

1. Caesarean section with in 24 (preferably 4) hours of ruptured membranes.
   Culture eyes, nose, mouth, urine, and stools at 48 hours.
   Treat with acyclovir if any culture is positive or there are signs of neonatal HSV*.
   Unavoidable vaginal delivery: Culture eyes, nose, mouth, urine, stools at 48 hours.
   Treat with acyclovir if any culture is positive or there are signs of neonatal HSV*.

* If an infant is to be treated with acyclovir, CSF analysis, culture and PCR for HSV DNA are indicated.

Preterm premature rupture of membranes (PPROM), caesarean delivery and use of antibiotics

The consequences of prematurity continue to result in neonatal morbidity and mortality. One of the causes of prematurity is preterm prelabour rupture of membranes in which there is evidence that sub-clinical infection plays a role. The effectiveness and the immediate and long-term safety of the effects of administering antibiotics to women with preterm prelabour rupture of membranes on maternal infectious morbidity, fetal and neonatal morbidity and mortality was analyzed by the Cochrane review in 2001[17]. The review concluded that the use of antibiotics following preterm prelabour rupture of membranes (pPROM) is associated with a statistically significant reduction in maternal infection after delivery prior to discharge and morbidity. There was a statistically significant reduction in the numbers of babies born within 48 hours and seven days of randomization. Neonatal infection (including pneumonia) and positive blood culture were statistically significantly reduced in the babies whose mothers received antibiotics as was the numbers of babies requiring oxygen therapy overall and at 28 days of age or older. One trial (ORACLE) found a statistically significant reduction in the use of surfactant. There was also a statistically significant reduction in the number of babies diagnosed with abnormal cerebral ultrasound scans prior to discharge from hospital. Overall, there was no evidence of adverse effect.

Intrinsically there are fewer data relating to specific antibiotics. When looking at the effect of beta lactum antibiotics (Augmentin) where two trials were included, there was a statistically significant reduction in the number of babies born within 48 hours and seven days of randomization. However, there was a highly significant increase in the numbers of babies with necrotizing enterocolitis in the Augmentin treatment group.

The effect of macrolide antibiotics (erythromycin), included four trials and found statistically significant reductions in the number of babes born within 48 hours of randomization but delivery < 7 days did not exclude unity. There was a statistically significant reduction in those requiring oxygen therapy and those with a positive blood culture.

The review concluded that there were sufficient data to recommend routine prescription of macrolide antibiotics in this clinical situation. The routine prescription of macrolide antibiotic (erythromycin) was recommended, as beta lactum antibiotics (Augmentin) are associated with a statistically significant increase in neonatal necrotizing enterocolitis.

Congenital malformations and caesarean delivery :

Congenital diaphragmatic hernia (CDH) and the EXIT procedure : CDH is most often a posterolateral defect in the left hemidiaphragm (88%) on one side, which leads to herniation of the viscera into the thorax, resulting in pulmonary hypoplasia and respiratory embarrassment[18]. Before 26 completed weeks of gestation, if the lung area to head circumference ratio (LHR) is less than 1.0, a tracheal plug is placed.

The fetus is delivered by the EXIT[19] (ex-utero intrapartum treatment) procedure. In performing the EXIT procedure, the hysterotomy is created away from the placenta using a uterine stapling device to prevent hemorrhage. The fetal head and upper chest are delivered. Fetal oxygenation is monitored with a pulse-oximeter applied to exposed fetal hand. Cardiac function is continuously monitored using transthoracic fetal echocardiography. Deep anesthesia is maintained by maternal inhaled isoflurane in oxygen, providing uterine relaxation, fetal anesthesia and preservation of uteroplacental gas exchange. During this period of placental support to the fetus, the tracheal clip is removed. The EXIT procedure also provides time for laryngoscopy and bronchoscopy if required.

The EXIT procedure has also been performed for giant fetal neck masses. The mean time on placental support in one study was 28 minutes.

Meningomyelocele and caesarean delivery: The major cause of morbidity in babies with meningomyelocele is the neurological deficit. Experimental and anecdotal data raise the possibility that exposure of the neural tube to amniotic fluid and to intrauterine pressure and mechanical stresses associated with labor and delivery can injure the spinal cord and worsen the neurological outcome. A study of 160 cases of meningomyelocele suggested that caesarean section before the onset of labor may result in better subsequent motor function than vaginal delivery or caesarean section after the onset of labor. Overall, infants' delivered by caesarean section had a mean level of paralysis which was 3.3 segments below the anatomical level of the spinal lesion, compared with 1.1 and 0.9 for infants delivered vaginally or delivered by caesarean section done after the onset of labor[20]. This variance is large enough to make the difference between the child's being ambulatory or wheelchair bound. Thus scheduled delivery by caesarean section before the onset of labor should be considered for the fetus with meningomyelocele, particularly if prenatal ultrasonography and karyotyping rule out the presence of severe hydrocephalus, chromosomal abnormality, or multiple systemic anomalies.

REFERENCES

1. International Guidelines for Neonatal Resuscitation: An Excerpt From the Guidelines 2000 for Cardiopulmonary Resuscitation and Emergency Cardiovascular Care: International Consensus on Science: PEDIATRICS Vol. 106 No. 3 September 2000, p.e 29.
2. Morrison JJ, Rennie JM, Milton PJ : Neonatal respiratory morbidity and mode of delivery at term: influence of timing of elective caesarean section. British Journal of Obstetrics and Gynaecology: 1995:102: 101-106.
3. John S McDonald, Jay J Jacoby: Anaesthesia for labor and delivery In: Fanaroff A A, Martin R J. Neonatal –Perinatal medicine 7th Edition. Mosby, Inc., Missouri, 2002 p 404-415.
4. American College of Obstetricians and Gynecologists: Fetal and neonatal neurologic injury. ACOG Technical Bulletin No. 163. Washington, DC, American College of Obstetricians and Gynecologists, 1992.
5. Ray O. Bahado-Singh, Ertug Kovanci: The Doppler cerebroplacental ratio and perinatal outcome in intrauterine growth restriction:American Journal of Obstetrics and Gynecology:Volume 180 • Number 3 • March 1999.
6. Barker DJP. Maternal nutrition, fetal nutrition, and disease in later life. Nutrition 1997;13:807-813.
7. Barker DJP. Mothers, babies and disease in later life. London: BMJ Publishing Group, 1994.
8. Moore VM, Miller AG, Boulton TJ, et al. Placental weight, birth measurements, and blood pressure at age 8 years. Arch Dis Child 1996;74:538-541.
9. Conduct of labor and delivery for the preterm infant: Gabbe: Obstetrics - Normal and Problem Pregnancies, 4th ed., Copyright © 2002 Churchill Livingstone,Inc.
10. Neil K Kochenour: Obstetric management of multiple gestation: In: Fanaroff A A, Martin R J. Neonatal – Perinatal medicine 7th Edition. Mosby, Inc., Missouri, 2002 p 325-329.
11. Twin-to-twin transfusion syndrome: New perspectives: Journal of Pediatrics:Volume 127 • Number 5 • November 1995.
12. Report of the National High Blood Pressure Education Program Working Group on High Blood Pressure in Pregnancy: American Journal of Obstetrics and Gynecology: Volume 183: Number 1:July 2000.
13. Neil K Kochenour: Fetal effects of autoimmune disease: In: Fanaroff A A, Martin R J. Neonatal – Perinatal medicine 7th Edition. Mosby, Inc., Missouri, 2002 p 320-324.
14. Richard B Wolf, Thomas R.Moore: Amniotic fluid and nonimmune hydrops fetalis: In: Fanaroff A A, Martin R J. Neonatal –Perinatal medicine 7th Edition. Mosby, Inc., Missouri, 2002 p 351-370.
15. The international perinatal HIV group: The mode of delivery and the risk of transmission of HIV type 1: NEJM vol. 340: 1999: no 13: p 977-987.
16. Kohl S: Neonatal Herpes simplex virus infection: Clinical Perinatology 24:129:1997.
17. Kenyon S, Boulvain M, Neilson J: Antibiotics for preterm premature rupture of membranes: Cochrane Review 2001.
18. Timothy M Crombleholme: Surgical treatment of the fetus: In: Fanaroff A A, Martin R J. Neonatal – Perinatal medicine 7th Edition. Mosby, Inc., Missouri, 2002 p 190-214.
19. Mychaliska GB, Bealer JF, Graf JL, et al. Operating on placental support: the Ex Utero Intrapartum Treatment (EXIT) procedure. J Pediatr Surg. 1996;32:227-231.
20. Luthy DA, Wardinsky T et al: Caesarian section before the onset of labor and subsequent motor functions in infants with myelomeningocele diagnosed antenatally, NEJM 324: 662-666: 1991.

12 | CHAPTER

Medicolegal Perspectives in Cesarean Deliveries

Nikhil Datar, Sanjay Gupte

FRAMEWORK

- Introduction
- Civil law in relation to obstetric practice
- Criminal law in relation to obstetric practice
- The domain of potential litigation in obstetric practice
  - The decision
  - Maternal morbidity & mortality
  - Missed congenital anomaly
  - Fetal morbidity & morbidity
  - Complications of anesthesia
- Avoiding litigations in cesarean section
  - Cardinal principles
  - Good communication skills
  - Documentation
  - The written informed valid consent
  - Exceptions to the law of consent
  - Setting up standards of care
- Protocols : Mortality after cesarean delivery
- Ethical Issues

INTRODUCTION

Obstetrics is a discipline, which involves a higher risk of litigation compared to other branches in medicine. Litigations are on the rise day by day and have become a necessary concern while practicing medicine. Understandably so, it is difficult to practice clinical obstetrics without a potential litigation in the backdrop. As a result, obstetric practice has become more defensive than in the past.

Cesarean section is one of the most commonly performed procedures in current obstetric practice. While the rising incidence of caesarean section all over the world is a matter of concern, on the other hand the feasibility of an elective cesarean birth based on patient's request is being entertained in some obstetric centers[1]. Thus caesarean section has raised many legal, ethical, moral questions for the modern obstetrician.

For various reasons, non-medical personnel sometimes view the cesarean birth as an "unnatural method of a natural event". It is unfortunate that patients look down upon cesarean section as "an unnecessary surgery advised by the obstetrician for monetary rewards". With this back ground when there is an unfortunate, unexpected, sudden complication during or after the surgery, the reaction from the relatives is usually that of outrage and anger.

Increasing litigation rates in caesarean section could be attributed to a multitude of reasons. The general perception is that the obstetrician deals with a natural event of parturition in woman's life. Thus, adverse events are less anticipated. It involves shouldering the responsibility of two lives instead of one. Obstetricians deal with "young and normal" women and hence a complication becomes unacceptable. The obstetric patient is at such a stage of her life that the loss of life or loss of "man hours" (such as breastfeeding the baby and taking care of the newborn etc) is perceived severely by the family and the relatives. The decision to perform a caesarean section is most often made under emergency circumstances wherein there is less mental preparedness; so much so that the patient and the relatives are not in a position to fully understand the consequences and the complications of surgery. Many of the complications of the surgery are very sudden and do not allow sufficient time for acceptance and assimilation. Thus even a minor complication may not be acceptable to the relatives and the patient. This is further compounded by the fact that in the era of consumerism, the untoward result of any treatment is considered to be due to medical negligence and not due to "natural consequence of the disease or surgery".

CIVIL LAW IN RELATION TO OBSTETRIC PRACTICE

The law in relation to medical and obstetric practice in particular is in the process of evolving slowly in India. When an unexpected obstetric complication occurs during the medical practice the patient most commonly would sue the doctor for "negligence". This negligence can be civil and criminal. Following the decision of the Supreme Court in IMA Vs V P Shanta, the doctor is considered as a service provider and the patient as a consumer[2]. Therefore a suit would lie in the jurisdiction of the consumer forum. The doctor patient relationship is based on the contract and hence the principles of Indian Contract Act become applicable. Medical negligence is a civil wrong and attracts the provisions of the law of Torts.

Let us understand the basic concepts of these laws to realize how the complaints are made and how defense is planned. Under the Contract Act the consent carries a great value. A good informed consent is the most important aspect of defense. With regard to the law of negligence, it is important that the patient succeeds in proving the following:

1) The doctor was legally bound to give the treatment.
2) That actual damage has been caused. (The patient would have to prove it and mere allegations would not suffice)
3) The doctor's treatment has been the proximate cause of the damage (causa causans)
4) The treatment of the doctor was below the accepted "Standard of care"

The doctor could contest the above stating that:

1) The damage was not due to the treatment of the doctor.
2) The patient was also negligent and had he/she not been negligent the damage could have been mitigated. (The commonest example: Not following the advice of the doctor)
3) The said complication is "Vis a major" (Act of God) and not due to negligence of the doctor
4) The treatment of the doctor was well within the standard established in the field.

These concepts must be employed in day-to-day obstetric practice. Meticulous record keeping with this insight of law can do wonders while contesting cases of medical negligence.

CRIMINAL LAW IN RELATION TO OBSTETRIC PRACTICE

In India, the Indian Penal code and Criminal procedure Code deal with criminal law. Most often when there is a death of a patient, the relatives are likely to lodge a complaint against a doctor. The complaint is lodged at the police station under section 304 A of Indian penal code.

This means that the patient could sue a doctor under :

1) The Civil law (Consumer law)
2) The Criminal law
3) The complaint can also be made to the respective state medical council, which in turn can initiate an inquiry against the doctor.

It must be remembered that the patient can complain to all the three authorities and in fact there has been an increasing trend of such situations in contemporary obstetric practice.

THE DOMAINS OF POTENTIAL LITIGATION IN CAESAREAN SECTION

The decision

Litigations in cases where the basic root cause of the litigation is the decision to do a caesarean section. The patient may state that the caesarean section was unnecessary or may state that it was necessary but not done.

Adequate communication and interaction with the patient could help to avoid such allegations. Careful and meticulous documentation in terms of verbal communication, partographic representations of the progress of labour and recording intrapartum fetal monitoring strips could medico legally support the decision to perform or not to have performed the caesarean section. Recording the accurate time of examination is also vital for every case.

Maternal morbidity and mortality

In particular situations wherever there is an increased risk of maternal morbidity like injury to the bladder or the bowel, wound infections and sepsis, thromboembolism, and postpartum hemorrhage, the doctor should carefully explain the likelihood of such complications to the patient and her relatives to increased prior mental preparedness and anticipation. The issue of maternal mortality has been discussed at length later in this chapter.

Fetal morbidity and mortality

Fetal morbidity may arise due to cerebral hypoxia, brachial palsy, fractures, and injuries to the new born while delivering the baby from the uterus. In such situations it would be more appropriate to jointly involve the neonatologist to explain the condition of the newborn to the patient and her relatives.

In cases of fetal morbidity or mortality, it is important to document the time required from decision to delivery.

Complications of anesthesia

It is a routine practice that the obstetrician and the hospital owner are both made a party to the case filled by the patient. The anesthetist is called upon by the surgeon or the hospital most commonly and has no direct contract of service with the patient. It is interesting to know how law looks at the relation of the obstetrician, anesthetist and the hospital with the patient. On understanding that the doctors who are not full time employees of the hospital with whom the patient has entered into a contract, Lord Denning said "The doctors and professionals who are not in full time service may not be called servants. If they are not servants then they are the agents of the hospital which undertakes to provide the service". The same principle was accepted by the Supreme Court in the case of B. S. Hegde versus Sudhanshu Bhattacharya[3]. The master is responsible for the acts and omissions of its servants and agents. This is called as the principle of vicarious liability. It must be noted here that the obstetrician and the anesthetist must continue to work as a team even in the medico legal scenario. Often cases, which could have been strongly contested, have been lost due to discordance between the anesthetist and the obstetrician.

It is the court that has to decide as to who is negligent and hence who should pay. With a gradual evolution of more clear cut Indian laws, the courts are now more clear on the issue of understanding the roles of the two professionals.

AVOIDING LITIGATIONS IN CESAREAN SECTION

Cardinal principles

Often steps, which are regarded as "minor", are forgotten. In retrospect they are viewed as a "major lapse" in the health care delivery system.

Recording a detailed history of past medical and surgical illnesses is very important. Drug allergies should be recorded. It is mandatory to review the basic investigations preoperatively. The history of oral intake prior to surgery especially in case of emergency Caesarean section is vital to reduce the risk of aspiration pneumonia - Mendelson's syndrome. Setting up the operation theater with proper sterile equipments needs no emphasis.

It should be a routine practice to have a mop and instrument count before the surgery and at the time of closure by the obstetrician or the responsible personnel. In an interesting study conducted by the association of medical consultants to find out what methodology is used to keep counts in the theater, it was found that the doctors relied only on their qualified and unqualified staff nurses for the same. We strongly recommend that there should be a black board in the theater for writing the counts and this should be stringently practiced as a "ritual". A mop or an instrument in the peritoneal cavity amounts to frank negligence and in most of the cases there is no defense available to the doctor.

Good Communication Skills and Patient-Doctor Interaction

The "consumers" of the health service i.e. the patients often have a demanding attitude. They have high expectations and the doctor could find it difficult to satisfy them. Unlike in developed countries counseling, patient education by qualified personnel is not very common in India. Hence the onus of counseling falls on the obstetrician. Thus it is important for the obstetrician :

1) Not to have an attitude of "do not ask questions"
2) Encourage a second opinion when the patient wants it and document such an opinion.
3) Explain issues to the patient in a language she understands and comprehends
4) Whenever there is a complication, make the relatives aware of all circumstances.
5) Discuss various alternative treatments available
6) If possible, document such communication in writing

To summarize, the obstetrician should involve the patient in the process of decision-making and simultaneously increase their accountability.

Documentation

Documentation does not only mean the record of the clinical findings.

The value of detailed clinical notes is unparalleled in the defense of negligence cases. The documentation also includes the nurses' notes, monitoring charts, the autoclave register, RMO's findings, prescriptions, and requisition slips. It is a good practice to document all the events transpiring between the patient, relatives and the doctor especially those, which show the demeanor of the patient and the relatives. Non-availability of relatives, indecisiveness on the patient's part, refusal to examination must be documented in the case paper. We are in the era of evidence-based medicine. Wherever possible, it is advisable to record vital parameters of the mother as well as the fetus and thus have more objectivity as regards documentation of management protocols.

In an anecdotal experience of the authors, there was a case where the doctor advised emergency caesarean section and the patient refused the same; the relatives of the patient were not available and hence they were called for. The relatives in turn convinced the patient for caesarean section. Due to this inordinate delay, the baby came out asphyxiated. The doctor's intelligent documentation of even non-medical facts came handy in the defense. Similarly when the patient does not follow the instructions of the doctor it must be mentioned on the indoor paper.

Lastly it is important to note that there should not be any discrepancy in the notes made by the concerned doctors treating the patients.

The Written Informed Valid Consent

When two parties understand the same issue in the same context they are said to consent. The doctor patient contract is based on the consent. In the words of Justice Cardozo "Every human of sound mind and adult years has a right to determine what should be done with his body" and a surgeon who performs operation without consent commits an assault[4].

Thus it is obvious that the consent of the patient is required and as far as caesarean section is concerned it must be a written consent and not oral or implied.

In India, the common practice of obtaining consent for medical treatment often means mere signing up of the forms without adequate verbal interaction. There have been unfortunate incidents where the patients have, retrospectively declined their own consent, simply because the signature was obtained when they were on the operation table and not in a relaxed or attentive state of mind.

The consent must be an "informed consent". This means that the doctor is duty bound to explain to the patient the following :

1) The nature of the procedure,
2) The risks and benefits of the same
3) The long term implications,
4) Alternatives available[5].

The consent is valid only when it is obtained form the person who is of sound mind. A consent given under the effect of sedation may be held invalid[6].

Consent by fraud, misrepresentation, undue influence is an invalid consent. We must remember that the consent of the patient (an adult of sound mind) suffices for the surgery.

Following issues should be practice

- One should never operate with the consent of the husband or relative and without the consent of the patient.
- The relative's signature is not a valid consent. Its use is only sufficient with as a witness. The witness's signature is helpful to prove that the consent was not obtained by undue influence or fraud.
- In an emergency situation if one has the consent of the patient who is major and of the sound mind then one need not wait for the relative. The authors would like to site a judgment in a case decided by the Maharashtra state redressal forum in Salma Khan V Parsee Lying in hospital[7]. In this case the obstetrician waited for the signature of the male member when there was an immediate need of caesarean section due to fetal distress. The court held that this was not a good practice. In teaching hospitals the superintendent or dean is informed but in private sector this may not be practical. There is a likelihood that the relatives and the patient later on may allege that the consent was obtained by unlawful means. Thus one needs toweigh the pros and cons while deciding whether to wait for the relatives who would sign as a witness or no.
- It is prudent practice to have a written consent form preferably in local language.
- It is a good practice to have a consent form for all patients in labour, which also contains detailed information about caesarean section. This is a contingent consent. When there is a need of caesarean section the patient can be explained about the decision and a consent can be obtained[8].
- A specific high risk if any must be particularly included in the consent form. e.g., risk of meconium aspiration in cesarean section for meconium stained liquor or risks of bowel or bladder injury in case of previous caesarean section or the risk of aspiration if patient is full stomach.
- A separate consent should be obtained for any additional operation or procedure performed besides a caesarean section e.g. a tubal ligation or ovarian cyst excision.
- Refusal of treatment is called a "negative consent"; the same must also be documented on the paper.

Exceptions to the law of consent

It is said that the emergency knows no law. Law does not condemn any step taken by the doctor in good faith to save the life of the person. The interest of the state to preserve the health of the citizens may override the right of self determination[9]. Though not in the context of caesarean section, it is interesting to note a medicolegal case relating to the law of consent. In the case of Manjuben, the patient was taken for MTP. For the excessive bleeding the surgeon ultimately had to perform hysterectomy as a life saving measure. The state commission examined the evidence laid down and found that the said surgeon after all alternative methods had also taken the opinion of two senior consultants[10]. The said surgery all though without documented consent was not held to be an assault.

Setting up standards of care

When any judge decides upon the case he has to arrive at a conclusion whether the treatment given by the doctor was in accordance with the existing standards. J. McNair in Boalm Vs Frien Hospital laid down the principle called as "Boalm's principle"[11]. The learned judge states that the standard of care for professional services is best decided by the body of professionals only. This emphasizes the need for the minimum standards of medical practice to be laid down by professional organizations like FOGSI/ICOG. In our country, these standards may differ from urban to rural areas but setting up the standards will go long way in preventing medico legal problems concerning surgeries like caesarean section.

The law cannot decide whether a graduate can perform caesarean section or one needs postgraduate training for the same. Every medical graduate is trained in basic surgical techniques and with due experience undertaking an apparently low risk case under supervision of a consultant may be a prudent practice. This is especially important considering the rural health care delivery system. It is important to note that what experience can be considered as "due experience". The authors recommend that a body of professionals could intervene in this issue and try set up standards for rural and urban India.

PROTOCOLS IN CASE OF MORTALITY IN CAESAREAN SECTION

1) Inform the police.
2) Complete all paper records. Sign on all the pages and make a photocopy.
3) Doubly check and preserve all ampoules of injection used.
4) Communicate the death of the patient to the relatives.
5) After giving a statement to police, make a brief note of what you have said.
6) Keep all the equipments in the operation theatre.
7) Help the police in conducting "panchanama" and hand over your papers if asked for. Do not forget to obtain acknowledgement of the same.

Whether a doctor can issue a death certificate in such cases, is difficult to answer. The obstetrician should judge whether he genuinely knows the cause of death and substantiate the evidence with the same e.g. sudden death on table after removing the baby in caesarean section. The commonest and the most probable cause of death is amniotic fluid embolism. However, this is a suspected cause and not proven cause. One should refrain from giving death certificate in such cases.

However, if the cause of death is known and can be proven a death certificate can be issued. The guidelines laid by the Coroner's Act (abolished) state that a doctor should inform the police when a death has taken place on operation table or within 24 hours of surgery[12]. If the doctor feels confident of certifying the death, he may write a death certificate and inform the police as well. The police in turn if satisfied may issue a disposal warrant or may send the body for postmortem. In cases of unnatural death following caesarean section the investigating police officer takes the statements of the doctors, relatives, staff. The postmortem report and the opinion given by police surgeon or Dean of a teaching hospital is an important piece of evidence. The most common charge leveled against the doctor is under section 304A (IPC). The said section deals with the death of an individual caused by rash and negligent act of another. Thus in the above context, the prosecution has to prove that the act of a doctor was so rash and negligent that it caused death of the patient.

The provision of the law states, that the investigating officer may arrest the doctor for alleged negligence. The offence under sect 304A is a bailable offence[13]. The bail is available as a matter of right. There is no need to go to the court, as the bail is available at the police station. The question of anticipatory bail does not exist, in such situations.

ETHICAL ISSUES

Caesarean section involves the issues related to health of the mother as well as the fetus. On many of the occasions there may be a conflict of interests. On one hand, the obstetric community is concerned about the rising incidence of cesarean births, while on the other hand, there has been an increasing trend on part of patients to demand an elective cesarean birth.

A consumer advocate states, "I do not believe that anyone has the right to demand women give birth vaginally". This view has been reinforced by the American College of Obstetricians in his editorial where he has called caesarean section as "life enhancing operation"[1]. Many doctors have to find out some false indication to convert patient's choice caesarean section into medically indicated caesarean section to fulfil insurance requirement. For a private practitioner, it becomes very difficult to honor the request of the patient to perform "caesarean section on demand". He is further worried that if a complication takes place whether his view will be accepted by the court. The authors feel that it is advisable that when there is a caesarean section on demand asked by the patient one should make the patient write down in clear words that there exists no medical indication for caesarean section, the risks of caesarean section has been explained, alternate options of pain relief such as epidural anaesthesia during labour have been discussed and the doctor is performing caesarean section purely on demand. There is a need to lay down guidelines in this regard.

It is not uncommon in clinical practice for a client refusing a caesarean section when it is indicated. The caesarean section may have been advised on the account of maternal risk. In analogous cases involving non-pregnant patients, the courts have expressed reluctance to allow an otherwise healthy person to refuse acute lifesaving care. The physician's ethical duty is difficult to determine in such situations. Ethicists who hold autonomy as the highest value argue that the patient should be allowed to die without attempts at legal intervention. Those who stress beneficence and the right of the state to act as parens patria for its citizens argue that the physician has an ethical duty to seek a judicial determination.

If this refusal is made during the first patient encounter, it presents the physician with the dilemma of whether to continue treating the woman.

The Indian courts have accepted the rule that life saving treatment needs no consent and it can be enforced barring few exceptions.

The question becomes still more complicated when the life of the baby is in danger. The law considers that every child begotten is a child in existence. (En Vetre Sa Mere). The question is whether the mother's right of self determination override the right of the fetus to healthy life? Neither the pregnant woman's husband nor her physician has the right to force her compliance by physical force or chemical restraint. The only way to challenge a woman's refusal of a Caesarean section is to obtain a court order. General medical-ethical thinking opposes the involuntary treatment of pregnant women who make a knowing decision to refuse medical care.

Many physicians ignore the refusal on the basis that the woman will change her mind if the section becomes necessary or in the hope that a section will not be required. This is a dangerous approach if an emergency section becomes necessary. Since there will be no time to obtain a court order, the physician must choose between respecting the woman's wishes or operating against her consent. Irrespective of the patient's expressed wishes, it will be difficult to defend allowing the patient and baby to die. The best that can be expected is a verdict based on the court's requiring the enforcement of a rigorously documented informed refusal of care. Conversely, operating against a patient's express refusal, without judicial authorization, is legally and ethically unacceptable[14].

In India there has not been any case law on this point and we even do not know which court one should approach in emergency. The authors feel that today the best way to tackle such problems is to involve senior family members to convince the patient for caesarean section. In odd circumstances it may be worthwhile informing police about such incidences. These cases raising ethical and legal dilemma are not all that uncommon. There is a great need to formulate guidelines on such issues.

REFERENCES

1. Leilah McCracken. www.birthlove.com : Lovine V,"The Girlfriend's Guide to Pregnancy".
2. IMA Vs V. P. Shanta.(1995) 3 CPJ 1 : (1995) 6 SCC 651.
3. B S Hegde Vs Sudhanshu Bhattacharya.1993 (3) CPR 414 : 1992 (2) CPJ 449 NCDRC.
4. Boalmschloendorff Vs Society of newyork hospital 103 NE 92.
5. Chatterton V Gerson (1980)BLMR 80.
6. Kelly V Hazlett (1976) 75 DLR.
7. TheGrasp Vol 29 Issue no 1 May 2000.
8. Medical and Public Health Law Site http://biotech.law.lsu.edu/index.htm.
9. Law of medical negligence & compensation r k bag second edition.
10. M V Patel V Dr H K Patel 1997 (3) CPR 264.
11. Boalm Vs Friern hospital management committee (1957) 2 All ER.
12. Appendix 3 Mason's text book on Forensic medicine edition 3.
13. Ratanlal & Dhirajlal The Indian penal code 28 th edition reprint 2002).
14. Marsden Wagner MD, The Lancet, vol 356, pp 1677-80, November 11, 2000.

13 CHAPTER

Cesarean Hysterectomy

Sarita Bhalerao, Trupti Pai

FRAMEWORK

- Introduction
- Historical aspects
- Incidence
- Indications
- Technique
  - Total hysterectomy
  - Subtotal hysterectomy
- Complications
- Discussion
- Conclusion and key points

INTRODUCTION

Caesarean hysterectomy, obstetric hysterectomy, peripartum hysterectomy are all terms used interchangeably to describe removal of the uterus in the peripartum period.

HISTORICAL ASPECTS

Cesarean hysterectomy was originally devised a hundred years ago as a surgical attempt to manage life threatening obstetric hemorrhage and infection. Emergency obstetric hysterectomy was first performed by Horatio R Storer in 1866 and later described by E. Porro of Italy in 1876[1]. The true Porro operation consisted of supravaginal amputation of uterus and pulling of the stump to the lower part of the abdominal wound and fixing it there with pins. With advances in modern obstetric surgery with its aseptic technique and excellence of anaesthesia and postoperative care, the indications of caesarean hysterectomy were expanded to include non-emergency conditions and even elective sterilization. M. Edward Davis in the 1950's introduced elective caesarean hysterectomy for sterilization as a logical advance in obstetric surgery but was vehemently opposed by most obstetricians[2].

INCIDENCE

Sheiner et al[3] conducted a population based study at a teaching hospital in Israel between the years 1988 and 1999 comparing all singleton deliveries that were complicated with peripartum hysterectomy to deliveries without this complication and reported an incidence of 0.048% peripartum hysterectomies in 117,685 deliveries.

Okogbenin et al[4] reported an incidence of 0.226% in a 14 year period at a University teaching hospital in Nigeria.

INDICATIONS

The most common indication is post partum hemorrhage occurring from uterine atony, or laceration of major pelvic blood vessels. Advances in obstetric care like use of prostaglandins, brace sutures and newer uterine packing procedures like the Shivkar's pack have reduced the incidence of Cesarean hysterectomy done for the classic indication of atonic post partum hemorrhage in recent times. Placental implantation disorders like placenta praevia and accreta and uterine rupture in cases of previous cesarean are newer indications for this procedure. Conditions where an elective cesarean hysterectomy may be planned are cases of severe cervical dysplasias, carcinoma in situ and invasive cancer of the cervix.

There are advocates of Cesarean hysterectomy who believe that the operation is indicated in patients where there is an indication for both cesarean and hysterectomy e.g. multiple fibroids but the policy in these cases differs from center to center.

TABLE - 1. INDICATIONS FOR CESAREAN HYSTERECTOMY

EMERGENCY	NON EMERGENCY
Placental disorders	
Placenta Accreta	
Placenta praevia	**Fibroids**
Post partum hemorrhage	
Atonic	
Traumatic	**CIN**
Abruptio placentae	**Invasive cancer of cervix**
Uterine rupture	
Spontaneous	
Previous cesarean scar	
Chorioamnionitis	

TECHNIQUE

Total hysterectomy is unquestioned today as the procedure of choice when removal of the uterus is required. There are times, however when this is not always practical; in the face of hemorrhage and poor condition of the patient, the subtotal operation is preferred because it can be done more rapidly. Also since less exposure is required comparatively light anesthesia will suffice. Pelvic pathology such as cul-de-sac endometriosis sometimes makes removal of the cervix somewhat more difficult. In all other cases, it is better to perform the total hysterectomy.

Technique of total hysterectomy

If an elective procedure is planned the abdomen is opened by a midline vertical incision and baby delivered by a classical incision on the uterus. Following delivery of the baby, the major bleeding vessels are clamped and ligated. The placenta is removed and the uterine incision can be approximated by either continuous or few interrupted sutures. Alternatively a few sponge holders can be applied to the edges of the uterine incision and if the incision site is not bleeding appreciably neither is required.

The uterus is readily brought out of the abdominal incision owing to the laxity of the supporting ligaments at this time. The right round ligament is identified, doubly clamped, divided and ligated. Similar procedure is carried out on the left side. The cornual structures are than clamped, cut and ligated on both sides close to the uterus. The ovaries are usually left behind, but this will depend on the indication.

The incision in the vesico-uterine serosa made to mobilize the bladder is extended laterally and upwards thru the anterior leaf of the broad ligament to reach the incised round ligament.

The posterior leaf of the broad ligament is divided inferiorly towards the uterosacral ligament. The uterine vessels are now 'skeletonised' by pushing the relatively loose areolar tissue away from them by means of a sponge on a ring forceps, clamped, divided and ligated.

The uterosacral and cardinal ligaments are doubly clamped systematically. Clamps are placed, as close to the cervix as possible and it is imperative not to include excessive tissue in each clamp.

In case of a stretched out or effaced cervix it is difficult to determine the lower limit of the cervix. In these cases an incision is made in the lower uterine segment, a finger introduced through this incision to differentiate the vaginal vault from the soft lower uterine segment. The last clamp is applied at the level of the vaginal vault and the uterus is removed from the vaginal vault by sharp dissection at this level. The vaginal vault edges are held with long Allis forceps. The closure of the vagina can be achieved by chromic catgut continuous interlocking suture. Others achieve hemostasis by a running lock suture around the circumference of the vault thus leaving the vagina open for drainage of secretions. Hemostasis is checked from all stumps. Peritonisation can be achieved with a continuous suture of 1-0 ccg by bringing together the two leaves of broad ligament burying the cornual and round ligament stumps on either side or approximating the vesico-uterine fold to the post peritoneum.

The abdomen is then closed in layers.

Technique of subtotal hysterectomy

The procedure is the same as that for total hysterectomy till the level of the uterine arteries. After this vascular pedicle has been clamped, divided and ligated, the cervix is held with a tenaculum and body of the uterus is removed by cutting across the isthmus with a scalpel. The cervical stump is closed by several interrupted figure of eight stitches of chromic catgut. The vesico-uterine peritoneum is drawn across the stump and anchored to its posterior wall.

COMPLICATIONS

The surgical complications of cesarean hysterectomy are not unique to this operation; however certain problems occur more often than with the usual gynecologic hysterectomy. Table II enlists the chief complications of Cesarean hysterectomy.

TABLE - 2. COMPLICATIONS OF CESAREAN HYSTERECTOMY

Hemorrhage

Bladder laceration

Ureteral injury

Fistula formation

- Vesico-vaginal
- Uretero-vaginal
- Recto-vaginal

Thromboembolic events

HEMORRHAGE

The hugely dilated veins of the pregnant pelvis make hemostasis imperative at every step. Serious hemorrhage may occur if these large vessels escape at any point of the dissection. As the round ligaments are clamped and divided, small branches of the Sampson's artery in the broad ligament, which are ordinarily unobtrusive in, the non-pregnant patient may require separate ligation or electrocoagulation. Special attention must be paid to the pedicle of the utero-ovarian ligament. Retraction of a vessel within a ligature around this thick pedicle is the most common cause of late postoperative intra-abdominal bleeding after cesarean hysterectomy. Transfixing the pedicle prevents vessel retraction to a large extent. The surgeon and assistant must be careful in manipulation of the clamps; pulling laterally on the clamps may separate a pedicle from the previous one and open vessels in an area in which the placement of further clamps may be dangerous. Vessels of Santorini, which are just lateral to the cervix close to the bladder pillars, are greatly dilated in pregnant patients. These vessels are avoided when the bladder is dissected in the midline.

Urinary tract injury

The most important surgical complication of cesarean hysterectomy other than hemorrhage is injury to the lower urinary tract. Both bladder and ureters are intimately associated with the surgical dissection and may be inadvertently damaged during the dissection or placement of clamps and sutures. Dense adhesions from previous surgery and hematomas from uterine rupture pose additional risks of urinary tract injury.

Inadvertent surgical cystostomy must be identified and carefully repaired. The operator should sufficiently dissect to visualize the complete extent of the cystostomy and free the edges of the wound for closure without tension. The bladder wall may then be closed with a continuous absorbable suture that encompasses all layers of the bladder wall. A second row of continuous interrupted sutures is placed to imbricate the first. The bladder is then drained by suprapubic or Foley's catheter for 5-7 days.

Unrecognized and unrepaired bladder injury can result in postoperative fistula formation. For these reasons we recommend filling the bladder with contrast material to check bladder integrity if there is reason to suspect bladder injury.

The ureter is subject to injury at several points in the cesarean hysterectomy: near the pelvic brim when the infundibulopelvic ligament is ligated, in the broad ligament if hypogastric artery ligation is performed, and at the time of clamping and ligating the uterine vessels and cardinal and uterosacral ligaments. The position of the ureter is not altered in relation to the pelvic structures in pregnancy except when pelvic tumors or hematomas change its course. The ureter is however significantly dilated and atonic in the pregnant patient which makes it more difficult to identify. Severance or significant injury to the ureter requires urologic consultation when ureteroureterostomy and ureteroneocystostomy are beyond the training of the operator.

DISCUSSION

Several authors have studied the obstetric risk factors for emergency peripartum hysterectomy. Sheiner et al[1] performed a population- based study in Israel from 1988 to 1999. They compared all singleton deliveries that were complicated with peripartum hysterectomy to deliveries without this complication. The authors reported that the indications in their study (in decreasing order of occurrence) were uterine rupture, placenta praevia, postpartum hemorrhage, cervical tears, placenta accreta, second-trimester bleeding, previous cesarean section and grand multiparity (more than 5 deliveries).

Osefo NJ[5] analyzed indications for obstetric hysterectomy over a 13-year period form 1973-1986 in a teaching hospital in Enugu, Nigeria. 71% of patients received no antenatal care in the index pregnancy. The majority were of high parity. Rupture uterus was the commonest indication, which resulted from obstructed labor in 73% of the patients.

Bakshi and Meyer[6] reviewed the risk factors for peripartum hysterectomy in a retrospective cohort analysis at a University hospital in USA. The authors concluded that cesarean delivery, prior cesarean delivery, placenta accreta and uterine atony were important risk factors in their study and abnormal placentation was the primary cause of cesarean hysterectomy.

Maternal morbidity and mortality following caesarean hysterectomy are serious concerns. Okogbenin et al[4] reported a maternal mortality rate of 12.5%. In their study, mortality was associated with torrential continuing hemorrhage and septicemia. The authors concluded that obstetric hysterectomy can have grave consequences and that availability of blood products, intensive monitors and limitation of family size is advised.

Caesarean delivery carries a higher risk of obstetric hysterectomy as compared to vaginal delivery. Baskett TF[7] in a population-based review of 142,634 deliveries reported a relative risk for caesarean vs. vaginal delivery of 18.32. Previous Caesarean delivery occurred in 47.4% of the cases.

With improvements in facilities for blood transfusion and intensive care, maternal mortality with obstetric hysterectomy is becoming rare. Chew and Biswas[8] reviewed cases of caesarean and post-partum hysterectomy performed over a 10-year period (1986-1996) at a teaching hospital in Singapore. There were 14 cases of caesarean and post-partum hysterectomy. Uterine atony was associated with 43% of cases. There were no maternal deaths in their series.

CONCLUSIONS AND KEY POINTS

- Caesarean hysterectomy and obstetric hysterectomy are often performed as life-saving procedures.
- In developing countries, obstructed labor is an important risk factor, whereas in the developed world abnormal placentation is the primary cause
- Hemorrhage remains the main cause of maternal mortality.
- High risk factors such as placenta praevia or placenta accreta should be identified antenatally and cesarean Section in these cases performed by a skilled obstetrician.

- High-risk cases are best managed in centers where facilities for blood transfusion are available and also facilities for intensive care.
- Detailed informed consent about the possibility of emergency peripartum hysterectomy should be taken in high-risk cases.

REFERENCES

1. Myerscough PR. Munro Kerr's operative obstetrics 10th ed. London : Bailliere Tindall; 2002 p. 316-318.
2. Plauche WC. Cesarean Hysterectomy : Indications, technique and complications clinical Obstetrics and Gynecology; 1986 June; 29 (2) : 318 – 328.
3. Sheiner E, Levy A, Katz M et al. Identifying risk factors for peripartum cesarean hysterectomy. A population-based study. J Reprod Med 2003 ;48(8):622-6.
4. Okogbenin SA, Gharoro EP, Otoide Vo, et al. Obstetric hysterectomy: fifteen years' experience in a Nigerian tertiary center. J Obstet Gynaecol.2003 23(4): 356-9.
5. Osefo NJ. Cesarean and postpartum hysterectomy in Enugu,1973-1986. Int J Gynaecol Obstet 1989. 30(2):93-7.
6. Bakshi S, Meyer BA. Indications for and outcomes of emergency peripartum hysterectomy. A five-year review. J Reprod Med.2000. 45(9):733-7.
7. Baskett TF. Emergency obstetric hysterectomy. J Obstet Gynaecol.2003 23(4): 353-5.
8. Chew S, Biswas A. Caesarean and postpartum hysterectomy. Singapore Med J. 1998 .39(1):9-13.

14 | CHAPTER

Forceps Application in Cesarean Section

Nozer K. Sheriar, Nagendra S. Sardeshpande

FRAMEWORK

- Introduction
- Difficulty in baby delivery during cesarean birth
- Indications for forceps applications
- Features of forceps for use in cesarean delivery
- Method of application
  - High floating head
    - Occipito anterior application
    - Mento anterior application
    - Occipito transverse application
  - Deeply engaged head
  - Aftercoming head of breech
- Advantages of forceps application
- Disadvantages of forceps application
- Alternatives of forceps application
- Authors experience

INTRODUCTION

"My father, brothers and I have by God's blessing and our own industry attained a way to deliver woman without prejudice to them or to their infants"

Peter Chamberlen, circa 1600

Since the introduction of the forceps by Peter Chamberlain in the 16th century, it has undergone tremendous modifications in its structure and application. The instrument itself has received both criticism and praise. However, it has withstood the test of time and, in recent times, witnessed a resurgence in use. While the history of the forceps goes back to four hundred years, the cesarean delivery has evolved and established itself in obstetrics only over the past century. The application of forceps for extracting the fetal head during cesarean delivery is a fusion of two diametrically contrasting techniques.

DIFFICULTY IN BABY DELIVERY DURING CESAREAN BIRTH

Although cesarean section has been introduced as a procedure to avoid or manage feto-maternal jeopardy, the surgery is not without its own risks and technical problems even in the hands of the most experienced of obstetricians. Difficulty in delivery of the presenting part can be encountered in the following situations :

1) *High floating head:* A floating head especially in a patient who is not in labor or in the latent phase with a thick lower uterine segment can be an obstetrician's nightmare. Good abdominal muscle tone such as that encountered in a primigravida can add to the difficulty. Desperate attempts at extracting the slippery head with even more slippery hands can lead to extension of the fetal head and uterine lacerations. The delivery of a high floating head may be especially difficult in cases of placenta previa where, in fact, a rapid delivery is most essential.

2) *Deeply engaged head:* Although a deeply engaged head is delivered by attempting to reach below it through the uterine incision, pushing it up vaginally or by the Patwardhan's maneuver, extensions of the uterine incision with lacerations of the bladder or the uterine vessels are common.

3) *Aftercoming head of breech:* Almost every breech pregnancy in today's era is delivered by cesarean section. Most operations are performed electively or early in labor. The poorly formed lower uterine segment can clamp down on the fetal neck. Attempting to maneuver the fetal head through the rapidly contracting incision can cause cervical vertebral injuries, brachial plexus trauma, oral injury and extensions of the uterine incision. Cutting the uterine incision further in a J-shaped or inverted T-shaped manner is often required thus compromising future obstetrics.

4) *Preterm cesarean section:* Liberal use of cesarean delivery for a preterm fetus often does not translate into reduced fetal morbidity and mortality. Delivering the fragile fetal head through the often narrow incision in the thick, poorly developed and contracting lower

segment exposes the fetus to the same compression-decompression forces that one is attempting to avoid by bypassing the vaginal route.

5) *Pfannensteil incisions:* In all the above-mentioned conditions and in case of ample-sized babies, a large incision is mandatory if easy manual extraction of the presenting part is to be performed. However a good muscle tone, especially in primigravidas, can create difficulty. Cutting or detaching of the rectii muscles may be required.

INDICATIONS FOR FORCEPS APPLICATION

1) *High floating head :* In case of a high floating head, a forceps application has the advantage of enabling flexion and controlled delivery of the fetal head and reducing uterine trauma[1]. The use of forceps in delivering the floating head is of importance in cases of cesarean section for placenta previa, as the amount of fetal and maternal exsanguination will be proportionate to the time lost in extracting the fetus which will definitely be shortened with forceps extraction.
2) *Deeply engaged head:* The obstetric forceps has also been used in delivery of a deeply engaged head by cesarean section as an alternative to the Patwardhan's maneuver which can cause severe lacerations of the uterine vessels or digital vaginal reposition of the fetal head into the uterine cavity which can be difficult in deeply impacted heads and has the potential for introducing infection.
3) *Aftercoming head of breech:* During a cesarean section for a breech presentation, a forceps extraction, in addition to providing a protective cage to the fetal head, is a better alternative to extending the incision on either sides or in an inverted T-shaped or J-shaped manner[2].
4) *Preterm cesarean delivery:* The contracting uterus and the narrow incision in an unformed lower uterine segment may result in a traumatic delivery. The forceps will act as a protective cage for the fetal head and allow an easy and gradual delivery of the fragile head of the preterm fetus.
5) *Small incisions:* Forceps extraction allows the controlled maneuvering of the fetus through a relatively smaller incision. The forceps itself requires less space as compared to the surgeon's hand. Retractors can pull the rectii muscles away on either side and can themselves act as levers to ease the fetal head through the incision.

FEATURES OF A FORCEPS USED DURING CESAREAN SECTION

The forceps should possess the following features:

1) Straight blades without a pelvic curve so that the toes of the blades do not dig into the uterine walls.
2) Wide cephalic curve of the blades which fit snugly around an often unmoulded head.
3) Short overlapping shanks to allow for the small distance between the fetal head and the abdominal incision and such that they do not stretch either the abdominal or the uterine incision.

4) Sliding lock to allow adjustment of the blades to bring the fetal head into alignment with the uterine incision.

One of the earliest instruments used was the Willet's forceps. It is a barbaric instrument never to be used in a live fetus. It causes scalp injury and, at times, scalp avulsion in premature babies. Most obstetricians prefer the long Simpson's type forceps for this purpose. Warenski has described the use of Kielland's forceps for the procedure while others have recommended the Haig-Ferguson forceps[3].

The Hay's forceps is one of the ideal instruments for this purpose. Its negative pelvic curve and parallel blades allow correct application. The thin flexible blades are unlikely to cause uterine trauma while lateral flexion of the fetal head can be easily achieved. The shanks can be extended after application. This is useful for the aftercoming head of a breech presentation[4].

METHOD OF APPLICATION

1) HIGH FLOATING HEAD:

There are two methods of application.

A) *Mento-anterior application:* The baby's head is rotated wih a finger inserted in the baby's mouth such that the sagittal suture lies anteroposteriorly with the chin anteriorly. The left blade of the forceps is applied over the left fetal ear followed by the right blade over the right fetal ear. Correct application is ascertained by checking that the head is grasped symmetrically between the blades with the fetal ears lying in the fenestrations and the fenestrae of the blades do not admit more than the tip of the finger. The handles are moved upwards to promote flexion of the fetal head (Fig 14.1a). Traction is applied to deliver the head followed by extension and delivery of the face (Fig 14.1b). In this application, the long anteroposterior diameter of the fetal head stretches the uterine incision vertically rather than transversely and can lead to laceration of the thinner lower edge of the incision[5].

B) *Occipito-anterior application:* The forceps can also be applied with the fetal head in an occipito-anterior position. Correct application should be ascertained as in a forceps application to an occipito-anterior head during a vaginal delivery - the blades are equidistant from the sagittal suture, the concave edge is about 3cm away from the lambdoid sutures and the fenestrations do not admit more than the tip of the fingers. However, extension of the fetal head can occur. As in case of the mento-anterior application, the long diameter of the fetal head stretches the narrow diameter of the uterine and abdominal incisions.

C) *Occipito-transverse application (Fig. 14.2):* The fetal head is grasped manually and rotated such that the sagittal suture lies transversely. Two C-shaped retractors on either side allow good exposure. The Doyen's retractor is removed. Slight fundal pressure pushes the head towards the incision. The blades are assembled after ascertaining the location of the occiput. The concavity of the pelvic curve should point towards the fetal occiput. The lower blade is applied first guided by the operator's hand and supported by the assistant.

This is followed by insertion of the right blade. After ascertaining correct application, the handles are moved to flex the head. The C-retractor on the side of the fetal face is removed while the other helps to lever the head through the incision. Traction is given gradually aided by fundal pressure till "crowning" of the fetal skull the abdominal incision occurs. The remaining C-retractor is removed. This is followed by controlled extension of the fetal head to deliver the fetal face. The blades are unlocked and removed, and the body of the fetus delivered[4].

Some authorities recommend the use of a single blade applied underneath the fetal head over the parietal bone. The blade is lifted and turned to guide the occiput upwards through the incision (Fig. 14.3). Although it is claimed that, by occupying lesser space, it is less likely to inflict trauma on the maternal uterus or abdomen, it is doubtful whether a single blade can achieve the controlled and precise delivery of the fetal head as effectively as a double bladed forceps application.

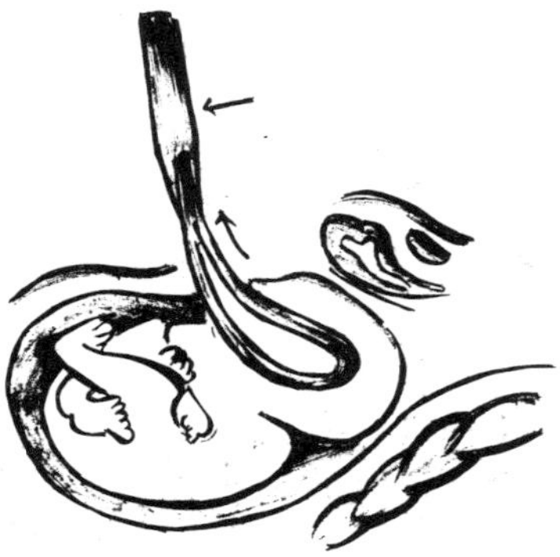

Fig. 14.1a : Forceps application in mento-anterior position and flexion of the head.

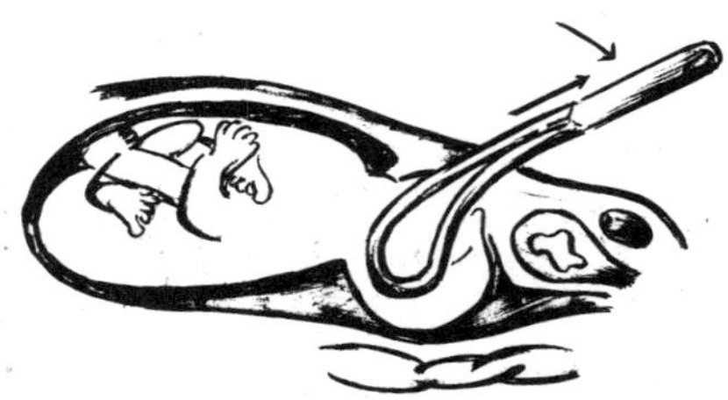

Fig. 14.1b : Extension and delivery of the fetal head in mento-anterior position.

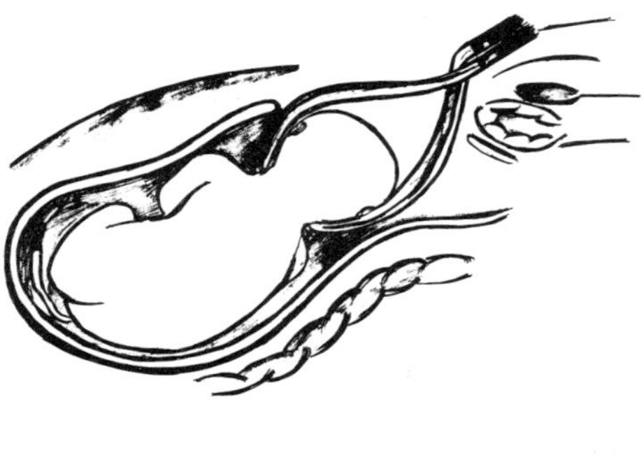

Fig. 14.2 : Forceps application in the occipito-transverse position.

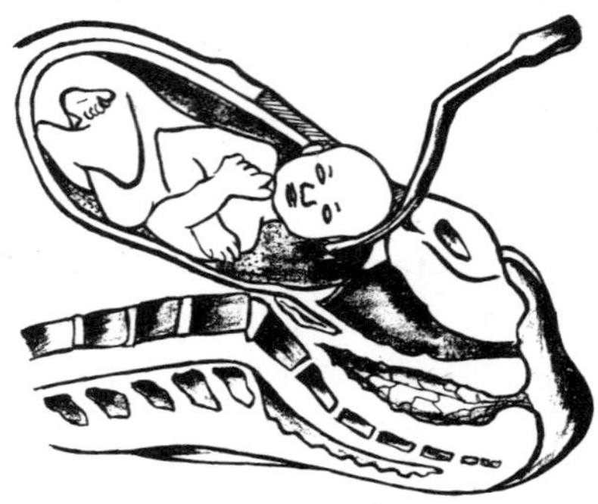

Fig. 14.3 : Application of a single blade of a forceps during cesarean section.

2) **DEEPLY ENGAGED HEAD :**

The obstetrician, by inserting a finger into the baby's mouth, rotates the saggital suture into the anteroposterior plane with the chin lying anteriorly beneath the pubic symphysis. The forceps is applied with the pelvic curve directed towards the pubic symphysis with the left blade passing over the left fetal ear and the right blade over the right fetal ear. Upwards traction helps to pull the fetal occiput above the sacral promontory. This is followed by depression of the handles towards the maternal abdomen to deliver the head by flexion through the uterine and abdominal incisions[4].

3) AFTERCOMING HEAD OF BREECH:

A forceps without a pelvic curve or a reverse pelvic curve such as a Piper's or Hay's forceps is suitable for such a case as it prevents hyperextension of the fetal neck. The occiput is kept anteriorly and slight fundal pressure is applied to fix the head. The left blade is applied over the right fetal ear followed by the right blade over the left fetal ear. Flexion of the fetal head is promoted by downwards traction of the forceps towards the maternal pubic symphysis. The body is supported in a towel and held slightly elevated. With traction, the fetal face is delivered. The body is then depressed and, with further traction, the fetal occiput is delivered.

ADVANTAGES OF FORCEPS APPLICATION AT CESAREAN SECTION

The introduction and removal of a forceps through an abdominal and uterine incision requires less space than manual extraction of the fetus. Additionally, manipulation of the fetal head is carried out with minimal relative movement of the shanks and handles. The delivery of the head is gradual and well controlled. All these factors allow the operator the luxury of a smaller abdominal incision. Although the uterine incision has to be approximately 15 centimeters in length, the inconvenience of an inverted-T or J-shaped incision can be avoided. Less fundal pressure is required and there is a reduced likelihood of uterine and fetal trauma.

DISADVANTAGES OF FORCEPS APPLICATION AT CESAREAN SECTION

Despite all the purported benefits, the fact remains that forceps application is a skilled procedure. Misuse and misapplication of this instrument can have disastrous consequences. Malapplication of the instrument can lead to its slipping over the head with resultant trauma to the fetus and added delay in delivery. Use of a forceps with divergent shanks causes vertical stretching of the uterine and abdominal incisions with resultant extensions and lacerations. Any instrumentation carries with it the hazard of infection although the exact additional risk posed over and above that of cesarean section is not known.

ALTERNATIVES TO FORCEPS APPLICATION AT CESAREAN SECTION

Use of the vacuum cup for extraction of the fetal head has been suggested as an alternative to forceps during cesarean section[6,7]. It is claimed that the vacuum occupies less space' is much gentler in terms of tractional force and compression of the fetal head, and is less likely to cause extensions of the uterine or abdominal incisions.

It must be remembered that a vacuum cannot be applied in cases of face or breech presentations. Its use is contraindicated in preterm fetuses as it can precipitate subgaleal, intracranial or retinal hemorrhage and unlike a forceps, it cannot protect the head from compression-decompression forces during abdominal or vaginal delivery.

In case of a deeply engaged head, the vacuum cup can only be applied after dislodging the head upwards by a hand inserted vaginally. Thus, the purpose of instrumentation is lost.

In case of a deflexed head, flexion of the fetal head is better achieved with a forceps. A vacuum cup may slip during an attempt to achieve flexion during abdominal delivery unlike a vaginal delivery where the flexion of the fetal head is mainly due its adaptation process to the pelvis rather than the effect of the vacuum cup.

Finally, the force required to deliver the fetal head through a thick lower segment, which may be the case in elective cesarean section or that performed early in labor, and through a narrow skin incision may not be achieved with a vacuum cup. The skin incision may have to be extended which once again defeats one of the goals of the procedure.

THE AUTHOR'S EXPERIENCE

In a prospective study by the author, 253 cases of forceps application at cesarean delivery were evaluated over a period of 10 years between 1988 to 1997. 50.6% of the patients were primigravidae and Pfannensteil incisions were performed in 79.1% of cases. The application was done prophylactically in cases of previous cesarean section, fetal distress or IUGR (35.2%), for a floating head (45.8%) or for an aftercoming head of a breech (19%). In cases with vertex presentation, the forceps was applied in the occipitotransverse position in 61.6% of cases and occipitoanterior position in 30.7% of patients. There was no forceps related fetal or maternal morbidity or mortality. Difficulty in application and delay in delivery was encountered in 6.7% of cases. This was experienced while attempting to flex the fetal head, slippage during traction or extension of fetal head during delivery.

CONCLUSION

Use of the obstetric forceps during cesarean delivery has definite advantages in certain difficult clinical situations. Hence, it is advisable for the obstetrician to be accustomed to this art by honing his skills by application in uncomplicated cases. The forceps should always form a part of the instruments on the operating trolley to be kept ready for unexpected use at cesarean section.

REFERENCES

1) Douglas-Stromme. Operative obstetrics (5th ed), Norwalk: Appleton Lange, 1988.

2) Penn ZJ. Breech presentation. In James DK, Steer PJ, Weiner CP, Gonik B (eds): High risk pregnancy-management options (2nd ed), WB Saunders; 58: 1025-50, 1999.

3) Warenski JC. A technique to facilitate delivery of the high-floating head at cesarean section. Am J Obstet Gynecol; 139: 625, 1981.

4) Purandare VN. The use of forceps during caesarian section. In Nargolkar SM: Hay's forceps-an atlas monograph (1st ed), Penham Inc; 224-5,1991.

6) O'Grady JP. Modern instrumental delivery. Baltimore: Williams and wilkins, 1988.

7) Pelosi MA, Apuzzio J. Use of the soft, silicone obstetric vacuum cups for the delivery of the fetal head at cesarean section. J Reprod Med; 29: 287-92, 1984.

15 CHAPTER

Extraperitoneal Cesarean Section - A Review

Nagendra S. Sardeshpande

FRAMEWORK

- Introduction
- History of extraperitoneal cesarean birth
- Indications
- Contraindications
- Principles of surgery
- Techniques of performing extraperitoneal cesarean delivery
  - Latzko's technique
  - Water's technique
- Advantages
- Disadvantages and complications
- Conclusions

INTRODUCTION

"The caesarean operation, as commonly performed, puts into such danger the life of the mother, that it is still a desideratum to ascertain some modification of it, which may diminish its fatality, and thereby inspire the profession with more confidence and promptness in undertaking it".

W.E.Horner, 28 September 1894[1]

Over a century ago, women who underwent a cesarean delivery were condemned to their grave either due to hemorrhage or, if they survived the surgery, from infection.

Simpson introduced anesthesia in 1847 to mark a significant advance in elimination of the agony of labor and cesarean delivery. Sanger, in 1882, described suturing of the uterine wound. Such an apparently simple step resulted in a dramatic decline in maternal mortality due to hemorrhage.

Despite all these efforts, infectious morbidity and mortality was a very common problem. Antibacterial agents and antibiotic prophylaxis was a relatively late development of modern surgery and medicine. The initial stumbling attempts at controlling or treating infection were outrageous ranging from confining the patient to barley water, thin gruel, tapioca and rennet whey to having her breasts drawn by glasses or puppies[1]. Among the more scientific changes included exteriorization of the uterus before opening it, shutting off the general peritoneal cavity before opening into the lower segment, packing off the peritoneal cavity and extraperitoneal cesarean section.

HISTORY OF EXTRAPERITONEAL CESAREAN SECTION

The credit for the concept that the uterus and vagina can be approached transabdominally without opening up the peritoneal cavity goes to Ferdinand von Ritgen in 1820. He derived his idea from the method of extraperitoneal external iliac artery ligation for an aneurysm developed by Abernathy and Cooper.

Ritgen planned his surgery by first pressing the bladder to the left with a male catheter. The assistant pushed the uterus to the right towards the surgeon followed by an elliptical incision through the skin from the right iliac crest to the pubic symphysis. During the incision of the underlying layers of subcutaneous tissue and muscle, the epigastric, abdominal and circumflex arteries were ligated and transected. This was followed by division of the cellular tissue between the bladder and peritoneum bluntly to approach the vagina, which was elevated with a bladder sound. An incision was made in the vagina, which was carried over to the right followed by vertical division of the upper vagina and cervix up to the edge of the body of the uterus. Following delivery of the baby, the vaginal incision was left unsutured while the abdomen was closed. Von Ritgen's assumption was that the uterine arteries and veins would stop bleeding by spasm of the former and tamponade with a sponge on the latter. This surgery is more appropriately called laparoelytrotomy or abdominal elytrotomy[2].

Dr. Physick (1822) made the first reference to extraperitoneal cesarean section and described anatomical relationships between the pelvic peritoneum, urinary bladder, cervix and pelvic cellular tissue. His views were endorsed by his friend, W.E.Horner, an anatomist from the University of Pennsylvania, during his communication with W.P. Dewees on 28 September, 1824[3].

However T. Gaillard Thomas of New York, unaware of these academic deliberations, which had occurred 50 years ago, performed an extraperitoneal cesarean section on February 1870, which ended in death of both mother and child. This was followed by another unsuccessful attempt by Alexander Skene in 1874 in a rachitic patient. Although T. Gaillard Thomas performed a laparoelytrotomy, he opened the abdomen with a lateral incision parallel to the Poupart's ligament[3].

Sellheim (1960) attempted and succeeded in performing an extraperitoneal cesarean section based on Physick's principle through a Pfannensteil incision[4].

Although Frank and Sellheim made modifications of this technique, Willhelm Latzko of Vienna revitalized the operation in 1909. He reported only 2 maternal deaths among 30 cases. Latzko reported his first case on April 26, 1908. The patient was a primigravida in good labor for 18 hours with membranes ruptured for 20 hours. The patient made an excellent recovery following surgery[5].

Following this, Kustner, in 1912, revealed his series of 72 cases with no maternal deaths[5].

E. G. Waters, in 1940, used the original technique suggested by Physick. This technique involves separation of the peritoneum from the dome of the bladder and downward displacement of the urinary bladder while Latzko's technique consists of lateral displacement of the bladder and peritoneum[6].

Following the revolution of penicillin and other antibiotics, and tremendous improvements in antenatal care and nutrition, interest in these techniques declined partly due to dependence on the efficacy of antibacterial agents and partly due to increasing rarity of cases of chorioamnionitis and prolonged labor due to liberalization of cesarean delivery.

INDICATIONS FOR EXTRA-PERITONEAL CESAREAN SECTION

Extraperitoneal cesarean section was primarily introduced as a safe method of delivery of the fetus in cases of suspected or frank chorioamnionitis which allowing fetal survival. Thus, it was a superior alternative to symphisiotomy, hysterectomy or fetal destructive surgery, which was prevalent in those times.

Traditionally, it plays a role in cases of proven uterine infection with symptoms and sign such as maternal and fetal tachycardia, uterine tenderness, fever, bacterial growth on culture of amniotic fluid or bacteria noted on amniotic fluid gram staining.

Its use has also been extended to cases with potential for uterine and pelvic infection such as in parturients in prolonged labor (more than 12 hours), prolonged rupture of membranes (more than 12 hours). In these cases, the ascending infection from the vagina as well as that carried into the uterus by repeated pelvic examinations can precipitate uterine infection[7].

Although its performance has rapidly declined with the advent of antibiotics, sporadic studies and case reports suggest that this operation may play a role in developing countries with their paucity of antibacterial agents and high incidence of neglected obstructed and prolonged labor, and possibly in developed countries, too, with the omnipresent danger of antibiotic resistance.

Hanson, drawing from his experience of 346 cases over a period of 10 years, suggests that avoidance of the peritoneal cavity is surgically sound and is a primary defense against infections that complicate cesarean section[8].

Durveniaskhi and Durveniashka reported their experience of extraperitoneal cesarean section in 151 cases of suspected or frank uterine infection and noted a great advantage of its use in such cases. All their patients recovered postoperatively without a single incidence of puerperal sepsis[9].

However, Wallace et al could not find any significant superiority of extraperitoneal cesarean section over a transperitoneal approach supplemented with antibiotics as a form of infection prophylaxis. In their study there was only an insignificant trend towards enhanced postoperative recovery with extraperitoneal section compared with those undergoing transperitoneal primary cesarean section[10].

Interestingly, E. G. Waters reports a case of a woman born with a persistent cloaca who underwent corrective surgery to produce a neo-rectovagina. At the age of 28 years, she conceived and underwent an extraperitoneal cesarean section followed by a repeat extraperitoneal section one and a half years later. The procedure was performed to prevent gross contamination of the peritoneal cavity by bowel content[11].

CONTRAINDICATIONS TO EXTRAPERITONEAL CESAREAN SECTION

This surgery involves dissection of the extraperitoneal fascial tissue. Scarring of this tissue as seen after previous cesarean delivery, surgery for genitourinary fistulae or urinary incontinence surgery increases the potential for failure of access of the vesico-uterine space, windowing of peritoneum and bladder trauma.

Large fetuses weighing more than 3.8-4 kg or involved in malpresentation can be difficult to deliver through the narrow space provided by this approach resulting in either delay in delivery, or bladder trauma due to extension of the uterine incision[7]. It must be noted that the cushion of perivesical tissue provided as a means of protection to the bladder is disturbed during dissection thus rendering the bladder more vulnerable to injury.

Similarly, an obstetrician attempting to deliver a fetus with a low-lying anterior placenta is likely to face difficulties.

Since this technically difficult operation does involve a longer delivery interval, a case of acute fetal distress is a poor candidate for the procedure. Although the occasional study e.g. Wang and Yang (1994), has suggested that the operation can be performed rapidly, the speed of performing the surgery has much to do with the skill and experience of the surgeon and very few obstetricians in this age have had the exposure required to achieve the requisite dexterity in performing this procedure[12].

Occasional studies and a few case reports have suggested that extraperitoneal cesarean section can be performed in the presence of some of the above mentioned contraindications[13]. However, the incidence of technical failure, and bladder, vascular and even ureteric injury is higher than that seen with a standard transperitoneal approach.

PRINCIPLES OF EXTRAPERITONEAL CESAREAN SECTION[1,14]

The lower uterine segment is formed by disappearance of the anatomical internal os, stretching out of the isthmus and its incorporation into the body of the uterus. The isthmus, from the fourth month forms the lower uterine segment.

The rectus sheath is deficient posteriorly below the arcuate line. The fascia transversalis, which lies in contact with the rectus muscle below this line, descends behind the symphysis pubis and frays out into the surrounding tissue.

The pubovesicocervical or vesical fascia extends from the front of the bladder (fascia vesicae anterior), over the dome of the bladder intervening between the bladder and the peritoneum (fascia vesicae posterior) and is reflected onto the lower uterine segment (fascia uteri or DeLee's fascia). The uterine fascia forms a loose membranous structure at term, which can be easily dissected as compared to the fascia vesicae, which is hypertrophied.

The fascia transversalis incorporates the preperitoneal pad of fat, which is most visible at the left superolateral aspect of the bladder thus defining the upper border of the organ.

The peritoneum, which is in close relation to the fundus of the bladder, is reflected onto the isthmus or lower uterine segment posteriorly (uterovesical fold). Laterally it is lifted away from the bladder onto the lateral abdominal wall (lateral false or peritoneal ligament). This potential space laterally (paravesical space or space of Bogrosi) allows dissection to be begun from the lateral aspect of the bladder safely.

During the course of dissection, the urachus is encountered in the midline with the umbilical arteries on either side. These structures have to be cut to approach the lower uterine segment. Dissection around the urachus in the area of maximum adherence of bladder to the overlying peritoneum entails the greatest risk of bladder injury (Fig. 15.1).

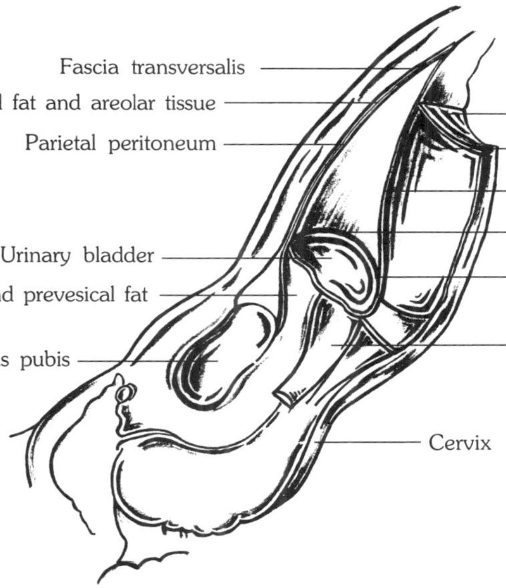

Fig. 15.1 Anatomy in extraperitoneal cesarean section

TECHNIQUE OF EXTRAPERITONEAL CESAREAN SECTION :

A) LATZKO'S METHOD OR PARAVESICAL CESAREAN SECTION[15]

This is the more popular technique. After anesthetizing the patient, 200ml of dilute methylene blue or indigo carmine (1.6% or 5cc of 0.8% indigo carmine in 1000ml of water as suggested by Norton) is instilled into the urinary bladder and the catheter is kept clamped.

The approach originally advised was a left paramedian incision although a transverse or Pfannensteil incision may be used. After dissection of the subcutaneous tissue and the anterior rectus sheath, the left rectus muscle is separated by blunt dissection from the underlying transversalis fascia and then retracted laterally. The deep epigastric artery running underneath the left rectus muscle is ligated and transected. The superior aspect of the left lateral surface of the bladder is identified by its covering of "chicken yellow" areolar tissue. The tissue is dissected bluntly to lift the transversalis fascia and anterior aspect of the perivesical fascia from the bladder. These layers are incised sharply. (Fig. 15.2 a & b).

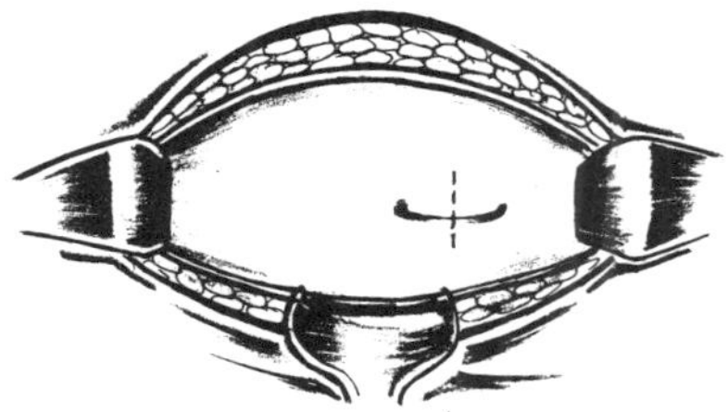

15.2 a. Incision on the transversalis fascia on the lateral aspect of the bladder.

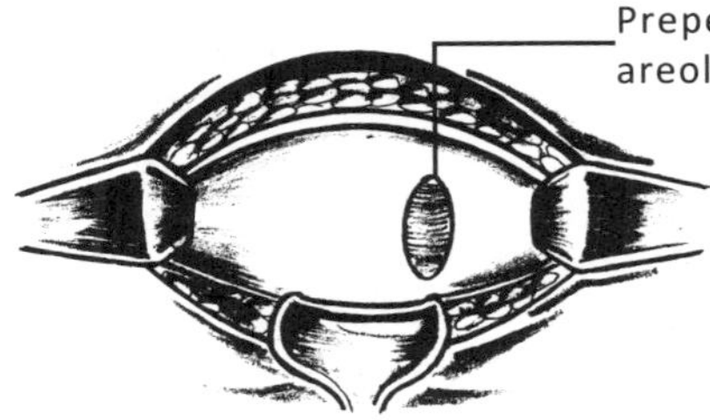

15.2 b. Incised transversalis fascia showing the preperitoneal areolar tissue

The bladder is partially emptied. The fascia connecting the left lateral aspect of the bladder to the overlying peritoneum is further dissected to expose a triangular area of the lower uterine segment. The upper border of this triangular area is formed by the reflected peritoneum, the lateral border by the parietal peritoneum, and the inferior border by the dissected upper surface of the left lateral part of the urinary bladder.

The fascia over the lower uterine segment is incised, the bladder pushed inferiorly to the right, the fascia to the left and the reflected peritoneum superiorly. The reflected peritoneum is covered by the transversalis fascia and the perivesical fascia. This layer is picked and pulled upwards to retract the underlying peritoneum. Simultaneous pressure on the bladder downwards will make the intervening connective tissue taut and amenable to incision for any desired distance till adequate exposure of the lower uterine segment is achieved. (Fig. 15.2 c & d).

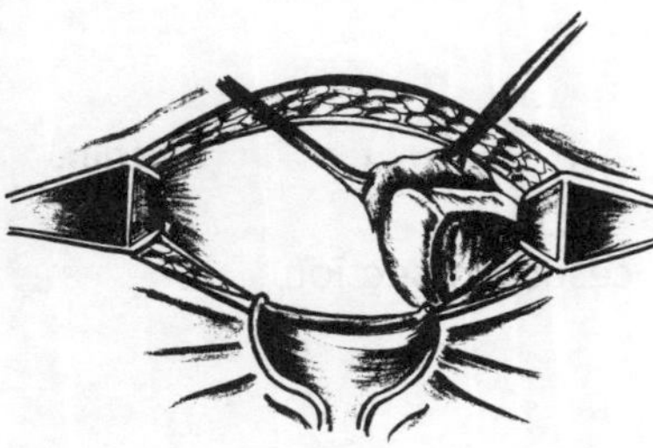

15.2 c. Further dissection of the transversalis fascia

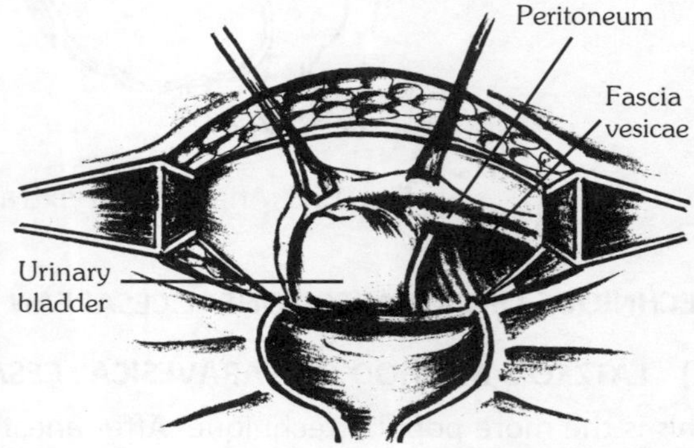

15.2 d. Dissection of the fascia vesicae

During dissection the terminal aspect of the left hypogastric artery (umbilical artery) may be clamped and cut. At this moment, the peritoneal fold is inspected for windowing. Any rent should be repaired. The bladder is drained completely. After exposing the lower uterine segment with retractors, the lower uterine segment is cut transversely or vertically. (Fig. 15.2 e).

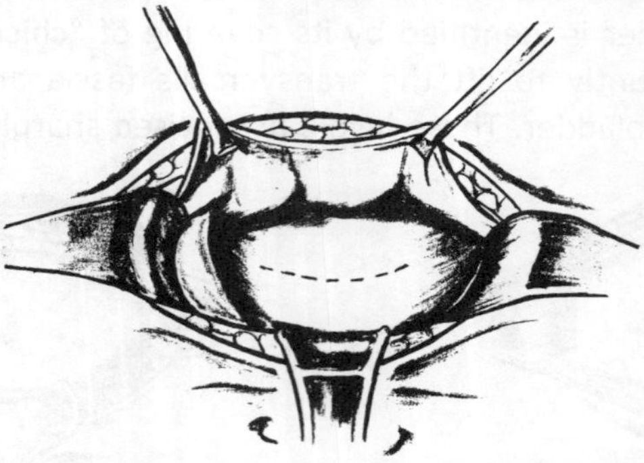

15.2 e. Incision on the exposed lower uterine segment

Fig. 15.2 Latzko's method of extraperitoneal cesarean section

After the fetus and the placenta are extracted, the uterine incision may be closed in one or two layers. While some authorities recommend placing a drain in the lower angle of the paravesical space, this is not mandatory. The peritoneum is allowed to fall back over the bladder. Its suturing is not essential. The abdominal closure is performed in the standard manner.

B) WATER'S OR THE PHYSICK-SELLHEIM TECHNIQUE OF EXTRAPERITONEAL CESAREAN SECTION (MEDIAN APPROACH)[4]

This technique, too, requires distention of the urinary bladder with 150-200ml of dilute methylene blue or indigo carmine. After an appropriate abdominal incision (classically the paramedian longitudinal incision or, alternatively, the Pfannensteil or transverse incision); a T-shaped incision is made on the perivesical and transversalis fascia overlying the fundus of the urinary bladder. (Fig. 15.3 a and b). The urachus has to be cut and the fascia overlying the dome of the bladder and intervening between the bladder and the reflected pelvic peritoneum is separated by blunt and sharp dissection. (Fig. 15.3 c). Thus, in the words of E.G. Waters, "the bladder is denuded of a fascial skull-cap which remains attached to the peritoneum from bladder fundus to the uterovesical pouch". The lower uterine segment thus exposed is incised, the fetus and placenta extracted and the uterine incision closed in one or two layers.

(Fig. 15.3 d). After this, the peritoneum is allowed to drop back over the bladder and the abdomen closed. As with the Latzko's operation, a drain in the paravesical space is optional.

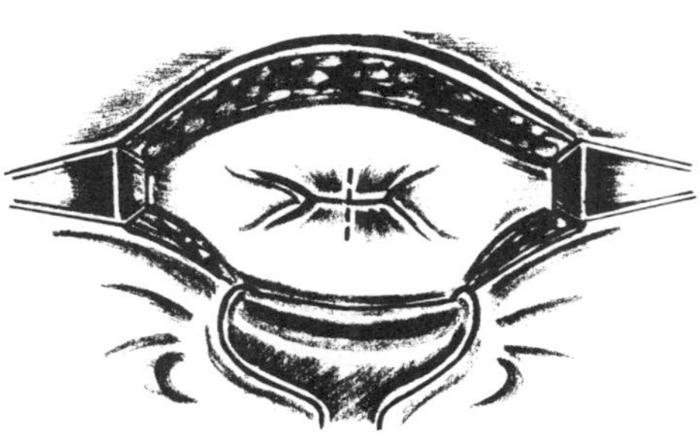

15.3 a. Midline incision of the transversalis fascia

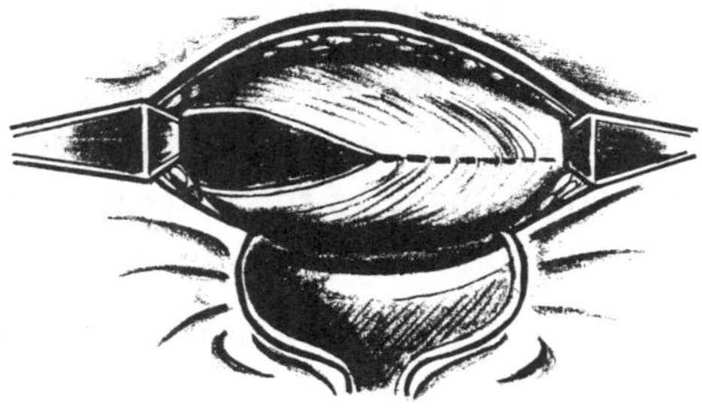

15.3 b. Dissection of the tranversalis fascia

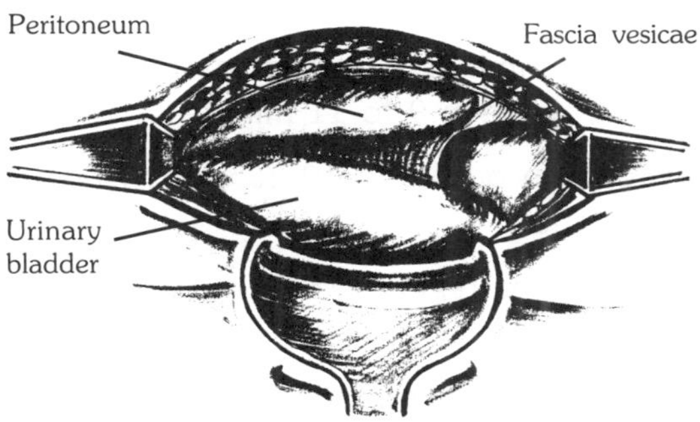

15.3 c. Dissection of the fascia vesicae

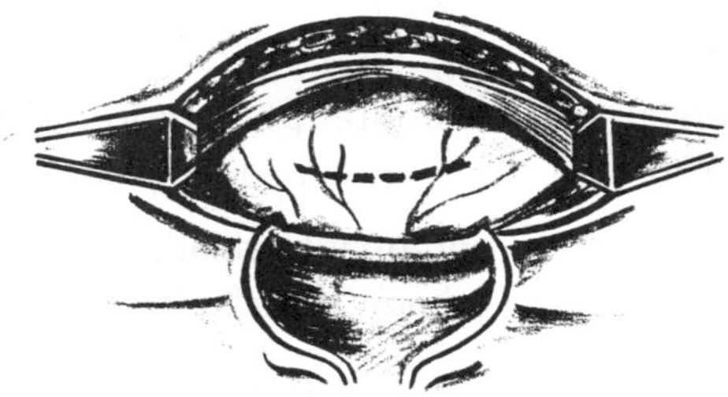

15.3 d. Incision over the lower uterine segment

Fig. 15.3 Water's method of extraperitoneal cesarean section

The disadvantage of the Water's operation lies in the fact that dissection is started in the area where the bladder is most densely adherent to the overlying peritoneum. There is greater danger of injury to the urinary bladder especially in the region of the urachus. If the dissection is carried out more towards the peritoneal aspect buttonholing is likely to defeating the purpose of the procedure.

ADVANTAGES OF EXTRA-PERITONEAL CESAREAN SECTION

Extraperitoneal cesarean delivery evolved in an era where suspected or frank cases of sepsis (especially with obstructed labor) were dealt with by either a hazardous destructive operation on the moribund or dead fetus, symphisiotomy or a cesarean hysterectomy.

Thus, the surgery proved unique in the fact that it could be carried out at any stage of labor when any maternal or fetal indication arose without allowing for complete cervical dilatation, which is a prerequisite for performing any of the above mentioned procedures. It also allowed survival of the fetus unlike a destructive operation[5].

Unlike a classical cesarean which was the more popular operation in an earlier era, this procedure could await an indication until the very last moment and thus never ran the risk of being performed unnecessarily[5]. In fact, in late labor, since the pubovesicocervical fascia is stretched out over the elevated bladder and the thinned out lower uterine segment, dissection is technically easier to perform.

Unlike procedures like symphisiotomy, it could be performed with greater control and relatively less probability of injury to adjacent structures such as the urethra or the bladder while avoiding damage to the bone or pubic symphysis with the subsequent problems of severe pain, abnormal gait and osteitis.

This surgery, in an earlier era, was definitely preferred to the classical operation in cases of frank and suspected chorioamnionitis since it did not breach the peritoneal cavity.

DISADVANTAGES AND COMPLICATIONS OF EXTRAPERITONEAL CESAREAN SECTION

This is a technically demanding operation. Due to the time required for extraperitoneal dissection, the incision delivery interval usually varies between 9 to 11 minutes[16].

The inevitable accidental perforation of the peritoneum occurs in 10-25% of cases thus compromising the extraperitoneal nature of the operation.[16]

There is definite potential for bladder injury especially in the region of the urachus. Ureteric injuries, too, have been reported.

The dissection also entails the risk of vascular injury especially to the inferior epigastric vessels, the uterine vessels and at times, the terminal part of the internal iliac artery.

Added to thus problem is the disadvantage of being unable to evaluate the pelvic viscera.

Haesslein and Goodlin noted that up to 57% of cases of unsuspected pelvic pathology would have been missed during an extraperitoneal cesarean section. The same authors as well other have also questioned the benefit of the surgery in modern obstetrics where prophylactic antibiotics apparently reduced any febrile morbidity[17].

CONCLUSION

As many as one in 10 women, following an elective cesarean section, develop a wound infection, fever or endometritis. The incidence of post cesarean infection varies from 0-86% for endometritis, 24% for wound infection, 1-34% for urinary tract infection and 0-66% for febrile morbidity[18]. There is a higher infection rate following emergency surgery especially following prolonged labor or prolonged rupture of membranes. Good surgical technique is an essential aspect of any attempt to reduce post-cesarean infectious morbidity. Although antibiotic prophylaxis has had a major impact in reducing infectious morbidity, antibiotics do pose the problem of adverse reactions and anaphylaxis. Added to this is the fact that, due to destruction of the commensal flora of the vagina by antibiotics, pathogenic bacteria tend to proliferate in the genital tract. There is also a major concern about the rapidly emerging widespread antibiotic resistance. In developing countries and mofussil areas, cases of neglected, prolonged and obstructed labor are often yet encountered. Additionally, these areas often face a paucity of good antibiotics.

With the emergence of penicillin, extraperitoneal cesarean section was thought to be dead and buried forever. However, with the concerns discussed above, this operation may yet find a place once again in modern obstetrics in selected cases. Due to reluctance of modern obstetricians to indulge in this operation, there are no properly controlled prospective trials available to evaluate the true worth of extraperitoneal cesarean section. The role of extraperitoneal cesarean section can be finally placed in its true perspective only after a scientific analysis and not by speculation. Science and nature has the ability to spring many surprises. This elegant operation, considered by many to be archaic, may yet face a revival.

REFERENCES

1. Dewees WP. A compendious system of midwifery, Chiefly Designed to facilitate the inquiries of those who may be pursuing this branch of study (4th ed). Carey & Lea, Philadelphia; 580-84, 1830.

2. Ritgen FA Von. Geschichte eines mit ungiinstigem Erfolge verricteten Baucsceidenscriittes and Folgerungen daraus. Heidelberg Klin Ann; 1:263-76, 1825.

3. Thomas TG. Gastro-elytrotomy; a substitute for the caesarean section – A paper read before the Yonkers Medical Association. Am J Obst. Gynecol 3:125-39, 1871.

4. Myerscough PR. Caesarean section: Sterilization: Hysterectomy. In Myerscough PR (ed): Munro Kerr's Operative Obstetrics (10th ed). Balliere Tindall, London; 22 (V): 295-319, 1996.

5. Speert H. Wilhelm Latzko and Extraperitoneal Cesarean Section. In Speert H: essays in Eponymy-Obstetric and Gynecologic Milestones (1st ed). The Macmillan Company, New York; 69 (IX): 594-603, 1958.

6. Waters EG. Supravesical extraperitoneal cesarean section. Presentation of a New Technique. Am J Obstet Gynecol; 49:739, 1945.

7. Perkins RP. Role of extraperitoneal cesarean section. Clin Obstet Gynaecol; 23: 585, 1980.

8. Hanson HB. Current use of the extraperitoneal cesarean section: a decade of experience. Am J Obstet Gynecol; 149 (1): 31-4, 1984.

9. Durveniaski KH, Durveniaska I. Our experience with 151 cases of abdominal extraperitoneal section in the Obstetric–Gynaecology Department of the Municipal Main Hospital in Ruse. Akush Ginekol (Sofiia); 30 (2):10-4, 1991.

10. Wallace RC, Eglinton GS, Yonekura ML, Wallace TM. Extraperitoneal cesarean section: a surgical form of infection prophylaxis? Am J Obstet Gynecol; 148(2):172-7, 1984.

11. Waters EG. Cloacal dysgenesis: related anomalies and pregnancies. Obstet Gynecol; 59(3): 398-402, 1982.

12. Wang JS, Yang MG. Clinical analysis of 36 repeat cesarean sections performed extraperitoneally. Hougua Fu Chan Ke Za Zhi; 29(8):461-2, 1994.

13. Rao R, Rao P, Rohidekar A. Extraperitoneal cesarean section. The Salem polyclinic experience. Obst Gynaec Communications; 1(3): 29-31, 1999.

14. Cartwright EW. Extraperitoneal cesarean section; Physick–Sellheim Principle. Wert J Surg; 57:509, 1949.

15. Norton JF. Paravesical extraperitoneal cesarean section technique, with analysis of 160 paravesical extraperitoneal cesarean sections. Am J Obstet Gynecol; 64: 899, 1952.

16. Hibbard LT. Extraperitoneal cesarean section. Clin Obstet Gynecol; 28:711, 1985.

17. Haesslein HC, Goodlin RC. Extraperitoneal cesarean section revisited. Obstet Gynecol; 55:181, 1980.

18. Murphy KW. Reducing the complications of caesarean section. In Bonnar J (ed): Recent Advances in Obstetrics and Gynaecology (vol.20); 9:141-152, 1998.

16 CHAPTER

Audit in Cesarean Deliveries

Sanjay B. Rao

FRAMEWORK

- Introduction
- Audit in current clinical practice
- Type of audit applicable to cesarean deliveries
- Development of audit standards
- Levels of evidence
- The audit cycle
- Conclusion

INTRODUCTION

There has been a public health concern for over 30 years about the increasing cesarean section rate[1]. Although a global phenomenon, there are marked differences in the rates of cesarean section in different countries across the world. In 1985, the WHO carried a consensus statement suggesting that there were no additional benefits associated with a cesarean section rate above 10-15%. This was based on an examination of the estimates of national cesarean section rates along with maternal and perinatal mortality rates from various countries.Developing countries like Chile and Brazil have the highest cesarean section rates in the world - 40% and 37% respectively[2]. In contrast, many European countries like Sweden, Belgium and Ireland have very low cesarean section rates - 5 to 12% and yet have much better maternal and neonatal outcomes[3]. Other countries such as the USA and Canada with high cesarean section rates (25% and 20% respectively) have initiated steps to reduce these rates[4].

AUDIT IN CURRENT PRACTICE

Audit in relation to cesarean section implies a "systematic, critical analysis of the quality of medical care"[5]. This includes the procedures used for diagnosis and treatment, the use of resources and the resulting outcome for the patient. The process of audit itself was originally developed by a multiprofessional and lay working group (Pilot Steering Group and Audit Working Groups) convened by the Royal College of Obstetricians and Gynaecologists[6].

Cesarean section has been viewed by many non-medical personnel as a "unnatural termination of a natural event". In the Indian context, there has been an increase in the number of elective as well as emergency cesarean sections over the past few decades. The accompanying morbidity has raised several questions justifying the need of the procedure. We are now in the era of consumerism. Any untoward complication following a cesarean section may be considered a "medical negligence" and not a natural consequence of the specific maternal condition or surgery. In the past, caesarean sections were performed for essentially absolute indications like a contracted pelvis or a transverse lie. However with the passage of time, technological advances in fetal surveillance and neonatal intensive care[7] has led to a rise in cesarean section. A preference to limit family size and an expectation of a healthy baby at the end of each pregnancy has further increased cesarean section rates. Often lack of skills for instrumental delivery, "an easy way out" for the attending obstetrician and some women "wanting" to deliver by cesarean section influence changing trends[7].

TYPES OF AUDIT APPLICABLE TO CESAREAN SECTION

A numerical audit is purely administrative and deals with figures. It is useful for demonstrating trends such as increase in rate of cesarean section. It can reflect the efficiency of case management as a whole. But a fall in cesarean section rates does not necessarily mean better obstetric and perinatal outcome. A case review audit is a randomised collection of case notes. It assesses the adequacy of history taking, investigations sent, diagnostic accuracy, intrapartum monitoring charts, indication for taking up the patient for section, decision to delivery interval and the subsequent perinatal outcome vis-a-vis the condition of mother and baby and any complications therein. An event based audit could be comprehensive, intermittent or randomised for e.g. perinatal and maternal mortality in cesarean section is an event based audit. A cost benefit audit could analyse the length of hospital stay, drugs used, total cost incurred by the patient and complications associated with cesarean in comparison with a vaginal delivery. This type of audit is of importance in terms of allocation of clinical budget.

Audit in cesarean section could evolve through 2 phases[6]:

Phase I :

1) To determine the frequency of Cesarean section in the hospital
2) To evaluate demographic, clinical and organisational factors associated with variations in section rates
3) To assess the quality of clinical care against established standards as published in literature

Phase II :

1) To survey maternal views, education and attitudes about Cesarean section
2) To explore the clinician's thought process and threshold for Cesarean section

The primary aim of any audit concerning caesarean section is to improve the quality of health care that the obstetrician offers the patient.In a wider perspective, it may also extend to other purposes such as service planning, resource management and cost-accounting.These activities may in the process of research, bring out some new and unexpected problems, which may introduce new difficulties, actually unrelated to audit.

It is important to identify who would be monitoring the audit and the manner in which it would be conducted. It is often impossible to exclude all biases. However there should be a detailed assessment of whether they could influence the study findings.

Interpretation of the results and their implications in further care of the patient is also important. It involves recognising deficiencies in the decision making process and proposal of specific solutions/standard management protocols for cases of a similar nature.

The ultimate aim of conducting the audit is to benefit the following:

1) Pregnant women and their families
2) Health care professionals viz. obstetricians and neonatologists who share in the caring of women during the process of childbirth and childcare
3) Public health professionals who are involved with the planning of maternity services
4) Those involved in the funding of maternity services

Audit methodology in the context of cesarean section would comprise of structure, process and outcome

Structure

Structure implies the organisational setup for the audit and would ideally include the obstetrician, nursing staff, anaesthetist, neonatologist and public health specialists working in tandem.

Process

This refers to the stages of management from the time the patient was referred to the hospital till the final obstetric outcome

Outcome

The denominator data indicates data collected in relation to birth of the baby. Data items to be collected:

1) Date of delivery
2) Mother's age
3) Total number of previous pregnancies of at least 24 weeks of gestation
4) No of prev LSCS
5) Mode of onset of labour
6) No of babies born
7) Presentation
8) Mode of delivery
9) Outcome of pregnancy (live or still birth)
10) Birth weight of babies

These would be available from reliable sources like hospital records or registers. Data collection should be complete to ensure a good quality and standard of the audit. It is equally important to ensure confidentiality by an appropriate coding system.

DEVELOPMENT OF AUDIT STANDARDS

For issues concerning therapy or treatment, the highest levels of evidence is a meta-analysis of randomised controlled trials or individual randomised controlled trials in the western world. The levels of evidence graded by the Royal College of Obstetricians and Gynaecologists is outlined in the table[6].

LEVELS OF EVIDENCE

Level definition

1a. Evidence obtained from meta analysis of randomised controlled trials

1b. Evidence obtained from at least one randomised controlled trial

2a. Evidence obtained from at least one well designed controlled study without randomisation

2b. Evidence obtained from at least other type of well designed quasi-experimental study

3. Evidence obtained from well–designed non-experimental descriptive studies, such as comparative studies, correlation studies and core studies

4. Evidence obtained from expert committee reports or opinions and/or clinical experience of respected authorities

The audit should be systematically structured using quantitative methods. It should be able to provide change wherever necessary and also should be with an inbuilt system of follow up and future change. The common goal of the audit should be to try and make the audit confidential, educational and non-disciplinary. The aim should be to review clinical management with reference to agreed professional standards. The members should be keen to modify management practices. The basic principles should be on RUMBA (relevant, understandable, measurable, behaviorally oriented and achievable concepts) and KISS (keep it small and simple). This would enable to complete the audit within a stipulated time limit so that results are analysed and known to all concerned[8].

THE AUDIT CYCLE

The audit team chalks out the audit cycle and decides the choice of the topic e.g.; the influence of the population and clinical characteristics of the study group in relation to cesarean section. Alternatively it could be a classification of the urgency of cesarean section - whether emergency, elective or semi-elective. An issue which was audited by the RCOG Clinical Effectiveness Support Group was the "decision to delivery" interval for emergency cesarean section. The overall conclusion was that the time limit should be 27 mins in cases of severe maternal and fetal compromise[5].

The audit of the quality of clinical care should be able to reveal the difference between the devised results and what was actually done. In a developing country like ours, there is still a lack of research based evidence to indicate standardised practice. Other issues which need an auditable standard include prophylactic antibiotic coverage to reduce morbidity from cesarean section. Labour ward facilities, competency of staff in practice drills for emergency cesarean deliveries and interpretation of electronic fetal heart monitoring are potential areas for audits in contemporary evidence based obstetric practice.

For the anaesthesia providers, it is important to analyse ideal practices like acid prophylaxis, the use of regional blocks, the availability of cross matched blood and post operative care. There should be uniform and regularly updated guidelines for anaesthetic practices in high risk pregnancies like cardiac disease, diabetes, pre-eclampsia and antepartem hemorrhage.

CONCLUSION

It would be worthwhile initiating genuine audits of cesarean section in developing countries like India. Use of interdepartmental audits especially in institutional practice, seeking a second opinion whenever required and use of standard management protocols would strengthen the practice of evidence based obstetrics. Audit has now emerged as an essential aspect of continuing education. It is a powerful tool to improve the quality of care and also protect the standard of the clinician. With a constant progress in the field of obstetrics, everyone concerned must accept the need for change.

REFERENCES

1. Notzon FC, Placek PJ, Toffel SM. Comparison of naticnal caesarean section rates. N Eng J Med 1987;316: 386-389.
2. Murray SF, Serani Pradenas F. Caesarean birth trends in Chile;1986-1994. Birth 1997;24:258-263.
3. Nielson TF, Otterblod Olausson P, Ingemasson I The caesarean section rate in Sweden: the end of the rise. Birth 1994;21:1(March).
4. Menard MK. Caesarean delivery rates in the US- the 1990s. Controversies in labor management. Obstet gynecol Clin North Am 1999;26(2):275-286.
5. Barron SL: Audit in obstetrics Br J Obstet Gynaecol 98:1965,1991.
6. The National Sentinel Caesarean Section audit report RCOG Clinical effectiveness support unit Oct 2001.
7. Asha Oumachigui: Changing trends in caesarean section. Obs and Gynae today Vol VII no 7:July 2002 377-381.
8. Chapple J: In Bonnar J(Ed) Audit in Obstetrics recent advances Obstetrics and Gynaecology 91,1995.

17 | CHAPTER

Contraceptive Options After Cesarean Birth

Mandakini Parihar, Rohan Potdar, Sarbjeet Kaur

FRAMEWORK

- Introduction
- The informed choice strategy
- Natural contraception
- Barrier methods
- Hormonal contraceptives
- Intrauterine contraceptive devices
- Permanent methods
- Emergency contraception
- Conclusion

INTRODUCTION

Millions of women would prefer to avoid becoming pregnant either right away or ever, but they are not using contraception. These women have an "unmet need" for family planning. In developing countries, over 100 million women who are married or in union have unmet need for spacing or limiting births. The MTP Fact File of India, shows there are about 6.7 million abortions every year, pointing towards the extent of our population's unmet need. In many developing countries, like ours, abortion remains a common way for women to control their fertility. The definition of unmet need has several layers. The first layer is to provide contraception to those who are not using it. The second is to provide a more effective, satisfactory, or safe method. The third layer is for safe treatment of contraceptive failure (or non-use), and the fourth is for such reproductive health services as infertility treatment and the prevention and treatment of sexually transmitted diseases. Today, we have one goal: population stabilization. This is the core issue in all our programmes and unless we realize this and act today we, as a country would be draining our resources and hampering our progress. National development and global health depend on fostering the full capacity of all citizens. An integral part of this development is the empowerment of women.

A good and effective contraceptive method implies that people are able to have a satisfying and safe sex life, and be able to decide freely and responsibly, the number of children and decide on the spacing and timing of their children. Today, with the incidence of emergency and elective caesarean deliveries increasing, we as practitioners need to educate the patients regarding the safe, effective, affordable and acceptable method of family planning during their post LSCS period. This chapter is aimed to provide important resource of information for counseling our patients on the best choice available to them for their contraceptive options during this period. Women must be empowered to make informed choices. Reproductive decisions are typically taken within the family and hence, every effort must be made to involve men in the promotion of reproductive rights.

THE INFORMED CHOICE STRATEGY

The principle of informed choice refers to decisions that people can make for themselves and not to a process that family planning programmes and providers carry out. Nevertheless, programmes, providers, and policy-makers can do much to support people's ability to make informed family planning choices. Programmes can do best by adopting a strategy that blends five areas- government policies, communication programmes, access to family planning, leadership and management, and patient-provider communication. This is where we as obstetricians can help and make a difference. We are the service providers and we can help by providing a "cafeteria approach" and allow them to make their choice[1,2,3].

1) Give our patients their desired family planning method unless it is medically inappropriate.
2) Provide clear, unbiased information on the advantages and disadvantages of the various contraceptive methods and explain correct use of the chosen method.
3) Tailor counseling and advice to each patient's expressed needs and personal situation.

4) Refrain from judging the patient and from holding preconceived perceptions about what is best for them.
5) Respect the patient's decision even if they choose a less effective method than your advise.
6) Respect the patient's decision to switch from one method to another.
7) Respect the patient's decision to refuse any or all services.

Contraception after a cesarean birth is of crucial importance especially since the uterus is scarred. An unwanted pregnancy would increase the risk to maternal health due to the potential complications of medical termination of pregnancy. This would also imply a delay in recovery or return to work. A careful counseling by the obstetrician would help to avert such situations. The Choice of contraceptive methods after a cesarean section would depends upon the time since delivery, infant feeding choice and desire of temporary versus permanent method.

Table 1 outlines the various modes of contraception which could be offered to women after a cesarean delivery

Table - 1. Cafeteria options for women after a cesarean delivery

1. **Natural**
   Lactational amenorrhea method (LAM)

2. **Barrier**
   a) Male Barrier
   b) Female barrier
      Diaphragm
      Cervical Cap
      Female Condom
   c) Spermicidal

3. **Hormonal**
   a) Progesterone only
      Mini pills
      Injectable contraceptives
      Implants
      Vaginal Ring
   b) Estrogen - Progesterone pills - not recommended during lactation

4. **Intra uterine devices**
   Copper releasing IUD's
   Hormone releasing IUD's

5. **Permanent methods**
   Tubal Ligation
   Vasectomy

6. **Emergency contraception**

NATURAL CONTRACEPTION

Lactation Amenorrhoea Method (LAM)

Breastfeeding and contraception have a paradoxical relationship. While lactation itself bestows a degree of contraceptive protection, this is not always independently dependable, though it often enhances overall efficacy of most methods. Lactation also requires consideration of the effects of contraception on milk constitution and the neonate. Choices of contraception may be limited for lactating women following cesarean section due to concerns about hormonal effects on quality and quantity of milk, passage of hormones to the infant and infant growth. Ideally, the contraceptive method chosen should not interfere with lactation. Additionally, because the return of menstruation and ovulation can be unpredictable in breastfeeding women, the timing of contraception initiation is important[1,4,5,6].
The advantages of the lactational amenorrhoea method are outlined in table 2

Table - 2. LAM

Efficiency is maintained if the breast feeding is done both day and night
At least 6 breastfeeds during day and two at night
Efficiency is decreased after six months even if patient is amenorrheic
Effective up to 6 months after child birth
Effective when patient continues to exclusively breast feed
Efficacy reduced if menstruation returns
Efficacy is 2 pregnancies per 100 women in the first 6 months of child birth.

BARRIER METHODS

During lactation barriers have proved to be reliable contraceptives with appropriate use. Though reported failure rates are generally high (female condom 5-21% and male condom 3-14%), these women experience lower failure rates at this time of reduced fertility. Barrier Methods helps both in preventing pregnancy and STDs. Most commonly, male barriers are used and they must be used correctly every time to be highly effective. The advantages are that there are no hormonal side effects and there are no effects on lactation. Female barrier methods are diaphragms, cervical caps and spermicides and soon the female condom will be freely available. The advantage is that they are safe, women controlled method and have no side-effects from hormones or any effects on breast milk[10].

They are suitable options for women following a cesarean delivery

Table - 3. Efficacy of barrier methods

Condoms	14 pregnancies per 100 women in the first year of use
Spermicides	26 pregnancies per 100 women in the first year of use
Diaphragm	20 pregnancies per 100 women in the first year of use
Cervical Cap	20 pregnancies per 100 women in the first year of use

HORMONAL CONTRACEPTIVES

Combined Hormonal Contraceptives and Lactation

Combined hormones definitely affect breast milk production, leading to decreased milk volume and changes in milk composition with decreased mineral content. However there are contradictory reports on slower infant weight gain ranging from equivocal to detrimental.

Breastfeeding and being less than 6 weeks postpartum are WHO Medical Eligibility Category 4 condition and the health risk increases unacceptably if used in this group. Combined oral / injectable contraceptives are hence to be avoided in this group of patients as a contraceptive option after cesarean section.

Progesterone Only Contraceptives[14,15,16,17,18,19,20,21]

Hormonal contraception is safe during lactation provided one uses progesterone only preparations. However the primary concern is when to initiate contraception, since Hartmann's theory hypothesizes that alveolar sensitization to PRL happens in response to fall in progesterone and there is concern of transfer of steroid to breastfed infants being greater with early initiation. Hence, the recommendation is to start progesterone only preparations after sixth week postpartum, particularly if the woman is partially breast feeding. There are many options available today in progesterone only preparations.

Table - 4. Progesterone only preparations

Progesterone Only Pill (Mini pill)
Injectable contraceptives
Implants
Vaginal Ring

Progesterone Only Pill (Mini pill)

The mini pill has long been accepted for safe use during lactation. A study comparing the use of desogestrel 75 ug/day (Minilon) with IUCD use during lactation, evaluated the quantity and constitution of milk with follow up of children up to 2.5 years. There was no change in amount or constitution of milk or affection of growth and development, confirming this to be a safe and effective contraceptive for lactating women. This acts by thickening cervical mucus and inhibiting ovulation and is an effective method for breast feeding mothers as the quantity &

quality of breast milk do not seem harmed. Also there are no estrogen side effects. Effects of progestin-only pill (POP) on ovarian activity during breastfeeding shows that POP does not suppress gonadotropins nor affect growth of ovarian follicles during breastfeeding. Thus, the contraceptive effect of POP is likely mediated through local actions at the endometrium and cervix in a manner similar to that in menstruating women.

Efficacy: 1 pregnancy per 100 women in first year of use in breast feeding mothers.

Progesterone Injectables

Multicentric studies of injectable progestogens have reported high use effectiveness (99.9%) and cumulative continuation rates (72.8%). While spotting, irregular bleeding and amenorrhea are the main reasons for discontinuation there is high acceptability and continuation with counseling. Also lactation amenorrhea masks the main complaints. It is highly efficacious and its efficacy rivals that of surgical sterilization. In addition it has no effects on lactation and no estrogen side effects especially after caesarian birth.

It is available as injection Depot medroxyprogesterone acetate (DMPA, Depo-Provera) given every 3 months & Inj NET-EN given every 2 months. Pharmacologically active levels of DMPA persist for 3-4 months following injection. A 150 mg dose is used most often for high contraceptive efficacy every 3 months.

Injectables act primarily by inhibiting ovulation, lowering the levels of follicle-stimulating hormone and luteinizing hormone. Approximately 50% of women using DMPA for 1 year report amenorrhea. Menstrual changes are the most frequent causes of discontinuation of injectables. In cases of heavy bleeding it is appropriate to undergo gynecological examination to rule out unrelated conditions, such as vaginitis, cervicitis, or cervical lesions. The use of conjugated estrogen (12.5-2.5 mg daily) for 10-21 days will minimize bleeding. Some women using injectables experience headache, dizziness, bloating of the abdomen or breast, and mood changes. Long-term use of DMPA or NET-EN can often result in 1-3 kg weight gain. The relative risk of breast cancer was 1.21, which was statistically not significant. Fertility returns in 70% of former users within 12 months; it is suitable for postpartum and lactating women, and provides other non-contraceptive benefits. They have been widely used in India and are particularly useful after cesarean birth.

Progestogen Implants

Contraceptive implants are a successful method for long-term prevention of pregnancy. Advantages of this contraceptive method include its efficacy, independence from user compliance and prompt return of fertility after removal. They have a good scope for use in women who have undergone a cesarean delivery.

The first progestin-only contraceptive implant placed on the market was Norplant, a multiunit system. Since then, several single- and double-rod implants have been developed, each using one of four different progestins: levonorgestrel, etonogestrel, Nestorone and norgestrol acetate. A new subdermal implant is in development in the U.S. It's already approved in several European countries. It's a single rod system. Unlike the existing system in the U.S. with six small rods, this has just one rod to insert and to remove. And the active ingredient is a progestin called 3-keto-desogestrel which has recently been renamed etonogestrel. It's approved for three years of use. The etonorgestrel implant (Implanon) was studied fully breast feeding mothers at 6 weeks postpartum. The volume of milk production was unaffected with no inter group differences in milk content of fat, protein and lactose, in timing and quantity of supplementary feeds and in infant weight, height or head circumference. Amenorrhoea and irregular menstrual bleeding though noted are less irksome during lactation.Occasionally women may experience headache, nausea ,breast discomfort and mood swings. The ideal time to implant is usually day 21-28 after a cesarean section.

Table - 5. Different Implants

Six Rods :

Norplant (Levonorgestrel)

Two Rods :

Jadelle (Levonorgestrel)

Norplant II (Levonorgestrel)

Single Rod :

Implanon - 3 year (etonogestrel)

Nestorone - 2 years (Nestorone)

Uniplant - 1 year (nomegestrol acetate)

Table - 6. Advantages of Implants

Efficacy: 0.1 pregnancies / 100 women in first year of use.

Extremely high efficacy, rivaling surgical sterilization.

It's a long term but immediately reversible method.

It does have the usual sort of hormonal side effects of progestin-only methods,

It doesn't require a skilled insertion and removal

Progesterone Vaginal Ring

Natural progesterone vaginal rings are a recent innovation in the western world. In a recent study, the ring (10 mg/day for 3 months) had a pregnancy rate of 1.5%, a continuation rate of over 50% at 6 months and 23.5% and amenorrhoea at 46% at 1 year postpartum. Lactation, health and infant weight gain were comparable with Cu T 380A use.

INTRAUTERINE CONTRACEPTIVE DEVICES

This is highly effective with no negative influence on lactation or infant growth. During lactation insertion is easier and less painful with fewer bleeding problems and pain, though special care is needed to minimize risk of perforation. In addition to the copper T-380A, we now have a levonorgestrel-releasing intrauterine contraceptive. A recent review of literature over 30 years reported the most effective IUDs in use to be the Cu T 380A (pregnancy rate < 2% at 2 years) and LNG-20 (pregnancy rate < 1% at 7 years). Increased failure rates were related to displacement[20,21,22,23].

IUD'S are less prefered option upto six weeks following cesarean delivery due to a potential risk of infection,perforation and migration.

The LNG IUS (Intra Uterine System) or Mirena is one of the newest forms of contraception. It is as effective as sterilization in preventing pregnancy. Apart from preventing pregnancy, the IUS makes periods lighter, shorter and less painful. When it's removed, fertility returns immediately. The IUS (Intra Uterine System) is a unique method of contraception combining the main benefit of the pill - effective birth control - with the main appeal of sterilization, "forget-ability'. The IUS also has an advantage over the Copper IUD (Intra Uterine Device) because it tends to make periods lighter and shorter which the Copper IUD does not. LNG IUS contains pure levonorgestrel in the vertical stem of this device which then leaches out at a rate of 20 micrograms per day into the endometrium. This method of contraception, like the injectables, like the implants, is tantamount to surgical sterilization. It is recommended that no IUD insertion be undertaken between 48 hours and 4 weeks due to uterine involution and an increased risk of expulsion. The levonorgestrel IUS (Mirena) insertion is undertaken after 6 weeks following cesarean section in keeping with the guidelines for progestogens[21,22,23]. The cost of Mirena may limit a large scale use especially in the lower socioeconomic strata.

Cu- releasing IUD's

CuT-200, Cu-T-380, Multi load,

Nova - T

Hormonal containing IUD

Progestasert, LNG IUS (Mirena)

Newer methods are in phase II and Phase III trials using frameless IUDs. Gynefix is Copper containing Framless IUCD and Fibroplant is LNG containing frameless IUCD releasing 14 micrograms of LNG per day (Contrel Research, Belgium). The results of this preliminary study suggest that the FibroPlant-LNG IUS, releasing 14 micrograms of LNG per day, is a safe and effective method. The absence of a frame is particularly advantageous in these women. The low daily release rate of LNG from the Fibro Plant-LNG IUS results in a virtual absence of hormonal side-effects[23].

PERMANENT METHODS

The decision for sterilization should preferably be based on careful counselling before caesarian section. Female sterilization (tubectomy) is convenient, cost effective with no negative impact on lactation provided the initiation is not delayed or intervals not prolonged due either the anesthesia or the procedure related discomfort. Male sterilization (vasectomy) could be offered and performed early, so that lactation amenorrhoea avoids the need for additional contraception till azoospermia sets in.

Vasectomy

Vasectomy is a permanent contraception for men who decide they will not want more children.

Almost all of the couples decided upon vasectomy during or immediately after a pregnancy. No man, however, expressed regret or reservation about undergoing the procedure. Most men in both focus groups reported never having considered vasectomy and did not envision doing so in the future. However, after having been provided facts about vasectomy, many men said that they may consider vasectomy as an option in the future. The researchers found prenatal and postpartum programs, well-baby clinics, and gynecologists, pediatricians, and family physicians offices to be important locations in which to provide information about vasectomy. They recommend that counseling and promotional materials on vasectomy focus upon the positive aspects of vasectomy and address men's fears, women's concerns, and cultural issues surrounding vasectomy[2, 6,7]. Vasectomy in the context of contraception following cesarean section is a good option in those women who have not undergone or not opted for a tubal ligation at the time of cesarean section.

Female sterilization

Female sterilization is the number one contraceptive choice among women in the India. Counseling issues include ensuring that the woman understands the permanence of the procedure and knowing the factors that correlate with future regret. It may be inappropriate to counsel women about sterilization at the time of an emergency cesarean section. However in developing countries like India, a large proportion of women often do not avail of antenatal care and report at the hospital only when they experience labour.

The cumulative failure rate of the procedure is reported to be about 1.85 percent during a 10-year period. Complications of tubal sterilization include problems with anesthesia, hemorrhage, organ damage, and mortality. The procedure can be easily performed during the cesarean section itself, if the couple chooses to[2,3,5,24].

EMERGENCY CONTRACEPTION

Emergency contraception has not been adequately researched in lactating women. It is appreciated that lactation amenorrhoea confers reasonable protection against conception. Advance provision of emergency contraception significantly increased use without adversely affecting use of routine contraception. It is safe and appropriate to provide emergency contraception to all postpartum women before discharge from the hospital especially after cesarean birth.

Recommended regimes would include levonorgestrel 0.75 mg within 72 hours, and 0.75 mg repeated after 12 hrs (prevents 85% of expected pregnancies) and IUD insertion within 5-7 days (prevents 99% of expected pregnancies)[25].

The postpartum distribution of written material about contraceptive options increases a woman's ability to make an informed decision regarding birth control after undergoing cesarean section.

CONCLUSION

Each year India adds the population of Sub-Saharan Africa to the earth. Improved obstetric services and child spacing could reduce maternal mortality in developing countries as they have in the developed world. The continuing practices of prolonged lactation and postpartum abstinence in rural areas have compensated to some extent for the absence of modern contraception. Limiting family size reduces both maternal and child deaths. In developed countries, 5-30 women die per 100,000 births, compared to 50-800 in developing countries. User based factors determining the type of contraceptive that is used most often. These are socio-cultural practices including religion, literacy, women's status and their role in decision making, men's status, misconceptions, and convenience of use. Service related factors include knowledge and skill of the provider, attitude of the provider, accessibility of family planning services, cost of the contraceptives, and quality of services. The mass media should be used to disseminate positive and accurate information on contraceptives. Temporary or spacing family planning methods should be popularized by positive reinforcement. The most cost-effective method is also the most popular method - sterilization. Even though female sterilization is more difficult to perform than vasectomy, it is more common than vasectomy. With a rising trend in cesarean deliveries in modern obstetrics,there is a concurrent growing need to limit the family size to safeguard the interests of maternal health.The best contraceptive options after a cesarean delivery could be tailored to suit the individual needs of the client. Contraception should become a people's movement rather than be forced upon the people. Family planning should come to mean "fewer babies - but better babies".

REFERENCES

1. Trussell J. contraceptive efficacy . In: Hatcher et al. contraceptive technology (17th revised edition) New york Irvington 1998. In press.
2. Dixon-mueller R, Germain A. Unmet need from a woman's health perspective. Plan Parent Chall. 1994;(1):9-12.
3. Moreno, L and goldman, N contraceptive failure rate in developing countries. Evidence from the Demographic and health surveys. International Family planning perspectivnes 17 (2) 44-49 June 1991.
4. WHO improving acess to quality care in FP- medical eligibility criteria for contraceptivw, use. Geneva , WHO, family & Reproduction health, 1996.
5. Technical guidance / competence working group, Recommendations for updating selected practices in contraceptiveuse, Vols 1, and 2. chapter Hil', North Carolina, Prog for int. training in health, university of north Carolina, 1994, & 1997.
6. Mikolajczyk RT, Stanford JB, Rauchfuss M. Factors influencing the choice to use modern natural family planning. Contraception. 2003 Apr;67(4):253-8.
7. Sharps PW, El-Mohandes AA, Nabil El-Khorazaty M, Kiely M, Walker T. Health beliefs and parenting attitudes influence breastfeeding patterns among low-income African-American women. J Perinatol. 2003 Jul-Aug;23(5):414-9.
8. Thapa S, Short RV, Potts M. Breast-feeding and birth spacing save lives. J Obstet Gynaecol East Cent Africa. 1988;7(2):51-3.

9. Nichols-Johnson V, Breastfeeding and Contraception, Breastfeed Abs, 21(2):11, 2001.

10. Khan ME. Situation analysis of the postpartum programme in India. Natl Med J India. 2003;16 Suppl 2:28-34.

11. Labbole, m. Cooney, k and Coly, s. guidelines; Breast feeding, family planning and the lact. Amerothea - LAM Washington DC eorgetonon university, institute for Reproduction health, 1994.18p.

12. IMAP, Statement on Barrier Methods, IPPF Med Bull, 35(4):1, 2001.

13. McCann, MF and Potter L.S. progestion only oral contraception. A comprehensive review Contraception 50 (6) (supplementI) S1-S195 Dec . 94.

14. Potter JE, Moore AM, Byrd TL. Cross-border procurement of contraception. estimates from a postpartum survey in El Paso, Texas. Contraception. 2003 Oct;68(4):281-7.

15. Perheentupa A, Critchley HO, Illingworth PJ, McNeilly AS. Effect of progestin-only pill on pituitary-ovarian axis activity during lactation. Contraception. 2003 Jun;67(6):467-71.

16. Blackburn RD, Cunkelman JA and Zlidar VM, Oral Contraceptives – An Update, Population Reports, A(9):5, 2000.

17. Bjarnadotti RI, Gottfredadottir H, Sigurdardittir K et al, Comparative effects of a progestogen only pills, Br J Obstet Gynecol, 108(11):1174, 2001.

18. Power J, Guillebaud J. Long-acting progestogen contraceptives. Practitioner 2002 May;246(1634): 332, 335-9, 341.

19. Bird S. Contraception failure and wrongful birth claims. Aust Fam Physician 2002 Oct;31(10):935-6.

20. Truitt ST, Fraser AB, Grimes DA, Gallo MF, Schulz KF. Combined hormonal versus nonhormonal versus progestin-only contraception in lactation. Cochrane Database Syst Rev. 2003;(2):CD003988.

21. Baldaszti E, Wimmer-Puchinger B, Loschke K. Acceptability of the long-term contraceptive levonorgestrel-releasing intrauterine system (Mirena(R)): a 3-year follow-up study.Contraception 2003 Feb;67(2):87-91.

22. Wildemeersch D, Schacht E, Wildemeersch P. Contraception and treatment in the perimenopause with a novel “frameless” intrauterine levonorgestrel-releasing drug delivery system: an extended pilot study.Contraception 2002 Aug;66(2):93-9.

23. Lahteenmaki P, Rauramo I, Backman T. The levonorgestrel intrauterine system in contraception. Steroids 2000 Oct-Nov;65(10-11):693-7.

24. Baill IC, Cullins VE, Pati S. Counseling issues in tubal sterilization. Am Fam Physician. 2003 Mar 15;67(6):1287-94.

25. Jackson RA, Bimla Schwarz E, Freedman L, Darney P. Advance supply of emergency contraception. effect on use and usual contraception—a randomized trial. Obstet Gynecol. 2003 Jul;102(1):8-16.

26. Johnson LK, Edelman A, Jensen J. Patient satisfaction and the impact of written material about postpartum contraceptive decisions. Am J Obstet Gynecol. 2003 May;188(5):1202-4.

27. Townsend S. Postpartum contraception: developing strategies for expanded services. Network. 1990 Aug;11(3):1,8-9,15.

INDEX